Headache Free

*Relieve Migraine, Tension, Cluster,
Menstrual and Lyme Headaches*

A Word to the Wise

This book is not intended to treat, cure, or diagnose your condition. Please discuss any changes to your healthcare regimen with your physician and get approval before beginning (or discontinuing) any type of drug therapy, medication, or dietary supplement. As with any book that applies to health, individual safety must be the top priority. So please be advised that my suggested nutrients (and dosages) are meant as general guidelines, not gospel. They are not right for everyone. The reality is that head pain is a serious, complex illness that sometimes requires immediate medical attention. The information in this book is not intended as any kind of treatment: It's purpose is educational, so you can hear about various options that you then discuss with your doctor. Follow your instincts and always comply with your physician's advice. It's okay to get second (and third) opinions when dealing with complex health conditions.

Headache Free

*Relieve Migraine, Tension, Cluster,
Menstrual and Lyme Headaches*

Suzy Cohen, RPh
America's Most Trusted Pharmacist™

Dedication Page

*To my wonderful parents, Helen and Bill Gurvich,
who to this day continue to graciously serve their
family, friends and community. I love you both dearly!*

Acknowledgement

Thank you Sam for letting me share your story with the world, you are an incredible man and the love of my life. I'm humble enough to know that I'd be nowhere without my friends in this industry. Thank you to Michael and Jo Len, Marty and William, Bob and Brent. Thank you to Dr. David Perlmutter and Dr. Joseph Mercola for the lovely book jacket quotes, your words mean the world to me. Thank you Mehmet Oz and Doug Kaufmann for putting me on your tv show all the time. Much gratitude to Mary Latsis and Natalie Tysdale. Hugs to my friend Erin Elizabeth, you always make me laugh. Thank you to my sweet friends and study buddies, Jill Carnahan, MD, Douglas Hall, MD, Jason Blalack, LAc, and Benjamin Lynch, ND, we nerds have to stick together. I love getting your emails with "You see this yet?" Cheryl Dial you are a numerical genius! Marita and Janet, my soul sisters, I adore and love you both.

Special gratitude for this particular book goes to my dear editorial friends who support and encourage me whenever I write books. These beautiful souls know what they've done, how they've helped organize my information, fix my typos, correct my "its" and provide generous advice at all hours of the night. Now that I'm done, you can all go to bed before 2am ;-) Thank you to my dear and sweet Alice Feinstein, you're eyes on my manuscript always make it better. Annie Gross, you're an impressive and thorough researcher. Also, special thank you Brooke Bouis, a triple threat, brilliant, intelligent and kind- you are my best medical researcher, and right there when I need you most. I love you Samara, Michael and Rachel, more than life itself. Danny, you are remarkable. Alex, Kelly, Sonia, hugs and love. Russell and Lesley, two special Angels in my life. Thank you to all the contributors and experts in my book, your input was invaluable. Big thanks to the following who I adore, in no particular order just to say I just love you guys: Merry C., Marty W. Jack S., Amy A., Alex and Kelly C., Dr. Michael W., Stephanie K., and Gerry C. Thank you to Traci and Sheryl. To Alan Butcher, my fellow pharmacist and rock climber :-) And so many others, forgive me that I didn't mention you by name, I appreciate you more than words can say ♥.

Headache Free
*Relieve Migraine, Tension, Cluster,
Menstrual and Lyme Headaches*

Table of Contents

Part I
The Headaches

Chapter 1

Why You Can Trust Me

There are one billion people in the world who have migraines. Add in all the other types of headaches and you have the makings for a health disaster of unfathomable proportions. It's taken me 2 years to complete this manuscript and get my book downloaded from my brain into your hands.

With all my heart, I hope this is the best and last book you ever buy on headaches! I'm going to cover it all in my book, so it doesn't matter if your headache is caused by hormonal problems, such as thyroid imbalances or over production of estrogen, exposure to environmental toxins, or the side effects from medications. You'll also find answers here if your headaches are triggered by food sensitivities, or even dietary supplements like green coffee bean extract. You may not realize it, but your headaches may be tied to what you are drinking during the day. The problem could be an infection that you have no idea that you even have. These and other causes for mind-blowing head pain are all covered in this book.

It's taken me years to figure out the best supplements and other remedies for relieving headache pain, including things that others (who have no clue whatsoever) call out-of-the-box or weird. I am not embarrassed to share any of these with you, I only ask that you check with your doctor about anything and everything you read here because I couldn't possibly know what is right for you.

My peers have told me I'm risking my reputation as America's Pharmacist™ to talk about non-drug options, I say to heck with that! You should not suffer another minute. I don't care what people think of my "weird" remedies if they happen to help you. I may be a pharmacist, but guess who I work for? I work for you! I only ask that you get permission from your doctors for whatever you want to try.

I have so much compassion for you. I know how difficult repeated bouts of headache pain are. I am aware of how it has possibly taxed your marriage and close relationships, perhaps cost you your job. Chronic pain can certainly make you feel irritable and miserable, bringing out a side of you that is not really who you are. Please do keep hope in your heart, for I am determined to help you get well. I want so much for my book to be your lifeline.

My Very Own Personal Story

Why can you trust me? I haven't experienced debilitating headaches myself, so this is a natural question. Because I have on-the-job training and I've seen chronic headaches up close. I have so much compassion for you because I've been there.

For many years of my life, I did nothing but eat, live, and breathe solutions for my sweet husband Sam, and then for you, the public who reads my weekly syndicated column and writes to me for help. Let me back up and share my journey because I want you to feel confident that you're holding priceless information in your hands, because you are!

When I graduated pharmacy school in 1989, I only had a few years of real life training in the trenches. I had to spend a little time interning in pharmacies. So as a graduating new pharmacist, I could name the next best drug for this and that, but I had little experience on how headaches could impact a person's life. Today I know they can destroy it.

For the first few years of my professional career, I worked as the manager of a large retail chain pharmacy in Florida, where I saw hundreds of people come in every month like clockwork. Many filled prescriptions for analgesics, and headache medicines like ergotamine or triptan drugs like Imitrex. Even though I didn't fully comprehend the amount of pain they were suffering, I still knew enough to triage my patients in our waiting room, and get them done and rung up as quickly as possible. The prescriptions they handed to me were almost always moved to the very top of my never-ending pile of scripts to fill.

Looking back, I was aware on some level that these folks needed to get home quickly. Many call me intuitive, and after resisting this label for years, I admit today, I really am. I can often feel the pain of others. This may sound silly, but I empathize so much that I avoid watching news on TV because it can move me to tears, or cause unnatural outrage at the injustices in the world... and neither of these emotions serve me. So I watch HGTV, Masterchef, travel channel, the history channel and reality shows like The Voice and Bachelorette.

Anyway, fast-forward to 1998, when I was raising 2 adorable toddlers from my first marriage, and I married my second husband Sam, a chiropractor in my town. He had mild headaches from time to time, no big deal. I didn't realize my life would change so dramatically when his headaches changed shortly after our marriage. His headaches took on a life of their own. They moved around his head. Sometimes they were disabling, and many days, he could not leave the house.

He would tell me he felt like ice picks were sticking into his head or eyes. I would push with all my might on his head because the pressure felt good for him. He'd hold his breath as long as possible in the pool, diving to the bottom in order to experience the relief the water pressure afforded. He wore baseball caps so tight that he went through them quickly, as the Velcro straps would break from the strain.

Over the next few years, during the early years of our marriage, he would experience migraines, cluster headaches, and headaches related to steroids or withdrawal of steroid medicine. There seemed to always be pain in his head, and frequently in or behind his eyes too. He took pain medications for a long time, including a strong one called oxycodone, along with high dose steroids, and anti-inflammatories, such as ibuprofen or celecoxib. He tried anti-nausea medicine, various eye drops, Beta blockers and anti-seizure drugs that supposedly help headaches. He had 6 MRIs, several CT scans, a PET scan, X rays, a spinal tap and every procedure you can think of. We flew across the country, we spent everything we had and then some. Long story short, nothing helped. Nothing. We were devastated.

These headaches later developed into something worse, as if it could get any worse for this sweet man, who even on his worst days, never uttered a harsh word to me, the kids or his patients. He was a chiropractor for many years, nicknamed "Dr. Sunshine" if that indicates his disposition. He started to experience a nerve pain syndrome called trigeminal neuralgia. This pain syndrome causes electrical shocks in your face! No kidding. I will tell you now, that trigeminal neuralgia is capable of stealing your soul, it is dubbed "the suicide disease."

All the while I was doing everything in my power to soothe and stop these headaches. It was horrifying to watch this big strong guy, all 6 foot 5 of him, reduced to helplessness because (above the neck) he was practically disabled. With an invisible symptom like this, people have a hard time believing it can go on for more than a few hours, or for days. But years? Yes, it can. You know it can too. Other people couldn't see the pain Sam was experiencing. And they can't see your pain either. There is so much judgment by others if they can't see your pain. You get more sympathy from wearing an ACE bandage on your knee than you do for a disabling headache.

I know how tough it is for you, especially when you look just fine on the outside, and no one can see your pain. And my guy definitely looked good on the outside. In fact, he is really easy on the eyes :-)

I'm thrilled to tell you that today Sam is headache free! Like most of us, he gets an ordinary, run-of-the-mill headache once in a blue moon, and it responds to ibuprofen. Eventually, we found out that all his different headaches and neuralgia pain, which spanned (ok, destroyed) 10 years of his life was related to an infection called Lyme disease. In fact, it was tied to Lyme, and a co-infection of Lyme called Babesia. For this reason, I've written a chapter on Lyme headaches, so you can discern if this fast-growing epidemic is behind your headache.

You may not think you have Lyme disease, but I want you to read that chapter anyway. To treat Lyme and Babesia-induced headaches, you have to kill the parasite. No amount of pain-relieving or anti-inflammatory medicine will ever fix the problem for more than a few hours.

As for Sam, he required strong antibiotics for a long time. I'll give you more details in that chapter, but here and now I want you to know that even the most horrific pain can be taken care of. Please don't do anything that you will regret. There is a solution, and it may be simpler than you think. It doesn't matter if you've had headaches for 10 days or 10 years, there is always hope for a solution.

Sam hasn't suffered with any serious headaches or facial pain for many years. He doesn't even like to talk about those days, and I had to twist his arm to get him to agree to let me tell you this story. But we realize there's a higher good. After all, I'm trying to help you and so many others put this nightmare behind you once and for all. I've seen them all, and spent many sleepless nights facilitating relief. Tips and tricks, I have many to share!

Up until that point in 1998 when I started seeing headaches up close in my own life, migraines and headaches meant little more than just another prescription to fill for a patient. I'd ring up the sale, and saying something like, "I'm sorry you are not feeling well. Take this medicine to help. Call me if you have any questions. I close at 10 pm." You see, to most pharmacists, medicine is the best, if not the only way to cure headaches. But I know (and you know) medications do not cure them at all! Therein lies the problem. Until headaches are part of your life, either your own life or someone you are close to, there is no possible way to understand the absolute hell caused by head pain, whether it is a migraine, cluster, tension headache, or nerve-based facial pain like trigeminal neuralgia.

I've helped my own husband recover from daily, intractable head pain where no physician could help him. And I've helped many others along the way because I am a syndicated columnist, lecturer and author. I met a woman named Marilyn at a book signing in Gainesville, Florida. She told me I saved her life with my tip on capsaicin, a chili pepper cream. Not even 3 surgeries had helped her, but a 10 dollar tube of cream did. I'll tell you more on how Marilyn resolved her pain in Chapter 5 "Trigeminal Neuralgia."

Call me fearless, call me crazy, but nothing is going to stop me from sharing everything I know with you. I only ask you check with your own doctor before trying anything. That's rule #1 and I'll keep reminding you of this throughout my book. I always want you to be safe. Not every tip you read is good for you. Okay? Okay, deal.

Read the testimonials which I've received over the years from fans who implemented my recommendations:

Dear Suzy

I have endured migraines almost all of my life, I am 22 years old. I read your article in 2009, which printed in my local paper, entitled, "Artificial Sweeteners Aren't So Sweet." You said that studies proved aspartame could increase frequency of migraines by up to 50 %. That blew me away because I had been drinking at least 2 cans of diet soda each day. My parents buy it by the case. I stopped cold-turkey and within 3 weeks my headaches went away. I no longer take any medicine, nothing at all, and I was able to enjoy my classes again. I joined the swim team, and I'm studying to become a dental hygienist. I cried myself to sleep so many nights from the pain, and now I am fine. You have changed the course of my life.

Robin

Dear Suzy

When you suggested riboflavin for migraines on your facebook page, I thought, "This is too good to be true, an over-the-counter B vitamin that costs $9 a month, this is what she's suggesting when I've spent thousands of dollars over the years on MRIs, doctor's visits and pain pills?" I tried it anyway, I had nothing to lose. Within 6 weeks of taking 200mg daily, I noticed they eased up. Now 3 months later, they are completely gone. Completely! I am both amazed and forever a fan.

Paul

Dear Suzy,

I took your suggestions to my doctor, who tested my hormones. Lo and behold, you are right. My estrogen levels are high, and my progesterone is low. He approved your suggestions of DIM (diindolylmethane), butterbur, and iodine. Because my migraines were caused by estrogen fluctuations (how did you even know that?) these supplements helped me reduce my headaches from 10 or 11 per month to just 1 or 2, and I can live with that. I'm going gluten free next month. You are better than Google, and for that matter, better than any doctor I ever paid.

Barbara

We all know that certain situations contribute to headaches, things like stress and tension, arguments with the boss or wife, eyestrain, hangovers, infections, hormonal imbalances, food additives. There are so many different causes, dozens, if not hundreds!

You as the reader are the detective faced with a mystery that you must solve with the clues that your body gives you. My book gives you the tools to help you do the investigation that will most likely reveal the culprit. I hope to pacify your pain while you sleuth out the underlying cause, which will help you fix this problem once and for all.

I plan to give you many quick and easy solutions, as well an understanding of the development of pain in each chapter. I have to tell you, though, headaches are a vast and complicated subject. If you are just looking to relieve your pain, I make that easy, with a "Plan of Action" and other solutions throughout each chapter. Focus especially on my "Script" section, so you get my suggestions about supplements and meds that can start helping right away. Naturally ask your physician if they are right for you. If you're not sure what kind of headache you have, you can turn to Chapter 7 "Mystery Headaches Solved" to find some relief along with directions on how to scope out the possible solution for your headaches.

If I were you, I would read each and every chapter so you don't miss a thing. Many tips for one particular headache apply to others. I wrote Chapter 12 which discusses how to "Reduce Pain-Causing Cytokines" primarily for health care professionals and it opens a window into what's new in the chemistry of pain. I list the cytokines that cause pain and inflammation. It'll be interesting if you are an acupuncturist, chiropractor, nutritionist, nurse, physician assistant, ARNP, pharmacist, or physician of any type. In fact, I hope to meet you at my favorite stomping grounds, like at gatherings for The Institute of Functional Medicine, Scripps, or the A4M group (American Academy of Anti-Aging Medicine). Those docs love science! Gotta keep everyone happy, plus I am a nerd at heart. If you want to skip Chapter 12 and all the science, I promise I won't be offended.

I've read other books that address pain, and I'm not in agreement with the authors who say to avoid a "quick fix" approach. They must not be a headache sufferer! It's easy to say that if you're a doctor writing a book. Try being the patient, or watching someone you love debate whether or not to continue living because of excruciating head pain. I see nothing wrong with the quick fix, so long as you are simultaneously taking measures to get rid of what I call "migrenades™" permanently. What I mean by that are things in your life that act like grenades in your body, sparking headache. For example, artificial sweeteners, dyes, and gluten could be considered "migrenades™." You have to take control of your situation, while reducing pain immediately with quick fixes.

No one should live in chronic, intractable pain. I just get highly irritated when I read other headache books, some popular ones, that call you a "victim" or blame you for being a "drug-seeker" or a "whiner." Have you been called names like this, or told your pain "is all in your head?" Shame on anyone who says this to you. Even if you've become dependent on pain-killers, there are still plenty of ways to help you. Once the headaches stop, or become less painful, you will be able to get off these drugs. I have faith in you. I believe you when you say you're hurting. I believe you when you say need the pills to get rid of the pain. That's why we have to hold each other's hand and decide what the best treatment options are for you. Option, options! Just dig in and you'll find plenty of options.

Please read through the entire book, especially if you're not responding as quickly as you hoped. Headaches are extremely complex, that's why there are so few authors willing to tackle the subject. Look on Amazon, you'll see a handful of books, not hundreds. Most all of them just say the same thing about avoiding caffeine and food triggers. You know that by now. As you read my book you'll find that it's more complicated than all of those currently available. I'm proud of that, I hope you see how much work and research I've put into this in order to help you. I am certain you'll uncover solutions within these pages, even if you have to read a chapter two or three times, or take it to your doctor to help you get tests and understand more. I have faith in your ability to learn, to incorporate meaningful changes and to ultimately reach your goal of living headache free. I am eager for you to begin reading the rest of my book, see your wonderful reviews on Amazon (if you feel led) and begin your own healing journey. You deserve more in life.

Like Jim Carey says, "Alrighty then!" Let's do this.

Chapter 2

Migraine Headaches

It floored me when I learned that more than 37 million Americans suffer from migraines. To make matters worse, fewer than half of those 37 million Americans are diagnosed with migraines by their healthcare providers! Instead, they may be told they have a "tension" or "sinus" headache. Easy for them to say! All the pain and discomfort translates to 157 million missed workdays annually. That data comes from the *National Headache Foundation* and to put it all in perspective, consider that the combined number of sufferers of asthma, diabetes and coronary heart disease adds up to 33 million people. That means an additional four million people suffer from migraines.

If you are new to my work, you should know that I'm a pharmacist by training and practice, that is my background. I am also a Functional Medicine practitioner (see: www.functionalmedicine.org) so I look at both mind and body as one living person. What a concept! I'm a detective and want to help you determine the cause for your migraines, which is just the name given to a basket of awful symptoms that occur in millions of people. It's just one name, "migraines" but it can be caused by a dozen different reasons. I want to help you figure out the reason for your migraine pain, and stop it.

I recall my days as a pharmacist in Florida where patients would come in to get their medications filled. I felt bad for them because I knew they'd be back soon to get more, and that nothing in my pharmacy held the cure. Some actually came in after the prodrome stage — that's the pre-headache time before the pain begins — and I would process their prescriptions (aka "scripts" in pharmacist lingo) as quickly as possible knowing they just wanted to get out of my pharmacy and go lie down in the dark! While writing this book, I saw websites saying that migraines are a "chronic" neurological disorder but I completely disagree with that perspective and I want you to wrap your head around the fact that you can cure yourself, and your migraines are not necessarily chronic or neurological. Here's why I say that:

Point #1:   You can have one migraine (or even a bunch over the course of a year) and never ever have another, so clearly they are not always "chronic."

Point #2:   It isn't "neurological" in some people, for example those whose migraines are triggered by food additives, artificial sweeteners, gluten or dairy allergies or a mineral deficiency.

Headaches can take the joy out of life and if you've ever had a migraine you know it! It's not the same as a garden-variety headache you get, the pain is much more intense and it usually affects one side of your head, not both your temples. A classic migraine can make you nauseous and sensitive to sounds, perfume and light. Risk factors include a family history. For example, if your sister or dad gets them, you are more likely to get them yourself. Being female is another risk factor. Some people even get migraines without any head pain.

Triggers for Migraine Vary

Many factors can trigger migraine attacks, especially if you are sleep deprived. For some, just missing a meal will bring on the pain. Any medications that cause a blood vessels to swell can induce a headache and bright lights, sunlight, fluorescent lights, can all contribute to a headache. Watching TV or working on your computer all day play a role. Even certain foods and excessive noise. For many of you, treatments to relieve stress, and reduce cortisol will help, see Chapter 9 "Adrenal Hormones and the Headache Connection."

Triggers don't necessarily always cause a headache, and likewise, avoiding a trigger doesn't keep them at bay for sure. As your resident nerd, I can tell you that this means something more is going on and it could be related to your morning bagel and cream cheese. I'm not kidding.

Gluten is a Migrenade™!

Can a cinnamon bun make your head hurt? I'm certainly happy to test that out with you! All kidding aside, gluten-containing foods like muffins, breads, pasta and cereal seem to affect some people's migraines, especially those with intestinal problems. Celiac is the autoimmune disorder tied to gluten, a protein found in wheat. For some of you, gluten acts like a grenade (a migrenade!) in your head.

In particular, people with Celiac seem to suffer the most. Celiac is an autoimmune disorder that causes the body to attack itself when you consume gluten. Researchers at Columbia University in New York discovered a strong correlation between migraine suffers and patients with celiac disease (and inflammatory bowel disease).

A recently published study in *Headache* (2013) found that patients with Celiac Disease had more migraines than those without celiac disease. Five hundred and two participants were given a questionnaire that asked detailed questions concerning their clinical, demographic, and dietary information. They were also asked to share details about their headache type and frequency. Celiac participants accounted for 188 of the total participants. Gluten sensitivity participants accounted for 25, Inflammatory Bowel Disease (IBD) participants accounted for 111, and there were 178 controls. The results found that 72% of celiac disease participants graded their migraines as "severe" compared to 30% of those with IBD, 60% of the "gluten sensitive" participants, and 50% of the control participants.

Scientists evaluated all the data from the participants and made some correlations regarding migraine type, severity, and frequency. The researchers found that migraines were more prevalent in the participants with celiac disease and irritable bowel disease than found in the control group. No surprise there, however, what is surprising is that there was no correlation between the *number of years* people followed a strict gluten free diet and the severity of their migraines. Apparently, it doesn't matter if you've been gluten-free 10 years, or 1 year, the severity of your headache will be the same, you're just less likely to experience the mind-blowing events if you eat gluten free.

Could you have Celiac and not even know it? Yes, of course, most Celiacs don't know they have it, they just have a lot of digestive upset, or neurological problems, or autoimmune diseases. Regardless of whether or not you have Celiac, nobody fully digests gluten. Lectins (beans, legumes) might be even worse, so I'd avoid them too.

A case study recently done by my good friend David Perlmutter, MD and Aristo Vojdani, PhD found that gluten is a trigger for migraine headaches. They evaluated the blood of a 60 year-old man who suffered for 30 years with debilitating migraine headaches; he found little to no relief from prescription medications. His blood showed antibodies (those substances in your body that fight against something specific, in this case the antibodies were fighting against proteins in certain foods) wheat, gluten and dairy proteins.

You know where I'm going with this. Once the gentleman began eating a gluten-free and dairy-free diet, he finally found some relief. And yes, you say, that is just a placebo effect, meaning he thought he would feel better by eating gluten-free. But the study confirmed a reduction in those antibodies against wheat, gluten and dairy, once he changed his diet. So not only did he say he felt better, but his blood proved it. Dr. Perlmutter is the author of many books, including his latest best-seller, *Grain Brain, The Surprising Truth about Wheat, Carbs, and Sugar—Your Brain's Silent Killers* (Little, Brown and Company September 2013).

While we're on the subject of food, and food additives like gluten, consider monosodium glutamate (MSG). It's well known to affect people, and cause various different types of allergies, mostly gastrointestinal reactions. It reminds me of one of my friends who gets a Chinese food reaction, and it triggers diarrhea and stomach problems for hours. Not all Chinese food outlets use the flavor enhancer of MSG, but some do, and if you're sensitive it could cause a headache to go with the potty problems. It's not just Chinese food, in fact, that's nothing! MSG is found in hundreds of thousands of foods, usually in refined, processed food. It can trigger headaches, to go with the GI problems in sensitive folks.

Dairy is Another Migrenade™!

I probably got your attention when I scared you away from gluten-containing muffins, bagels, doughnuts, pasta and bread. Please don't hate on me, I'm only trying to help you. I'm about to dash your dreams for pizza now. Because of the dairy with the gluten! I'll leave pizza alone for the moment, let's just isolate the cheese because it's made with cow's milk, another migrenade™! Dairy is implicated in approximately 37% of migraine cases. That's nothing to sneeze at (although sneezing is one hallmark sign of dairy allergy!)

When you take dairy (and gluten) out of your diet, the headaches usually get better or dare I say, disappear for some. Yes, for some! Try it, you have nothing to lose. A gluten-free, dairy-free diet comes close to a Paleo diet, or Phase One diet. That is what I recommend. Can I prove your headache will go away if you ditch the gluten and dairy (and all grains)? No, but you can prove it to yourself.

This reported relationship between migraines and reactivity to wheat and gluten, and dairy is difficult to prove since the diet-triggered headache is not consistently confirmed by standard testing, such as a skin-prick test, or IgE antibody titer (blood test). Therefore, an alternative to IgE testing, such as IgG and IgA antibody testing (yes, a blood test used to see your reaction to food antigens) in combination with an elimination diet, where you eliminate the offending foods would just be the best way to go. And I might add that MSG, and artificial sweeteners would have to go to! Sorry, I'm not trying to be an ogre, you have to just trust me on this. It won't hurt you to try, it's free, and it could very well help. Nothing ventured, nothing gained. Clean up your diet for just 1 month and then send me your 'love note' via email. I know this will help some of you!

MSG The Hidden Migrenade™

New research has found that a single dose (intake) of monosodium glutamate (MSG) is enough to cause headaches and muscle pain in patients. Temporomandibular Disorders (let's call it TMD for ease), affect around 10% of the entire population. Diet has been identified as a significant life-style factor that could contribute to muscle pain in those who suffer with TMD. Certain foods have been identified as triggers for craniofacial pain. MSG (a taste enhancer) has been suggested as a leading cause of this type of pain and may trigger headaches as well as an elevation in systolic blood pressure.

Recently, researchers published a double-blind, placebo-controlled cross-over trial examining the relationship between MSG and headache and peri-cranial muscle pain.[38] Fourteen folks volunteered for the trial, and to anyone's knowledge, they did not have any documented allergies to MSG, no diarrhea, no stomach problems, no visible reactions to the MSG; no uncontrolled hypertension either. So they had a clean slate at the outset of the trial.

I can't tell you I'd ever do this myself, but these lovely folks consumed five doses of MSG in the form of 75 to 150mg/kg from a sugar-free lemon soda. They drank this for one week and then drank placebo. Various types of pain were measured; spontaneous pain, pressure pain thresholds, and tolerance levels for the masseter and temporalis muscle, side effects, and blood pressure. These measurements were evaluated before MSG consumption and then at 15, 30, and 50 minutes after consuming it. Saliva samples were taken before administration and 30 minutes after MSG intake to evaluate glutamate concentrations. Glutamate is just an amino acid that is measurable but in excess glutamate is an excitotoxin (harmful).

Point is, researchers found headaches occurred in more than half, to be exact 57% of participants! Salivary glutamate concentrations and blood pressure were both significantly elevated after MSG intake as well. This study suggests that individuals who consume MSG in their diet are more apt to have headaches and masseter muscle sensitivity, and both of those are associated with facial pain like temporomandibular joint syndrome, or trigeminal neuralgia.

Typically, the body is perfectly capable of breaking MSG down into GABA, a neurotransmitter that has a calming effect. What happens if you consume so much MSG that your body can't break it down fast enough? It builds up. You accumulate excessive amounts of glutamate, and you can't break it down fast enough to calming GABA. So you are out of balance, in an excitatory state because glutamate is excitatory. Imbalanced, you have excess glutamate as compared to GABA, so you are wired, prone to headaches, seizures, insomnia, anxiety, and everything that goes with a ratio of high glutamate to GABA. If you're not sensitive to MSG I'd say no worries, but if you're a migraineur, I'd avoid this additive, and avoid artificial additives and colors too.

More initials coming, as if MSG and TMD and GABA (Gamma-aminobutyric acid) aren't enough! Sorry, but I want to help you and need to relay it, your doctor can help you understand but here's the deal: Some of you (who have autoimmune disorders) have such an issue that your body attacks larger enzymes such as GAD (Gutamate decarboxylase).

This GAD enzyme converts MSG into something calming and relaxing, GABA! If your body attacks the GAD enzyme, you are stuck with a lot of glutamate, and again, this puts you into a pro-inflammatory cycle, where you have an excess of glutamate (as compared to GABA), and that can add to the migraine challenges. Think of glutamate as a loose cannon in the body, it's what I call a "migrenade™" as in, grenade that triggers a migraine! That's glutamate, whereas it's calming, soothing sister GABA helps you relax and sleep because it's an inhibitory hormone. Too much of that and you feel like a walking sleepy zombie, it's all about balance. To see if you are one of these rare individuals with autoantibodies to GAD enzyme, just have your doctor order blood tests aimed at identifying GAD antibodies; you can also look for gene snps which show a predisposition, and that requires saliva through 23andMe.com, and you can order that one by yourself online if the FDA doesn't close them down for selling genetic tests.

Migrenades

So many ordinary, everyday things can trigger migraines. Things that are no big deal to most folks for others open the door to hours of pain:

- Anxiety or emotional stress
- Bright lights or loud noises
- Certain odors or perfumes
- Physical exertion
- Lack of sleep (or oversleeping)
- Inhaling smoke or smoking
- Skipping meals
- Alcohol
- Estrogen fluctuations
- Tyramine (wine, cheese, smoked fish, chicken livers, figs, some beans)
- Monosodium glutamate (MSG)
- Nitrates (found in some bacon, hot dogs, salami, etc)
- Other foods such as chocolate, nuts, peanut butter, avocado, banana, citrus, onions, dairy products, and fermented or pickled foods.
- Gluten, dairy, eggs and other sensitizing foods
- Environmental toxins and POPs (persistent organic pollutants)
- Vitamin D in sensitive people (read more page 24)

Anatomy of a Headache

For the approximately 30 to 40% of migraineurs who are lucky enough to get a warning, food cravings, fatigue, frequency of urination, neck stiffness, diarrhea or feeling suddenly irritable or tearful marks the moment that you know your migraine is coming on. Why would I say "lucky" enough to get a warning? Because it gives you a chance to abort what's to come with medications or supplements. By no means do I mean to be flippant.

The Aura

The "aura" happens next in about 20% of sufferers and can last up to an hour. The symptoms are scary, especially the first time you experience them:

* Visual disturbances - Flashing lights, wavy lines, spots
* Partial loss of sight, blurry vision
* Visual snow
* Hallucinations of various odors or sounds that aren't there
* Tingling or numbness of the face or your side
* Difficulty speaking (easily mistaken for a stroke)
* Confusion
* Hearing loss
* Vertigo or dizziness
* Paralysis (temporary)
* Reduced sensation to touch
* Hypersensitivity to being touched

The Headache

Then the actual headache begins, and may include the symptoms in the aura, plus a variety of other discomforts. You know you're into this phase because of the head pain, sometimes termed *hemicranial* pain. This is pain that occurs on one side of your head, but it can move to the other side, or become bilateral (both sides). Sometimes there is a sensation of an earache to go with sound sensitivity (and light sensitivity), plus nausea, vomiting, diarrhea or sinus problems.

After the Headache

The post-drome (or "after" the "syndrome" that is a migraine headache) is the final part, as if the aura and headache weren't bad enough. This phase is best described as a hangover feeling combined with unnatural feelings or mood changes. These include either melancholy or depressed mood, or for some people, a weird sense of euphoria. Overall weakness or fatigue, inability to concentrate or poor comprehension can occur as well. From start to finish a migraine can last anywhere from 4 hours to several days, it's very individualized. It can be different for you each time you have an episode!

Why the Pain Begins

The experts can't agree why migraines happen, though many feel they are the result of blood vessel enlargement. New research shows that some migraines occur with no vasodilation though, but we'll talk about it because for some of you, this is a factor. To describe a migraine fully, I would need another 100 pages because it's really rather complex. I'd much rather focus on remedies than on details about nitty gritty stuff like this.

Research confirms that IL-1ß (a pro-inflammatory cytokine or chemical you make in your cells) is involved in the development of pain, but it's just too complex to explain here, it might literally give you (and me) a headache! Read Chapter 12 "Reduce Pain-Causing Cytokines" if you crave more of the nuts and bolts. If you crave 'real people' advice, turn to Appendix IV to read "Facebook Friends Helping Friends."

Regardless of what chemical activates the pain, it's fair to say that some experts, see it as a 'squeezing off' or vasoconstriction in an artery, sometimes in the occipital area (back of your head). This cuts off blood flow and reduces the normal level of neurotransmitters in the brain giving you the "aura." In response to the vasoconstriction, your body sends out platelets which get together (or "aggregate") with lymphocytes and leukocytes (white blood cells) and so the inflammatory "cascade" -like one domino pushing over the others- begins.

All this results in the release of serotonin and glutamate, biochemicals that increase your sensitivity to pain. Different cranial nerves are affected, depending on the type of migraine you have, and what area is affected (like your eye, temples, trigeminal area).

Once vasoconstriction starts in an area of the brain, your nervous system responds and forces the opposite situation, vasodilation (opening wider of the arteries; like "dilated" pupils) so that your brain doesn't starve from any lack of blood flow or oxygen. The increased blood flow from the vasodilation is what causes throbbing. Some migraines occur without vasodilation.

So during the flare, an artery (eventually) enlarges or "vasodilates" and it happens on the outside of your skull (not deep inside your brain). Most often it is just under the skin of the temple, the temporal artery. This action causes the release of chemicals which trigger pain and inflammation. That is why you will read about medications that narrow or constrict blood vessels such as the triptans (and ergotamine drugs. These prescription medications offer a good strategy, at least for temporary relief because they constrict the blood vessels. Ah, but if it were only that easy.

Your body has a mechanism that notices what is happening in the skull, and it notices the dilation of the artery and the engorgement of blood. In response to a migraine headache, your sympathetic nervous system (which in this case has no sympathy whatsoever) does what it's supposed to do. It produces compounds that make you feel queasy and throw up. There is a complex fluctuation in your neurotransmitters during this entire process, which causes many of the aura symptoms. Some of the symptoms associated with migraine are due to changes in dopamine, norepinephrine and various cytokines.[7] Other studies have shown serotonin deficiency to be a factor in migraine headaches.

As I said earlier, the experts can't agree why migraines occur, some don't even think it has much to do with blood vessel dilation. I would fall into that class, meaning I think migraines have more to do with mitochondrial dysfunction and what compounds your cells are pumping out. By that I mean, are they pumping out pain-causing cytokines? Are they pumping out enough ATP (your energy molecule)? Wrap your head around this type of thinking because it will allow you to embrace new ideas that alter the way your cells work, and that could mean you reach your ultimate goal, becoming headache free!

The Life & Times of Mitochondria

If you could put a microscope deep into your body, all the way into your cells, you would see the mitochondria suffering or dying. Your mitochondria are your energy generators, or "powerhouses" you have trillions of them throughout your body. People lose function of these precious mitochondria or "mito" for short. What poisons kill these mito? It could be environmental toxins, metals and residues of pesticides. You can read about all those in Chapter 8 "Detoxification Matters."

Your mito can be destroyed by viral or bacterial infection. It could be chronic lyme (even if undetected) so you should read Chapter 6 "Lyme Headaches." It could also be excess estrogen that you get from prescriptions, or using products with xenobiotics. Read Chapter 10, entitled "Estrogen & Progesterone Connection to Hormones" for solutions to hormonal-related headaches. Your mito might be damaged allowing migraines to occur if you are malnourished, or you have excessive oxidation from free radical damage, which you get from smoking, drinking alcohol, eating refined food, and saturated fats.

Serotonin and Migraines

Another reason migraines occur is because of serotonin breakdown, which leads to a deficiency in the body. The story goes like this. Back in the 1960s, researchers found a lot more 5-HIAA (5-hydroxyindoleacetic acid) in the urine of patients having a migraine.

At first they assumed this meant the person had an excess of 5-HIAA, so it was spilling into the urine. But with more recent research, we now know that the increased 5-HIAA in the urine is due to increased breakdown of serotonin in the body. It's breaking down faster because of increased activity of an enzyme called monoamine oxidase (MAO). Migraine sufferers actually have low levels of serotonin in the tissue because of the overzealous effects of MAO.

You need serotonin to minimize headaches, but too much is just equally bad. How do you get too much serotonin? Combining triptans with supplements that make more of it, like 5HTP or rhodiola, sold over the counter. Yeah, it could happen, I've seen it.

So you need serotonin for your nerve cells and brain to function. But too much serotonin causes symptoms that can range from mild, shivering and diarrhea, to severe symptoms like muscle rigidity, fever and seizures. Severe serotonin syndrome can be fatal if not treated.

Avoid or be extremely careful about combining multiple vasoconstrictive (artery-narrowing) drugs within a 24 hour period. I wouldn't do it unless I had my doctor's permission. An example of this type of combination is a triptan plus an ergot drug. Another example would be two triptan drugs. You'll read about those medications shortly. The concern is that you will excessively narrow your blood vessels (think TIA or stroke). You really don't want to cut off blood flow to an important area because that tissue can die, if it's an artery that leads to your brain for example, and you cut off blood flow, that is called a TIA ("transient ischemic attack") or stroke.

This becomes a point of contention at the doctor's office, because many of you don't want to admit you're taking a higher dose than you should (or combining drugs that shouldn't be) and while I understand you may be in terrible pain, the interaction that results and consequences that befall you may not be worth it. When your physician asks you what medication you take, be honest. If what she/he prescribed isn't working, say so. This is a good time to remind you that if you're not responding to the strongest medications of our time, then maybe something else needs to be uncovered, like a food allergy or infection.

Popular SSRI Antidepressants
Selective Serotonin Reuptake

Chemical Name	Brand Name
Citalopram	Celexa
Escitalopram	Lexapro
Fluoxetine	Prozac
Paroxetine	Paxil
Sertraline	Zoloft

The hope is that these SSRI antidepressant medications will reduce the frequency (and severity) of migraines, but SSRI drugs are not a cure. They do work for some people, and your prescribing clinician must find just the right dose. They don't work for everyone though. In fact, the authors of a study published in 2005 found that even after two months of treatment with SSRIs, they were "no more efficacious than placebo in patients with migraine."[8]

So in my book, migraineurs should always include restoration of mitochondrial (cell) health, and reduction of pain-causing cytokines. This can be done with supplements in most cases, and is perfectly reasonable to do even if you are taking antidepressant medications, presuming, as always, that you check with your prescribing clinician first.

Bacteria Can Cause Headaches

What if migraines were caused by a germ? With Lyme disease, that's exactly what causes them so it's not far-fetched to me. I think bacteria, fungus, viruses and parasites are pretty much the cause for all diseases and inflammation.

Years ago, Drs. Barry Marshall and Robin Warren were considered practically insane when they said ulcers were caused by bacteria called Helicobacter pylori (aka *H. Pylori*) instead of by stress, which all the other doctors said was the cause of ulcers. Today, we know that eradication of *H. pylori* does in fact resolve peptic and duodenal ulcers, whether you are stressed out or not. It is tied to a germ. Reducing *H. pylori* is good to do anyway, because it reduces your risk for gastritis and stomach cancer. Those crazy scientists by the way, were awarded the 2005 Nobel Prize in Physiology or Medicine.

How crazy would you think I was if I told you that *H. pylori* (the same bug tied to ulcers) is associated with migraines? Well it is! A randomized, double-blind placebo controlled study proved it in 2012, and that was not the first study to examine bacteria, parasites, worms and virus as a cause of migraines. Some experts believe that migraines are more likely to occur if you have a dead tooth (as in chronic bacterial toxins that get out from under your root canal). The only way around that is to extract the tooth (ouch) and I'm not necessarily recommending it, unless it is your last resort.

Anyway, the 2012 study I mentioned earlier was published in *Pain Physician* and researchers concluded *"H. pylori eradication may have a beneficial role on migraine headache."*

They came to this conclusion by performing what's called a "randomized, double-blind, controlled study" with 64 people, which essentially means they gave the same questionnaire about their symptoms to all participants, without knowing which person was getting the treatment to eliminate the *H. Pylori* bacteria, and without the participants knowing if they were being treated or not.

The quick fix for *H. pylori*? Something called "Triple Therapy" which your doctor prescribes. It consists of a proton-pump inhibitor for acid reduction and two antibiotics that you take for a week or sometimes two. There are slower ways, that are natural such as zinc carnosine, mastic gum, probiotics and broccoli sprouts. I wrote about this topic and you can read that article by visiting my website, *www.DearPharmacist.com* and searching for the article entitled, "Advice for Ulcers and H. Pylori Infection."

Vitamin D May Be a Trigger

I can't put my finger on why vitamin D affects a subset of you, I just know that it does. If you've started to notice more migraine attacks, with or without aura, photosensitivity, or if you've noticed left eye aura or one sided headaches, temporary vision loss in one of your eyes . . . anything to indicate less stability in your head, it could be your vitamin D. Now, that is contradictory to what some experts say, they want your levels to be very high. I'm one of them, I know that higher levels of vitamin D, around 70 - 90 ng/ml can lift depression, improve autoimmune disease and reduce risk of leukemia and various cancers. But there are some of you who should not attempt this because the D triggers a migraine. Also, testing for vitamin D is confusing. You can take a blood test, and it may come back as "low" but the active, body-ready version of D (which is really a hormone) is sky-high.

I know you want to know more about vitamin D testing so I'll share that here. Some people get this test: $1\alpha25(OH)_2D$ but that's not what I recommend because it may be elevated even if you have a deficiency. I prefer this test: The 25(OH)D or "25 hydroxy vitamin D" test, that's the only one that will tell you what is really going on inside your body. Now, just because it's low doesn't mean you should take vitamin D. Like I said, some of you will react negatively to this nutrient, and get more headaches, or halos.

So if you've been taking vitamin D supplements, and your headaches have changed for the worse, this not your imagination. I don't think it's any of the fillers in the vitamin D, I think it's the actual D. The good news is that if you've been taking D for a long time and you stop now, the migraines should retreat. You don't have to wean off D; it is a vitamin that can be suddenly stopped.

Suzy's "Migraine Script" for Pain Relief

Before you take any of the following supplements, you must ask your doctor(s) if they are right for you. My intention here is to educate you about possibilities and options. Do not misconstrue my ideas for medical advice. I have no idea what is right for every individual reading this so take my list to your practitioner(s) to ask if they're right for you with your medical history. Dosages are also just basic guidelines, some people tolerate different dosages than others.

    Magnesium glycinate
    CoQ10
    Riboflavin
    Acetyl L carnitine
    Alpha Lipoic Acid
    Butterbur

How This Helps You Become Headache Free

Magnesium. I think it's time I came clean and just said it out loud, magnesium is my *favorite* mineral. And for me to say that when I've been deficient in iron for years speaks volumes. I can't help it, I really love magnesium, it's your natural chill pill. We're all deficient in this one baby! Especially if you drink coffee, a known drug mugger. The mineral is an antioxidant and works all over your body. You're deficient if you have constipation, heart palpitations, anxiety, menstrual cramps, bad PMS, muscle cramps or insomnia. When your system is tight or irritable (you are sensitive to light or sounds, have a nervous stomach, twitches), you are probably low in magnesium. You can test if you want, but testing fails many. The best way is a red blood cell level, termed an RBC magnesium. But I have to tell you, this can be within normal ranges in the face of a total body deficiency. Unfortunately, there isn't a better test than an RBC magnesium just yet, you may just have to try it and gauge response. Treatment with magnesium is my number one choice for migraine sufferers, and it may be all you need.[12,13] When buying magnesium, choose glycinate, aspartate, malate, citrate, chelate or taurate salts. Avoid magnesium oxide, it's a strong laxative. In fact, magnesium citrate can be a laxative too, if you are sensitive, but it's still among my preferred forms of magnesium.

CoQ10. This one supports mitochondrial health. Remember how I explained your mito are sick as one new theory behind migraines? Well CoQ10 feeds your mito. It's an antioxidant that you make in your liver under normal circumstances. Estrogen-containing drugs (birth control, menopause drugs) as well as statin-cholesterol reducing medications (Lipitor, Zocor) can interfere with your body's ability to make CoQ10. Those medications are drug muggers of CoQ10, and the longer story regarding that is in my *Drug Mugger* book (Rodale Press, 2011). The big deal is that a deficiency of CoQ10 affects mitochondrial health, and harms you. CoQ10 is the most studied substance for the treatment of mitochondrial disorders. There's a pretty tight connection between CoQ10 and headache relief. One study presented at *The American Academy of Neurology* annual meeting in 2004, found that CoQ10 can stop 50% of migraines,[14] Another found that CoQ10 is able to reduce IL-2 and TNFα (two pro-inflammatory compounds you can read about in Chapter 12).[15]

A study from 2002 published in *Cephalalgia*[16] did an open label trial for CoQ10 as a preventive nutrient. The study concluded that 61.3% of participants in the trial found at least a 50% reduction in the frequency of migraine attacks (over 4 months). Data suggests that it make take a minimum of 1 month to achieve this 50% reduction, and possibly as much as 3 months. Still, I'd wait it out 3 months if I had to in order to get that kind of relief. It helped both types of migraines, those with auras and those without. Studies show it can be given to adolescents as well as adults without concern for side effects. The dosage is about 150mg daily, but that differs with each individual.

Riboflavin. Riboflavin all by itself is helpful to migraineurs, but when taken along with CoQ10 it is even better in preventing headaches, as demonstrated by a study published in the journal, *Headache*, in 2012,[17] and another study published in the *European Journal of Neurology* in 2004,[18] which concluded, "We could demonstrate a significant reduction of headache frequency following riboflavin treatment."[19]

In addition, the number of abortive anti-migraine tablets was reduced. In line with previous studies our findings show that riboflavin is a safe and well-tolerated alternative in migraine prophylaxis. The researchers also wrote that riboflavin is a "safe and well-tolerated alternative" in prevention of migraines! High-dose vitamin B2 (400mg riboflavin) was given to 23 people, aged 20 to 65 and their symptoms, pain intensity and duration of pain were tracked for 3 months. Those receiving riboflavin noticed a 50% reduction in headache frequency, going from 4 headaches per month to 2. Headache duration was shortened, although intensity remained the same.

Riboflavin is pretty safe, the only side effects that may occur include diarrhea and a harmless discoloration of urine (it will turn your pee bright yellow orange). The dosage varies, some experts say the best range for headache relief is 50mg taken 4 times daily (for a total of 200mg daily) while others feel that high dosages are vital, as in 200mg twice daily. I cannot say what's right for you, but I believe that you should experiment and always take the lowest effective dose for you.

Acetyl L-carnitine. This is an activated form of the amino acid "carnitine" which is used to transport fatty acids. Acetyl L-Carnitine revs up the mitochondria producing more energy. If you take high doses of this, and you might need to for your personal condition, you will want to take a little alpha lipoic acid (discussing that one next). The reason is that Acetyl L-carnitine causes a little oxidation, kind of like cellular rusting. Don't be concerned about this, just bring in the Alpha lipoic acid (or R lipoic acid) to prevent the damage (oxidation). The two together are fabulous for your general health anyway, and as an added benefit, acetyl L-carnitine happens to turn into acetylcholine in your brain, and that is one of your primary memory molecules. Relieve headaches and remember stuff better with this one supplement, but again, take a little alpha lipoic acid with it too.

One other little-known action that is important is Acetyl L carnitine's ability to sweep ammonia out of the brain. This could help clear brain fog too. In fact, right now (at publication time) researchers at the prestigious Norwegian University of Science and Technology were recruiting adults for a placebo-controlled study to look at the efficacy of Acetyl-L-carnitine as a preventive for people who have suffered from migraines in the past. Stay tuned on their progress . . . see: http://clinicaltrials.gov/ct2/show/NCT01695317.

Alpha Lipoic Acid. This is a powerful antioxidant that (just like CoQ10) crosses the blood brain barrier, gets into your brain cells and nourishes your precious mitochondria. It's important to take this if you happen to take Acetyl L carnitine as explained in that section. A trial found that ALA all by itself was helpful in reducing migraines too. Alpha lipoic acid reduces MMPs (inflammatory compounds that your body makes). To read more, refer to chapter 12. The headache Research Unit of the Neurology Department of the University of Liège, in Belgium, studied 54 patients with migraines (with and without auras). They were given 600mg ALA (total daily dose) to prevent migraines, and the researchers (conservatively) concluded that the ALA did in fact help prevent migraines.[20]

Butterbur. Known botanically as *Petasites hybridus*, this shrub has been used for centuries to treat asthma and cough, but it also supports healthy blood vessel tone and blood flow in the brain, and clinical studies cite its effectiveness in preventing migraines. One of the active ingredients in this herb is petasin which inhibits production of leukotrienes in eosinophils and neutrophils (those are some cells in your immune system).[21] Excessive production of leukotrienes causes many allergy symptoms as well as pain and inflammation so butterbur puts a stop to some of that misery. Another ingredient called petasites reduces smooth muscle spasm.

Leukotrienes are harmful pro-inflammatory compounds when produced in excess. Dr. Levin, of the Dartmouth Hitchcock Medical Center in New Hampshire, wrote, in his 2012 study, "Butterbur and feverfew are the 2 herbal oral preparations best studied, and they seem to have real potential to help many patients with migraine and perhaps other headache types."[22]

ThyroScript™

This dietary supplement supports a healthy thyroid gland, energy production and metabolism. I'm proud to say it is my own personal blend of natural herbs and vitamins. I developed ThyroScript™ based upon my studies and every ingredient has scientific research to support a beneficial effect. Read Chapter 11 for more on the thyroid connection to migraines. www.ScriptEssentials.com

Butterbur is a remarkable plant-based tool in the fight against migraines (and seasonal allergies). Burping was the only side effect noted in a study published in the December 2004 issue of Neurology, where researchers studied some 230 people who experienced migraines, and concluded, that a standardized *Petasites hybridus* extract 75mg taken twice daily (aka "BID" in pharmacy speak) is both effective and well tolerated as a preventive therapy for migraines.[23]

This trial was a three-arm, randomized group that examined dosages of 75mg, 50mg and placebo. Two hundred and forty-five patients ranging in age between 18 and 65 were entered into the study and they all had 2 to 6 migraines per month. Over 4 months, researchers found migraine attack frequency reduced by 48% in the butterbur 75mg bid group. The data also showed a reduction of 36% in migraine frequency in the butterbur root extract 50mg bid group and a 26% migraine frequency reduction in the placebo group.

No one left the trial due to adverse side effects, although burping was seen at a higher incidence compared to placebo. Hmm, let me ponder that for one second, burping or migraine headaches? I'll take burping any day. The results show that butterbur root extract at 75mg twice daily is a safe an effective preventative agent. Another study examined the effectiveness of the 75mg dose for 12 weeks with 60 people, and made the same conclusion, as reported in *Phytomedicine* in 2006 in an article by researchers at a headache center in Zurich, Switzerland.[24]

Why No Niacin?

For most people, the B vitamin niacin is just fine. But it's not for everyone!

High dose niacin is often prescribed to lower cholesterol. And some people take it as an over-the-counter supplement. Some studies suggest niacin can help a migraine, even stop it altogether during the aura phase. That is definitely possible for some of you. Even the 2003 edition of *Mayo Clinic Proceedings* reported that niacin can be effective for preventing migraine headaches.

So what's the problem? It is true that the vasodilation abilities of niacin may prevent or abort certain migraines, while in their aura phase. However, once the body has started increasing blood flow during the painful part of the migraine taking niacin at that point may simply contribute to the pounding pain! That's why I don't recommend it for everyone. If you are curious, certainly you can try the non-sustained release form of niacin. (The kind that causes a flush.) But if you are among the unlucky ones who feels worse on niacin, don't call me at 2 in the morning when your head is pounding. I'll just say, "I told you so."

Get Rid of Migrenades™!

Along with all the supplements I want you to consider, there are a number of things you should eliminate because they can act like grenades in your head and trigger migraines:

Artificial sweetener packets for coffee and desert (aspartame, sucralose, etc)

Diet soda (because of the artificial sweeteners)

High fructose corn syrup

Artificial dyes

Chewing gum (those that contain artificial sweeteners)

MSG (monosodium glutamate sometimes disguised as "natural flavor")

Deli meats containing nitrites

Dried fruit (that contains sulfites)

Tyramine-containing foods (cheese, chocolate)

Foods which commonly cause sensitivities like dairy, gluten, soy, corn, eggs, etc.

Excess weight

Vitamin D

A Potential Nutricure

I looked in my trusty book "Nutricures" written by my good friend Alice Feinstein and I found a simple remedy that could work for some of you, if you sense the pain approaching. Follow this recipe (get your doctor's blessings for anything you try):

1,000 - 2,000mg vitamin C powder
400mg of magnesium powder
Mix in a glass of water or juice.

This remedy may lessen the intensity of your headache. If you use poorly absorbable forms of magnesium, you could get diarrhea, so use high quality brands.

I'm a Pharmacist, Let's Talk Medicine

A great many medications can help reduce the incidence of migraines or stop one from progressing. They are not foolproof, nor are they without side effects. Nevertheless, they can be a godsend for some people.

A variety of drugs are designed specifically to relieve migraine pain, and you can buy them over-the-counter, or with a prescription. Let's look first at the pain-relievers that you can buy over-the-counter.

Headaches and Weight

Researchers at Johns Hopkins analyzed data from nearly 4,000 adults and concluded that your odds for headache go up with excessive weight. If you are obese, your odds of getting headaches are actually 80% higher.

Over-the-Counter Pain Relieving Medications

The most popular over-the-counter medications are ibuprofen (Advil, Motrin, others), naproxen (Aleve, others), all of which belong to the NSAID class, pronounced "N-said") and it stands for non-steroidal anti-inflammatory drugs. Another pain relieving drug sold over-the-counter is acetaminophen (Tylenol, others). You can also find medications sold at pharmacies nationwide that combine these ingredients along with some caffeine (Excedrin Migraine).

Dosage. Follow label directions on the package you buy. For acetaminophen, be very careful not to combine different products that contain it (for example, multi-tasking cold formulas with a sleep aid) because the maximum daily dosage is 4,000mg. Always try to take the lowest effective dose of any medication.

Caution: They may take up to an hour to kick in, assuming they are going to even work (some people get relief, others don't respond). This category of drugs is not effective for severe migraines. Medications containing acetaminophen can harm the liver if taken in excess, or long term, or in combination with wine and alcohol. Acetaminophen is a drug mugger of glutathione. NSAIDs are harmful to the stomach and esophagus. The NSAIDS have a knack for attacking the gastrointestinal

(GI) lining and in sensitive individuals they can lead to ulcers, stomach or intestinal bleeding and rebound headaches. In fact – big red flag here:

   A study in *Therapeutics and Clinical Risk Management* in 2010 noted NSAIDs are responsible for over 100,000 hospitalizations, $2 billion in healthcare costs, and 17,000 deaths in the US each year, and has been the case since 1999.[25] To avoid this side effect, a compounding pharmacist can make you a suppository form, but your physician will have to phone that prescription in and it could take a few days to fill. You can also take acetaminophen if you have an existing ulcer, that should be safer for you than another type of NSAID such as ibuprofen or naproxen. Acetaminophen doesn't appear to harm the GI tract as much as those two drugs can. Of course ask your prescribing clinician what is right for you. One more caution for you, in case you have already suffered a heart attack. Using NSAIDs is not advised, I recommend you use acetaminophen or some of the preventive supplements in my Script section. Why? Because studies suggest it increases your risk for another heart attack, regardless of how long it has been since you had the first.

Aspirin

The oldest over-the-counter medicine for pain is aspirin (around 1829, when scientists discovered salicin in willow plants), but I can't promise it will help reduce your migraine frequency, I read the average reduction with a baby aspirin a day is about 10% lowered reduction.

Prescription Pain Relieving Medications

If you experience frequent migraines, you'll probably have prescription pain relievers on hand instead of relying on OTC relief. Here's the big picture:

The Ergots
Examples: DHE, Ergotamine

These are a very old class of drugs that have fallen out of favor since the advent of triptans (discussed next). When I first graduated pharmacy school in 1989, this was pretty much the gold standard for migraine sufferers, and my customers would complain the drugs didn't work for them and try to get refunds (which they weren't given). The best of the ergotamine-type drugs is DHE short for dihydroergotamine. Brand names included

D.H.E.[45] or Migranal, and these are more effective with fewer side effects than plain ergotamine (brand Cafergot). DHE related drugs are useful for migraines (with or without aura) as well as cluster headaches.

Caution: Always be careful combining medications — I really can't say that often enough. In this particular case, life-threatening side effects such as ischemia of the extremities, or even stroke have occurred when DHE was combined with certain anti-microbials such as protease inhibitors (medications used for HIV), macrolide antibiotics (erthyromycin, clarithromycin, troleandomycin) and others.

Triptans.
Examples: Zolmitriptan, sumatriptan, frovatriptan

These prescription drugs constrict blood vessels in your brain and relieve the swelling. Classified pharmaceutically as "serotonin receptor agonists," they lift levels of serotonin. They also seem to have other properties, not fully identified, that treat migraine symptoms. Triptans come as a tablet, a lozenge, an injection (sumatriptan), or nasal spray (zolmitriptan). Some drugs come in nasal sprays offering intranasal delivery of the drug, meaning it gets into your bloodstream through the vessels in your nose. That's pretty cool if you're nauseous.

Triptans work quickly to minimize headache pain, and in some cases abort it altogether. They help reduce sensitivity to light and noise, while also reducing the urge to vomit (if that is part of your migraine scenario). Even though there are several medications in this category, some work better than others for each individual. You will have to try a few of them before you find out which works best for you. Regardless of which medication has the best effect for you, triptans work most optimally when you take it immediately when the headache starts.

Meet the Triptans	
Chemical Name	**Brand**
Almotriptan	Axert, Almogran
Eletriptan	Relpax
Frovatriptan	Frova, Migard
Naratriptan	Amerge, Naramig
Rizatriptan	Maxalt
Sumatriptan	Imitrex, Imigran
Zolmitriptan	Zomig

You can still take them after the attack has begun, it's just that they won't work quite as well. Sometimes taking a triptan with an over-the-counter analgesic (acetaminophen for example) makes it work better. Common side effects include drowsiness, dry mouth, lightheadedness, feeling hot or cold, or feeling "strange" in some way, muscle aches or cramps, racing heartbeat, soreness or burning at the injection site, or in the nose (if you use the shot or nasal spray). Interestingly, some of the side effects of triptans reek of a migraine itself: light sensitivity, fatigue, dizziness, nausea/vomiting, numbness, weakness and neuropathy. Not everyone gets these side effects, and they seem to go away over time, especially if you take the medications long enough.

Calcium Channel Blockers (or CCBs)
Examples: nifedipine, felodipine, amlodipine and verapamil

These do nothing to abort pain, because they take a long time to work. These drugs narrow (constrict) of blood vessels during the initial phase of a migraine headache. They reduce the frequency of migraine, but not alter intensity or duration. If you are prone to hypotensive (low blood pressure) episodes, don't use calcium channel blockers.

Side effects: constipation, headache, tachycardia (abnormally rapid heart rate), dizziness, drowsiness, flushing, swelling of the legs or feet, tremors, mood changes, depression, and weight gain.

Caution: Avoid grapefruit juice when taking these medications or levels of the medication could spike dangerously high.

Algae Does a Migraineur Good

Natural astaxanthin is a protective antioxidant, derived from the microalgae as *Haematococcus pluvialis*. How they get "astaxanthin" from that I just don't know! Whatever you call it, think of this protective antioxidant as something similar to beta carotene but stronger. It's a carotenoid just like beta carotene, and we already know how well that nutrient supports vision. Astaxanthin is no different. The Japanese are leaps and bounds ahead of the rest of the world in terms of research on astaxanthin and eyestrain. A 2002 study included 13 people who received 5mg astaxanthin every day. They enjoyed a 54% reduction in eye fatigue complaints.[42] Another study that same year,[43] found that critical flicker fusion improved by 46% when participants were given 6mg astaxanthin daily. Flicker fusion is defined as "the point or frequency at which all flicker of an intermittent light stimulus disappears" according to the *United States Library of Medicine*. This study evaluated it in order to understand how well the participant's vision improved.

This is pretty important stuff because natural astaxanthin is made from a simple algae, it's red in color and it can support healthy vision, joint health and skin integrity. In 2004, just 2 years, 49 volunteers were given 4mg astaxanthin every day for a month, and more significant improvements were noted.[44] See where this is going yet? Astaxanthin might very well be a migraineur's best friend. Results from two other studies[45, 46] showed how well the nutrient which is actually a red dye . . . it what 'puts the pink in pink flamingo' can reduce eyestrain which occurs from fatigue, soreness, dry eyes and blurry vision. What's

Wrinkle Drug for Migraines?

In October 2010, the FDA approved Botox (botunlinum toxin) for migraines. This is the same drug that is used to take 10 years off your face by smoothing out wrinkles. Up to 31 shots around your head may be injected, depending on the severity.

Botox is preventative, not abortive. It helps reduce frequency, as well as pulsing and throbbing pain.

My husband Sam tried it years ago, and only noted mild relief; however, his headaches were due to infection. I did, however, receive this letter from Lenice in Oklahoma who said this, *"I too have suffered for years [with migraines] as did my dad and his mom. I tried everything and someone mentioned trying Botox shots in my forehead. I am headache free. I get them every 6 months."*

so interesting to me is that astaxanthin can help prevent the eye fatigue.[47] This research proved that people were able to recover quicker than the control group after dealing with a big visual stimulus. And there are other studies too, but you get the point. If there's one eye-loving nutrient that could support eye health, it's astaxanthin. Because I am one of the Scientific Advisors for one of the makers of astaxanthin, I was able to obtain a coupon for you, for 25% off this (in fact, any purchase) from their site, www.Nutrex-Hawaii.com Use coupon code "suzy" for 25% off BioAstin astaxanthin; it will also work on your entire product purchase. I think this will work anytime you use the code, not just for initial purposes. You can try the 6mg or the 12mg, take it once daily.

Serotonin Syndrome

Most migraine medications increase serotonin. Watch for the possibility of "serotonin syndrome" if combining 2 triptan medications, a triptan with an SSRI drug such as Zoloft, or SNRIs like Cymbalta. Don't combine with MAO inhibitors or cough medicine (dextromethorphan). Serotonin syndrome can occur when you increase dosages or take dietary supplements with your triptans such as St. John's wort or 5-HTP. Here are some symptoms:

Tachycardia	Seizures	Overactive reflexes
Hypertension	Muscle stiffness	Poor coordination
Hallucinations	Diarrhea	Feeling hot
Anxiety or panic	Nausea/vomiting	

If you have a severe case, the physicians at the hospital can administer benzodiazepine drugs like lorazepam (Ativan) or diazepam (Valium) which help with muscular issues and seizures, as well as agitation. Cyproheptadine (Periactin) can also be given which is a serotonin blocker.

When Medicine Backfires: Medication Overuse Headaches

You can overdo it and give yourself "rebound headaches." That's what they are called, also more technically known "Medication Overuse Headaches" or MOHs,[29] and the headaches occur almost daily when you take too many analgesics (painkillers). These are a more common cause of chronic daily headaches than you might imagine. A transformation of sorts takes place over the course of time, usually months. You go from getting episodic migraines for example, to chronic daily headaches, from the excessive use of acute headache relieving medications.

MOH is a serious disabling and well-characterized disorder that is a recognized by the ICDH classification "International Classification of (Headache) Disorders." The tricky part is defining "overuse," as that could be different for every individual. The current definition of overuse is the following:

- Greater than 10 days per month for ergotamine, triptans, opioids or combo medications
- Greater than 15 days per month for more than 3 months for simple analgesics such as anti-inflammatory drugs (ie ibuprofen, acetaminophen, others).

The best way to cure yourself from MOH is through gradual reduction of the medications, and while doing so, using preventive herbs and supplements. See pg. 341 for a list of drugs that may trigger migraines.

Think Outside the Doc Box

Acupuncture is based on 2,500 years of Chinese medical tradition and helps improve the flow of chi (our life force) through specific meridian points on the body. It increases circulation and endorphins. The largest study examining the relationship between acupuncture and migraine was published in the March 2006 edition of *The Lancet Neurology*. Scientists determined that "47 percent of participants in the traditional acupuncture group . . . experienced a reduction of migraine days by 50 percent or more." That is just amazing, considering there are no side effects to acupuncture, and when done by a professional it is virtually painless, if not relaxing! Try it weekly for 2 months and note if your baseline improves.

Weirdest Pain Relief Yet!

How 'Bout Tonight? Yes please, I have a headache! Having sex is more fun than taking Tylenol! According to a German study published in *Cephalalgia*, migraine sufferers find relief through sexual activity. We've known this for years (anecdotally), but researchers from the University of Münster in Germany wanted to test the hypothesis. They mailed a questionnaire to people, 800 of whom suffer with migraines, and 200 more with cluster headaches. I don't know about you, but you'd have to catch me on a really good day to get me to answer questions about my sex life, whether or not I partake with a headache, and the impact of orgasms on my head pain. Chutzpah! But anyway, the researchers actually got a little more than 40% of the people to answer this questionnaire.

About a third of all people surveyed said they did have some sort of sexual experience during a migraine (or cluster headache). Two thirds of those surveyed didn't have any sex at all during headaches, but surprisingly, a third of them did. (I'm thinking their headache couldn't have been that bad!) The most intriguing thing is this. Sixty percent said their migraine pain was relieved afterward! Do you realize this is about the same efficacy as the most common prescription drug category used for migraines, the triptans. Those drugs work 60 to 80 percent of of the time. But back to this study. Keep in mind, about 60% reported an improvement of their migraine attack (70% reported moderate to complete relief). About 33% worsened.

Those who had sex with a cluster headache raging didn't get that lucky (well, it depends on how you define "lucky"). Only 37% of them reported improvement and 50% got worse. Most people avoid sex when they have a headache, you know the proverbial comment, "Not tonight honey, I have a headache!" From this study, we see that sexual activity, more specifically an orgasm, relieves head pain in some individuals. And since we're not looking, we don't care how you get to the Big O, the point is your relief may be an orgasm away. It works because your body releases endorphins when you're enjoying sex (or exercising). Endorphins, as you know, block pain. Next time your honey asks how about tonight, say "Yes please, I have a headache!"

Know the Difference

Most of you reading this chapter are reading it because you have a history of migraines, but some of you are just reading my book cover to cover because you've been a fan of my syndicated column or facebook page. Whoever you are, I need for you to know the difference between a migraine (should one ever happen to you) and a transient ischemic attack (TIA) or a stroke. The symptoms run slightly parallel because of the severe headache, the visual problems or double vision, but here are some of the other signs you need to just be aware of in case it is a stroke. Call 911 immediately if you think you're having a stroke:

Numbness, weakness or paralysis of face, arm, or leg (usually unilateral)

Sudden blurry vision

Confusion or trouble understanding

Slurred or garbled speech

Trouble walking

Dizziness or clumsiness

Severe headache

Drug Muggers that deplete pyridoxine (Vitamin B6)

Some medications rob your body of vitamin B6 and this could affect your brain's ability to produce serotonin, raising your risk for migraines. Also, vitamin B6 supports mitochondrial health, and without enough B6, or enough folic acid, B12, and magnesium, your mitochondria will starve to death, increasing risk for migraines.

Antacids & Acid blockers

Antibiotics

Blood Pressure Medications

Hormone Replacement Therapy (HRT)

The Pill (as in birth control pills)

Non-steroidal Anti-Inflammatory Drugs (NSAIDs)

Drugs Cause Migraines

Did you know that medications you take have the ability to cause head pain? Common offenders are nitroglycerin, warfarin, steroids, decongestants, antihistamines and some hormone replacement drugs. Refer to Appendix III.

For a comprehensive list of medications that zap B6 from the body (or folic acid, B12 or magnesium) thus increasing your risk for migraine, please refer to my *Drug Muggers* book (Rodale, 2011).

Diabetes and Headaches?

Yes, there's a connection but before you actually get diabetes, where your fasting blood sugar goes up, you will see a rise in insulin. High levels of insulin as measured through a blood test, is termed hyperinsulinemia. And it appears that insulin is higher in people with migraines. Is it the chicken or the egg? I think it's the egg, meaning I think the insulin rises (due to sedentary lifestyles, consumption of high fructose corn syrup, refined foods, blah blah blah :-) and then you get more headaches. I don't think it's the other way around, meaning the headaches cause your insulin to go up. Science agrees with me.

A study published in the journal, *Cephalalgia*, found patients who suffered with migraines also have insulin sensitivity or insulinemia. Insulin is a blood sugar lowering hormone that regulates carbohydrate and fat metabolism in the body. Research has shown when patients have insulinemia (abnormally large concentration of insulin in the blood) they are more at risk for developing high blood pressure, stroke, and/or other serious blood vessel disorders.

In this study, researchers evaluated and studied insulin sensitivity in 30 participants who suffered from migraines and 15 control participants. All of the participants had comparable blood sugar and insulin levels before the study began. After the participants were given a high-sugar beverage, data showed the blood sugar levels of the migraine group were dramatically higher than those in the control group. These blood sugar elevations continued for up to 3 hours after consumption of the high sugar beverage. Researchers also noted that the insulin sensitivity was also impaired in the migraine group compared to the control group.[35]

This study found that insulin sensitivity is impaired in patients with migraines and also suggests a link between insulin resistance as comorbidity between patients with migraines and vascular disorders.

Migraines & Strokes

Brand new research published in the journal Neurology shows that the brains of those who have had many migraines look like the brains of those who might have had some minor strokes.[34] These images show what look like scar areas in the brain. We also know that migraines can specifically affect brain volume and cause white matter abnormalities. While migraines are not strokes, this new research sure makes me want to urge you to nip those regular migraines in the bud.

Your Plan of Action: A Dozen Ways to Minimize the Pain

If you feel a migraine headache coming on, here are some ideas. For the supplement or medication ideas, you need to get permission from your practitioner:

1. Get hydrated. Drink a full glass of water, preferably with a squeeze of lemon or lime to alkalize it.
2. Take pain-relief meds like an anti-inflammatory or anti-headache medicine or one of the natural remedies I suggest in my "Script" section, earlier in this chapter.
3. Reach for anti-migraine supplements such as 200mg magnesium and 200mg riboflavin.
4. Relax. Lie down in the dark, preferably where it's quiet.

5. Take in some air. Breathe deeply, take an extra 'sip' at the top. Many times, headaches are caused by poor oxygenation so nice deep belly breaths can reduce the intensity, if not abort a headache.

6. Take on even more air. Since some acute migraines are due to poor mitochondrial dysfunction, I see no problem with inhaling oxygen. You can buy hand-held oxygen canisters at REI, or at camping or army stores. Living in Colorado, where you can hike fourteeners (14,000 foot mountains where altitude sickness can quickly ensue), I can attest that these oxygen gismos are pretty cool. They're sold everywhere where I live. With a few inhalations, over the course of 5 minutes, you might feel your headache completely abort, or the severity lessened.

7. Chill. Try an ice pack to your head, or cold washcloth.

8. Find a happy place! You need more silence, or perhaps calming music.

9. Try acupressure. Find the meaty part just above the webbing of your hand, between your thumb and index finger. Using your other thumb, squeeze the muscle by pressing down hard. This is an acupressure point that sometimes helps to relieve head pain.

10. Visualizations help. Imagine yourself doing something pleasurable, or a happy time. If you spiral into the scary place of how this migraine is going to take you down for 3 days straight now, and how you're going to throw up all over your bed again, and everything else that goes with it, these terrible things are harmful to your emotions. Do as best your can to mentally transport yourself to a happy place, if nothing else, it serves as a good distraction, and it may ease the situation at hand.

11. Call upon Mother Nature for herbs. If your or someone home, can help you make peppermint tea, do it. Sip that every few minutes. If you can't make the tea, then sniff it. Essential oil of peppermint is a powerful home remedy. It's also ok to try rubbing a peppermint lotion on your temples, or forehead. If you're allergic to peppermint or don't like it, an alternative is ginger tea, another strong anti-inflammatory.

12. Follow up. As a long range plan, consider implementing any or all of the supplements recommended in my "Script" section,

on page 25. Teasing out why you get a migraine is critical to you ending the pain, that's why you should keep track of your symptoms in the Headache Log in Appendix II. If you notice a pattern, you can intervene more efficiently. Migraines occur for many reasons, as you've just learned. They can happen from nutrient deficiencies, such as magnesium, or from the retention of toxins. Opening up your detoxification pathways is crucial, I know many people who cured their headaches by relieving constipation or by improving the functioning of their respiratory or urinary systems. When these elimination pathways are opened up, your body lets go of stored poisons that could otherwise cause a headache.

In fact, anyone who experiences migraines on a regular basis needs to pay careful attention to detoxifying. Eliminating poisons from the body is essential. Teasing out why you get a migraine is critical to you ending the pain, that's why you should keep track of your symptoms in the Headache Log, Appendix II. If you notice a pattern, you can intervene more efficiently. Migraines occur for many reasons as you've just learned. They can happen from nutrient deficiencies like magnesium, or from the retention of toxins. Opening up your detoxification pathways is crucial, I know many people that cured their headaches by relieving constipation or improving their respiratory or urinary system. When these elimination pathways are opened up, your body let's go of stored poisons, getting you one step closer to becoming headache free.

Also, I can't finish this chapter without sharing some pretty amazing stuff, there's one common genetic issue that may be an underlying factor in your migraines. That's coming up now, along with a possible solution to the problem.

Homocystex Plus: The Solution for Poor Methylators

An often overlooked and unknown link to migraines with aura is a common genetic mutation that affects 45% of the population mildly and 20% significantly. This means that, at minimum, one in five people reading my book has a significant genetic personality that causes migraines with aura. And the quick fix includes natural B vitamins! Could it be that simple? Yes it can! And I'll get to that shortly.

First let's take a look at this gene situation. We need to talk about it more because this simple genetic problem with an easy fix is making so many people so very miserable. You can test for this mutation with a simple blood test from www.directlabs.com/suzycohen.

This genetic mutation is found in the gene called **M**ethylene**T**etra**H**ydro**F**olate **R**eductase. I'm serious; that's what it's called. We abbreviate that sexy beast as MTHFR. I discuss more biochemistry for my fellow geeks, in "Detoxification Matters," Chapter 8, but right now the take home point is simple: If it turns out that you have this gene, you can easily overcome this quirk in your genetics. And that will allow you to be untethered from your pain meds.

So I want you to get tested for this MTHFR gene mutation. I tell you where and how to get tested in "Test for MTHFR Gene Mutation" in Appendix I on Labs.

The whole situation becomes especially important if your blood levels of homocysteine are elevated AND you have this genetic mutation or "snp" as it's called (pronounced "snip"). Honestly, I'm jumping out of my skin right now, because I'm excited to tell you it may very well be the explanation you've been dreaming of! Now that I think about it, you should order the blood test that includes your homocysteine level along with the MTHFR gene.

I am in your head already, and I can hear you saying, *"My doctor will want proof that my migraines are tied to this genetic mutation."* I'm one step ahead of you. Feel free to share information about this study[40] that was published in the journal, *Headache*. In the study researchers noted: "Determination of MTHFR C677T polymorphisms and homocysteine levels may be useful to identify patients with a high risk of suffering from migraines with aura."

What is the solution if you have this MTHFR snp? Medications? No, I can tell you that with confidence because I'm a seasoned pharmacist, and I know my drugs inside out. So I asked the man who studies methylation day in and day out. He's a researcher, naturopathic physician, and good friend, Ben Lynch, ND, from Seattle, www.MTHFR.net.

I got him alone for an interview and he explained, "The solution is to optimize your homocysteine levels and go around the MTHFR gene mutation. When I say 'go around,' I mean one must improve their lifestyle habits, increase uncooked leafy greens in their diet, reduce environmental exposures, and consider targeted supplementation which can help you overcome your genetic defect."

Dr. Lynch is dead serious. Did you catch that? There's no mention of triptan or ergotamine drugs. No recommendation for addictive opiates or NSAIDS either! Just a simple supplement . . . can it really be that simple? Let's look at a 6-month randomized, double-blinded placebo-controlled trial published in the journal, *Pharmacogenetics and Genomics* published in 2012. This study looked at over 200 women experiencing recurring migraines with aura. The treatment was vitamin supplementation—just vitamin B6, folate, and vitamin B12. Nothing else!

The results were rather significant (P less than 0.001 for you research nuts). People taking the supplements experienced reduced homocysteine levels along with reduced severity of migraines compared to the placebo group.

So it's not medication, and it's not folic acid, like everyone buys at the health food store. It's a simple, inexpensive combination of three essential nutrients in a highly absorbable, body-ready form. Imagine that, natural ways to control migraines with aura, without expensive drugs and bad side effects! I love simple. And I love science. If you want to read more, look at the well-designed study[41] published in *Pharmacogenetics and Genomics*, October 2012, and you'll see that migraine disability was significantly reduced with nothing but key vitamins!

Dr. Lynch concurs: "Not only do these three nutrients reduce the severity of migraines with aura, they also support your immune system, mood, energy, DNA, and your ability to move toxins out of the body. The benefits, collectively speaking, reduce the severity and frequency of your homocysteine and MTHFR-related headaches, if not eliminate them altogether, all the while supporting cognitive function and mood."

If you want to try and see if your headaches improve from taking these three nutrients, buy HomocysteX. It offers these same three nutrients in the best forms used by your body. Need something stronger? If you know your homocysteine is quite high or you need some extra support, the expert on methylation, Dr. Lynch, also designed HomocysteX Plus. This offers the same three nutrients found in HomocysteX but has two more key nutrients that help reduce more stubborn and elevated levels of homocysteine. You can find both

HomocysteX and HomocysteX Plus at www.SeekingHealth.com. Use coupon code "Headache Free" to save 15% off your order of one or both or of any item you like on that website.

I personally use Homocystex Plus because it supports the MTHFR gene defect which up to 45% of us have! Why? Because I have the MTHFR defect! You know what?! So does Dr Lynch! And so does my hubby Sam and so does my best friend. It's really more common than you think!

Please take the time to learn more about this common gene defect, MTHFR, I highly recommend you visit Dr Lynch's website because it's dedicated to it, www.MTHFR.Net and get his free newsletter.

Test for MTHFR Gene Mutation

The best test option, because it's simpler and less expensive, is to go for a cheek swab. Go to www.SeekingHealth.com and buy the "MTHFR Test Molecular Laboratory Test." It's an oral swab, no blood draw required. No doctor, no insurance company, no headaches.

The kit is currently $150 dollars, but because I'm friends with Dr. Lynch, I've negotiated a 15% discount code for you, on any purchase from his site. Use the code "Headache Free," and it will lower your price. The kit will be mailed to your home. You swab your cheek in the privacy of your own house, put your sample back in the kit as directed, seal it up, and mail it as instructed in the pre-paid envelope. Then, if you're results come back to you as positive for MTHFR, you can try HomocysteX or HomocysteX Plus.

Testing is also available at many labs as a simple blood test; however, I need to warn you that at about $1,500 the blood test is expensive. And I can't vouch for whether or not your insurance will reimburse for this! So if you and your doctor opt for the blood test, make sure you call your insurance company in advance and ask specifically if "MTHFR genotype testing" is covered. When they put you on hold, I suggest you put the receiver down, go out, have a nice dinner, and catch a movie. By the time you get home, hopefully you won't have to wait too much longer before they pick up and say, "Your call is very important to us." Don't be surprised if they say no.

You can try a specialized lab, like www.directlabs.com/suzycohen. My understanding is that they're pretty straightforward in their billing system, and since your insurance company isn't involved, you pay them directly. I don't know their price. Once you get their kit mailed to you, you will then require a laboratory's assistance to take your blood, treat it correctly, and mail it off in a timely manner. Hopefully, your doctor can help you get all this taken care of.

Why Medicine Fails

Genes actually influence response to triptan migraine meds. Your response is based upon little tiny parts of your DNA that contain information, called your "snps" pronounced snips. We just say "snips" because it's easier than saying "single nucleotide polymorphisms." Snps occur due to errors in DNA replication at some point during evolution, usually an environmental factors. If you have the "T allele" of the snp of rs5443 in your genetic code, you are 3 times more likely to respond to triptans than if you didn't have this genetic personality.[28]

The lab test offered by 23andMe tests for many snps. I did that test for $99, and according to my genes, I have the CC allele of this snp. Translated into English, this just means I'm less likely to respond to a triptan compared to a person who is TT or CT. You'd have to take the 23andMe test to fully understand the genetics of all this. I just want you to know that if you are unresponsive to triptan medications, it's because of your genetic make up. Blame mom and dad if you want to. Interestingly, this same snp (rs5443) also makes men respond to Viagra![39]

If you are homozygous for MAO A gene snp, you should NOT take zolmitriptan and rizatriptan because those drugs are metabolized via that pathway and if you take them (and can't break them down properly) they will build up in your blood stream and cause more side effects. I'd recommend something else.

Now, if you are homozygous for certain genes in the CYP450 category (and there are easily 36 genes for this), you should not take eletriptan, frovatriptan and naratriptan because those drugs need that CYP enzyme to be broken down.

The gene snps determine how safe a particular drug is for you. Before we leave the topic of genetics, let me say one more thing, the variant COMT gene (Val158Met) is *not* associated with migraine. I know this is a lot to take in. One of my purposes in including this information is to inform physicians who buy my books and use my information in their practice. A good physician will be able to sort all this out for you, do some tests, and if nothing else, do trial and error with the triptans to see which work best for you. I'm certain some of you know which ones work for you, and which don't. You can also subscribe to my free weekly newsletter to get updates and more down-to-earth explanations. (www.DearPharmacist.com).

Chapter 3

Tension Headaches

Tension headaches are the most common type of headache and I'm willing to bet you've experienced one yourself. Approximately 1 to 3% of adults in the United States suffer with chronic tension headaches.[1] That's millions of people.

It can add more to your stress levels and miserable mood than you imagine. It can cause depression, even if you are a happy-go-lucky person. Chronic pain can do that to anyone. The tenderness and pain associated with tension headaches are frequently the result of muscle contractions in the head, shoulders or neck (*National Headache Foundation*). If you are like me, and sit in one position for many hours (like right now, I've not moved out of my chair for 6 hours solid because I'm writing this book), then you are apt to have your head 'locked' in one position for a long time. Also, if you are a sound sleeper (as opposed to a thrasher) then you have your head in one position for a long time. These are triggers for tension headaches. So is grinding or clenching your teeth and sitting/standing with poor posture. You're about to learn surprising causes for tension headaches, and how you can control them.

Tension headaches are almost always diagnosed by the absence of migraine-like symptoms, which is called a "diagnosis of exclusion." If you don't get an aura, the nausea or halo with the head pain, boom, you are slapped with the diagnosis of CTTH (chronic tension-type headaches). The reason I wrote this book is because I think you are dealing with headaches the wrong way, why do you think you keep getting one?!

One thing for sure, there's oxidative stress (free radical damage) from all those pro-inflammatory chemicals continues in between migraine headaches, whereas in CTTH, you are free and clear of these dangerous cytokines in between your bouts of pain.[4] For CTTH sufferers, take heart because that is some good news. Another piece of good news is that generally speaking, the degree of free radical damage is higher in migraineurs than it is in tension headache sufferers, so basically your brain is turned on a lower flame with CTTH as compared to migraine headache sufferers. You can read all about the dangers of chronic pro-inflammatory cytokines in Chapter 12 "Reduce Cytokines and Live Headache Free."

Easily, 70% of the population has had a tension headache at some point or another and if you haven't had one yet, give yourself a little more time. The pain can occur in the back of the head, the neck, your temples, forehead or scalp. According to the WHO, tension headaches affect three women to every two men.[1]

Tension headaches can be episodic or chronic. Episodic headaches are defined as those that occur less than 15 times per month. Chronic headaches are more constant, defined as *more than* 15 headaches per month for 3 months or more.

Episodic and chronic tension headaches differ in more ways than their frequency. Research suggests that chronic headaches are mediated by central pain mechanisms inside your nervous system. Episodic tension headaches are mediated by peripheral pain mechanisms, meaning the pain is driven by forces and chemicals outside your nervous system.[3] It's not completely understood, but at least tension types of headaches are a little easier to manage as compared to clusters or migraines. They often respond to non-addictive pain-killers like ibuprofen or naproxen, or non-invasive therapies which help release trigger points.

Allergic to Your Bedding?

There's such a thing as an allergy headache. Do you sleep with feather down comforters, pillows or old pillows laden with dust mites? My son called me to tell me he was waking up with headaches, and sneezing fits all of a sudden.

"Did you eat a pint of ice cream before going to bed last night sweetie?"
(He's allergic to dairy, like me)
No mom!

Then it dawned on me, I had just sent him a fluffy new down comforter for his college apartment. He only had it a week. I told him to remove all the new bedding and use a 100% cotton blanket (and take a Claritin), and luckily, the symptoms went completely away in 3 days. It's okay to reduce histamine for a few days with natural quercetin, about 500mg three times a day, or an over-the-counter antihistamines.

Risk factors include scoliosis, or uneven leg length as that will aggravate muscle tension in the body. Heavy lifting, sitting in front of a computer monitor all day or sleeping in hotel rooms also put you at risk. It's not uncommon to go on vacation and wake up with a headache, if your mattress is uncomfortable or you've slept poorly because you're in a new time zone or environment.

Life Situations Can Cause Headaches

Tension headaches are more common among people dealing with stressful, unhappy relationships, difficult co-workers or unfulfilling jobs. We've all found ourselves there, and it's tough making important decisions about your relationships and career. I can't make those for you.

I know for myself, when I made changes in my relationships and career in my early thirties, I became the healthiest and happiest I'd ever been because of the change. It's tough weighing out the risk to benefit of life changes but your health is at stake. If you have headaches all the time, listen to your body. If you can't make a change yet, do something joyful in your life to balance the stress you deal with. You must learn to rank relaxation and happiness just as important as your other commitments.

Have a little fun, whether that is painting, beading, gardening, or writing that book you've been wanting to write for the last 20 years. Anything that makes you smile and preferably something that allows you to breathe deeply. It will give you a better perspective on life. Sometimes it's just a walk in the park, or a picnic at the river. Perhaps a hot luxurious bath with the doors locked so you can have 10 minutes to yourself without your husband hollering, *"Honey, where's my favorite T shirt with the hole in the sleeve?"*

(The one you threw out 2 weeks ago).

Yeah! Lock the door, breathe. You deserve it, even if it's just 10 minutes of the day, do it because it could reduce the frequency of your headaches. Make sure you avoid emotional conflict as much as possible since anxiety is a common cause for tension headaches, as well as a variety of other chronic illnesses. For some good motivation, read Chapter 9 "Adrenal Hormones and the Headache Connection."

There's An App For That!

It's called "My Pain Diary" and there's a one-time charge for it, at the time of this writing it was $10 but it varies a little bit. You can download this app for your droid, iPhone or iPad. My husband downloaded the original app for testing purposes and he says it's worth every penny. Now the developers actually have one specifically for headaches and migraines called "Headache & Migraine Tracker."

It's amazing how much technology is used in doctors' offices. Four out of five doctors now use mobile devices to call up patient records and consult treatment guidelines. The Pain Diary app was designed by a man who had chronic pain from an injury and a background in web design. I think he really hit it out of the park with this. It allows you to enter and track your personal symptoms while simultaneously tracking medications, meals, exercise, mood and weather, which is a stroke of genius! You can click a picture and immediately attach images for each day if you want to, it's easy. Everything is color coded, and you can create bar graphs. It allows you to print reports for your doctor. In 2013, My Pain Diary became the #1 paid medical iPhone app in the United States. www.chronicpainapp.com You can also put this into youtube, and watch a demo video: "Headache & Migraine Tracker iPhone App Teaser" and the trailer will pop up.

If you're just not the techy sort, or don't have a smart phone, turn to Appendix II where I have created a Headache Log for you. Cut this out, copy it and you can use a pen to keep track each day. You can also buy a big calendar for the year, and keep track. For example, jot down what you ate on a big calendar, who you spoke with or worked with and the severity of your headache. A pattern may develop over time (ie head hurts more on Mondays after executive board meetings, or did yoga today and no headache . . . or whatever).

Sex Pills and Headaches

Recent studies, even one printed in the respectable *Lancet,* suggest that nitric oxide plays a role in sparking chronic tension headaches.[5,6] The supplement called L-arginine will go on to form nitric oxide in the body. Nitric oxide should not be confused with nitrous oxide (an anesthetic gas). Nitric oxide increases blood flow to your brain and also to your sexual organs. That's why its precursors like L-arginine are commonly found in supplements for erectile dysfunction and heart disease.

A little bit of it is fine, in fact desirable for many conditions. My friend Dr. Nathan Bryan has a product called NEO 40 which may be useful for some people. That said, it's a supplement, with powerful effects especially on the heart (considered helpful) and so I want you to ask your doctor if this, and any supplement I mention, is right for you. Excess nitric oxide (as opposed to healthy physiological levels) spells trouble in the form of headaches, there is heightened sensitivity to muscle and skin pain. Excess nitric oxide has been implicated in chronic tension headaches.

So it's a question of too much or too little with headaches. Arginine-containing supplements will backfire if you take too much, or there aren't enough co-factors to reduce it to an innocuous form.

Nitric Oxide is supposed to be removed within seconds but some of it may morph into peroxynitrites and those are nasty wicked compounds associated with heart attack and stroke. So I rarely recommend one take L-arginine by itself. For the same reason, I beg you not to eat bologna, salami or other cured meats high in nitrites. And if you want to measure peroxynitrites, you can take a lab test, see Appendix I "Labs."

Anatomy of Tension Headache Pain

These are not as severe as migraines, nor are they quite as disabling. Unlike migraines which are often due to food sensitivities hormone imbalances or mitochondrial dysfunction, tension headaches seem to be closely tied to stress levels. That's good news because reducing stress levels is often under your direct control. To further differentiate tension headaches from migraines, it's a blessing that they do not include those frightening symptoms of auditory hallucinations, blind spots in your vision, or vomiting (which goes with the territory if you have migraines). Tension headaches feel more like there's a tight rubber band around your head, and the pain may spread into the neck. Rarely, they are accompanied by minor sound or light sensitivity. Most of the time, they only last a a few hours, and can frequently be relieved by sleeping, or by taking over-the-counter pain-killers. There are an unfortunate few who experience *both* migraines and tension headaches.

For years we thought it was just due to tight muscles, but emerging studies suggest CTTHs are tied to an over-stimulated nervous system firing excessively and resulting in trigger points occurring in the back of the head, shoulders and neck. These trigger points refer pain up into your head. Think of trigger points as knots in the muscles. Researchers in Spain who study headaches printed this in their study,[11] *"An updated pain model has suggested that CTTH can be explained by referred pain from trigger points (TrPs) in the cranio-cervical muscles, mediated through the spinal cord and the trigeminal nerve nucleus caudalis."*

This is just a complicated way to explain tight neck muscles, and while this study says it's mediated by a nerve cluster, the end result leaves you with tension headache. And you know what that feels like. Hashtag ouch!

Tension headaches often involve muscle contractions and tenderness in the head, shoulders and neck, according to the *National Headache Foundation*. Activities that lock your head in one position for a long periods of time, such as typing or sleeping in an awkward position can trigger a tension headache. Clenching your jaw, grinding your teeth, teeth grinding and having poor posture add to it.

I want to talk about your posture for a moment because your head weighs about the same as a bowling ball, maybe 10 pounds (4.5 kilograms). Now stick your hand out, and imagine you are holding that 10 pound bowling ball two feet out in front of you. It would get heavy pretty fast and your arm would drop quickly. That is what your neck has to deal with all day long, it has to hold that up and it gets especially hard if you are hunched over. It may cause your neck muscles to tighten or even spasm, restricting blood flow to the back of your head and creating more trigger points. Your muscles get microscopic tears and large chunks of muscles start to hurt. They usually patch up over time but adopt this bad habit of slouching long enough, and it may create some scar tissue.

There's a good deal of chemistry involved (isn't there always when you're dealing with me?!) Your immune system T cells and macrophages secrete a chemical called interleukin 6 or IL-6 during infection, or after you get burned, or have some other injury. It helps repair tissue, and acts as an anti-inflammatory. With tension headaches, where your muscles are tight, more IL-6 will be made. IL-6 is technically a "myokine" because it's made in the muscle, and it's elevated in response to muscle contractions.[7] You can imagine how IL-6 goes up during exercise. I know I said IL-6 can be helpful, but like any good thing, too much is a problem because it goes rogue on you and elicits pain. My research tells me that people who suffer with chronic tension headaches do happen to pump out more IL-6.[8] Certain nutrients reduce IL-6, such as magnesium, CoQ10 and glycine, that's one of the reasons I've included them in my "Script" to help you get well.[12, 13, 32]

Do You Need An Adjustment?

Don't underestimate the power and relief that could be yours for simply sitting up straight with your head held up in a normal upright position. Routine chiropractic adjustments can be helpful, and I recommend gentle "Activator" method, or other gentle manipulations that help your craniosacral spine.

I'm not personally a fan of manual manipulations of the neck or any rotational techniques in that delicate area. I know there are skilled chiropractors that do these techniques, but I'm used to an Activator so I'm biased toward gentle techniques, nevertheless, a good chiropractor might be able to help you, especially if you combine that therapy with massage.

Add More Therapy to Your Massage Therapy

Some of you may like it gentle, while others will like deep tissue massage. No matter how you like it, it's still therapeutic. You can get more out of your massage by asking your therapist to put slather on her lotion with one or two of these goodies:

Arnica gel or oil relieves inflammation and soothes muscles. You can buy this at any health food store. Boiron makes a good brand and there are others, I've seen this at my local Vitamin Shoppe.

Menthol offers a cooling sensation. If you're using BioFreeze brand, make sure you get the new and improved one that is free of parabens and synthetic dyes. It's sold online and many chiropractor or physical therapy clinics. www.biofreeze.com You can buy all sorts of copycat formulas at your local pharmacy too but they may not be as strong.

Salonpas Deep Relieving Gel contains menthol, camphor and a skin-penetrating form of aspirin which gives it a dual action. Your massage therapist may not want to do this because the aspirin will go through his/her hands. Perhaps this one is better for self-treatment. You get instant cooling from the essential oils of menthol and camphor, and for hours you have benefits of aspirin which takes down pain and swelling like any anti-inflammatory drug. Salonpas makes this in patch form so you can wear relief hours at a time. www.salonpas.us

Magnesium cream or oil Just a little bit, it feels tingly going on. Magnesium relaxes muscles and goes right through the skin wherever you put it. Ancient Minerals makes a good brand of this. www.ancient-minerals.com

Capsaicin creams contains chili pepper and causes a mild burning, stinging or heating sensation. Better for self treatment since massage therapists often have clients back to back. Have someone give your tense trapezius muscles and neck a little massage with this. You may have to dilute it with another lotion if it is just too prickly for you, or you can buy the lowest dose which is 0.025% sold at any pharmacy. Creams like this works by interfering with pain signals (Substance P) that would normally transmit pain. I think repeated applications, like two or three times a week would be perfect in the beginning. If you're the sensitive sort, test your skin first, it contains a chili extract, capsaicin. This is a great option for people with arthritis too. Wash hands thoroughly after applying capsaicin. Popular brands include Sombra, Zostrix, Capzasin. You can also wear the warmth, as in a patch. My favorite one here is "Salonpas Hot." It lasts about 8 hours, and it didn't burn me when I tried it, it felt very nice and I remember thinking, "I should slap this baby on when it hits 10 degrees outside!" a common occurrence in Colorado where I live.

Kink-Ease® MSM Salve by Stages of Life was developed by my friend David Klein, MD a pain specialist in Orlando, this contains a high dose of MSM (methylsuflonylmethane), as much as 10 times the active ingredient of MSM compared with other popular brands. It also has some menthol. It can ease any kink in your body, hence the name. www.stages-of-life.com

---

Signs & Symptoms of Tension Headache

Pain, usually both sides of your head

Pressure, constant, not throbbing

Sensation that your head is in a vise

Dull or aching pain at temples, forehead, between the eyes

Neck pain, or back of head

Pain may come on slowly or suddenly

Triggers for Tension Headache

Drinking or eating cold foods like ice cream or smoothies

Stress

Grief or depression

Arguments

Skipping meals

Muscle strain

Poor posture

Insomnia

Fatigue

Overworking yourself

Intense work outs

Clenching or grinding teeth

TMJ (temporomandibular joint) syndrome

Caffeine or nicotine withdrawal

Eyestrain at the computer

Alcohol withdrawal

Suzy's "Script" for Tension Headache Pain Relief

Before you take any of the following supplements, you must ask your doctor(s) if they are right for you. My intention here is to educate you about possibilities and options. Do not misconstrue my ideas for medical advice. I have no idea what is right for every individual reading this so take my list to your practitioner(s) to ask if they're right for you with your medical history. Dosages listed anywhere in this book are basic guidelines, some people tolerate different dosages than what is stated here:

Rhodiola rosea

Magnesium

CoQ10

Hops

Glycine

Traumeel® Homeopathic gel

How This Helps You Become Headache Free

Rhodiola.

Since tension headaches are commonly associated with stress, I'll assume for the moment that your stress hormone (cortisol) is high and if it's not high, it could be a flat-line because you've totally exhausted yourself. Stress causes weight gain from the constant carb consumption, blood sugar swings, belly fat, rolls in the neck and face, bone loss, erectile dysfunction and hypertension. Having Rhodiola in your system may lift depression and reduce anxiety, while helping you cope with stress. That's why rhodiola is termed an "adaptogen" as it helps you adapt to situations better. I think it could be a wonderful herb for you if you have chronic tension headaches. It may be okay for some migrainers too, because it helps lift serotonin, a neurotransmitter in the brain. That's what triptan drugs do too, but via a different mechanism than natural rhodiola. Some active constitutents in rhodiola include including rosavin, rhosavidin, rhodiolosid, salidrosid.

Rhodiola herb is a plant-based adaptogen, it offsets high cortisol and helps you deal with stress. Perfect for people with a lot of mental stress, emotional conflict or anxiety. Rhodiola may provide remarkable relief for you if you feel like you have muscle weakness, chronic fatigue, low motivation or just feel sluggish and want to sleep. This Siberian herb helps your body handle stress and it calms the sympathetic (fight or flight) part of your nervous system. Because rhodiola removes ammonia and lactic acid from your blood,[9,10] I feel confident it could help reduce muscle fatigue. There's more about rhodiola's action on the body, and how it helps with all sorts of other conditions in Chapter 9 "Adrenal Hormones and the Headache Connection."

Caution: Because it has not been studied in pregnant or nursing women, I'd recommend not using it. Also, if you have bipolar disorder it is not advised. If you start to have insomnia or bad dreams it could be from the stimulating effects of rhodiola, I would back off the dose, or stop it for 2 weeks and then start again. In fact, that's how some clinicians dose it, cyclically. On for a period of time, then off and so forth. There isn't a clear defined way to dose it or I'd tell you, this is entirely up to you and your physician. About 100mg is the dose to shoot for, per capsule.

Magnesium.

Magnesium relaxes your muscles. You can take a bath with it (ie Epsom salts), slather some on in lotion or oil form, and even take it by supplement. I recommend this for anyone dealing with any kind of headache or facial pain. I recommend it for millions of other people who take any of 200 prescription medications which mug it from your body leaving you more susceptible to headaches and muscle aches and pain. I recommend magnesium for people who drink coffee because coffee is a drug mugger of magnesium.

A few popular medications that suppress magnesium levels include heartburn medications, diuretics and estrogen-containing drugs. The heartburn medicines called "proton pump inhibitors" or PPIs are dangerous to your magnesium levels, there's even a warning that drug companies have to place to warn people, called a "black box" warning. I told you about this many years ago, and in fact there are hundreds more medications that rob you blind, the list is in the magnesium chapter of my *Drug Mugger* book[23] so please refer to your copy of that.

There's an epidemic of magnesium deficiency in this country. Some signs and symptoms of that include headaches, migraines, constipation, depression, anxiety, heart palpitations, menstrual cramps, bad periods (pre-menstrual syndrome), spasms, fibromyalgia-like pain and tenderness, muscle cramps, insomnia and much more. When your system is tight or irritable (you may be sensitive to smells, sounds or light, or you could have diarrhea, a nervous stomach, muscle twitching), you may be magnesium deficient. You can take a blood test but it's not always accurate. The best way is a red blood cell level, termed an RBC magnesium or "RBC Mag." I need to warn you, levels of RBC mag may fall into "normal" range in the face of a total body deficiency. Sometimes the best way to tell is by your clinical presentation of signs and symptoms, and your response to supplements.

Caution: Some forms of magnesium will give you diarrhea so be picky. If you take magnesium oxide (sold at all pharmacies) you are likely to experience cramps and diarrhea. To get high quality forms of magnesium go to the health food store or online and look for magnesium malate or magnesium taurate, or chelated magnesium. A brand of magnesium that tastes good is a powder (and you mix it with water) called "Calm" and this has my stamp of approval as well. Great for kids with attention problems too. If you have kidney impairment, and many people with diabetes do, you will want to stick to the lower end of dosages listed on the label.

But if you are fine, and your doctor agrees with my recommendation of magnesium for you, then I think about 600 - 800mg per day would help you (divide the dose up during the day, don't take that all at once). And if you want to eat more magnesium, it is found in leafy greens like kale, spinach, salad, chard and so forth. Whenever I say that in lectures, inevitably an alpha male finds his way to the podium to hammer me about why not meat? *You can eat meat!* Just not cured meats like bologna or salami that are high in nitrites (remember that forms peroxynitrite and sparks headaches). But eating clean, grass-fed hormone-free meat is fine by me, I'm just saying eat greens too because they are high in magnesium. So go ahead, eat like a rabbit, you'll get fewer headaches.

CoQ 10.

This vitamin-like nutrient ranks at the top of my list for good health because it is an antioxidant and it gets into every cell of your body. You make it, so the whole time you're thinking of this as a supplement, it's being cranked out of your liver. It is needed by every cell of your body, particularly the muscle cells.

I've included CoQ10 in my "script" for tension headache pain relief because it helps stabilize the pain-causing pathway NFκB, which if you read Chapter 12 "Reduce Pain-Causing Cytokines" you'll learn how NFκB pathway opens the floodgates to a bunch of pain and inflammation causing cytokines. CoQ10 feeds and nourishes your muscles while putting a clamp on the NFκB pathway reducing IL-6 and other compounds[32] that become elevated during tension headaches (and migraines).

Muscles use up CoQ10 all day long! Aside from that, people with tension headaches are often under stress and that takes a toll on your health at the cellular level. CoQ10 improves muscle and brain function.[14] It sparks energy by feeding your mitochondria (your powerhouses) and this in turn creates cellular energy or ATP. For you it translates into help with chronic fatigue and a sense of well-being and endurance. I want you to feel your best and I think CoQ10 is the best muscle food for you. A prolonged deficiency of CoQ10 can contribute to significant muscle pain, not just headaches.

One more thing, your heart, it is a non-stop working muscle (well, we hope!) If your heart stops working it's bad news. CoQ10 is the most well-researched nutrient for heart health so you get that added benefit. Statin cholesterol drugs mug CoQ10 from your body, as do hundreds of other medications. This can add to the underlying cause of tension headaches, and it's often overlooked by doctors. After all your physician is focused on your headache pain, and which analgesic is best for you, whereas I'm less concerned with temporary bandages, I'd prefer to uncover the root cause (and treat that). Keeping that in mind, I'm concerned with mitochondrial (mito) respiration, the way your powerhouses work for you. It's the way your cells 'breathe' and these poor little overworked mito need CoQ10 to produce ATP and 'breathe.' A shortage causes muscle pain and cramps anywhere in the body. Ring a bell for you? If your headaches are due to missing nutrients, like if you are taking a statin, (ie Lipitor, Zocor, etc) or one of the other 200 drugs listed in my *Drug Mugger* book[23] and you have more headaches, that could be the reason. CoQ10 can help.

Caution: CoQ10 is very good at reducing blood sugar, consider it an added benefit but watch out if you inject insulin or take diabetic medicine. They will start to be more effective and your sugar may drop. I could say the same exact thing for people with high blood pressure. CoQ10 reduces blood pressure so be careful combining it with your anti-hypertensives. Once in a blue moon, I hear of an allergic rash, which I suspect has more to do with a filler than CoQ10 (because we make CoQ10 in our own bodies). Other miscellaneous reactions include stomach upset, nausea/vomiting, or increased light sensitivity.

Hops or Humulus lupulus.

Hops is best known as a flavoring agent in beer. I'm not suggesting a Bud, I'm suggesting the herb, hops. Well known for it's ability to manage hot flashes, and protect against breast cancer, hops is also a natural muscle relaxer.[15,16,17] You can drink tea any time you feel nervous or anxious. Supplements in higher dosages can be used to help you get a good night's rest; if sleep is the name of the game, take this with the glycine which I discuss next, otherwise, I'm thinking of mild, gentle dosages, not those that put you to sleep. Hops can reduce histamine levels in your body, and histamine is a cytokine that contributes to headaches and migraines. You may know histamine better if I tell you that's one of the compounds that causes allergic fits and rashes. Dosages vary depending on the concentration of the herb.

There are many brand you can take so please follow label directions for your particular brand. The one I trust to be pure and extracted properly is made by Reservage and the dose for that is 500mg one or two capsules nightly. Another good option is the liquid herbal extract by Nature's Answer. This one is concentrated, it's like 2,000mg per 56 drops. The dosage is 28 - 56 drops (1,000 - 2,000mg) once or twice daily. The reason for the disparity in dose between this dropper formula and the Reservage capsule is just the concentration and blend of herb, this is why I always tell you to follow label guidelines for your particular product and I generally avoid giving dosages; it differs with the product.

Caution: Hops have been shown to contain one of the most potent *in vitro* estrogenic substance known from the plant kingdom. It has estrogenic properties but don't worry if you're a guy, it won't make you less manly. It should not be combined with sleep medications, or alcohol; stop taking it a week or two before surgery. Hops is thought to exacerbate depression but this is quite debatable. Ask your doctor if it's okay for you.

Glycine.

Amino acid that is needed for relaxation and normal muscle function. It is considered one of the most important "inhibitory" neurotransmitters in the CNS (along with GABA) meaning it slows things down in your brain, and all over your body. That's good, with headaches there are enough excitatory and inflammatory compounds circulating! Glycine may even help with memory, over time. Glycine helps your body make glutathione, an important antioxidant you need to clear your body of toxins and one that may be deficient if you are a poor methylator. Poor methylators have lots of headaches, read Chapter 8, "Detoxification Matters" for some critical information on that. Sometimes opening up that methylation pathway is all you need.

I'm recommending glycine because it naturally relaxes your muscles, nourishes them and simultaneously improves feelings of tension and anxiety. It works pretty fast possibly with the first dose, unlike other remedies that need days to weeks to kick in.

Caution: Glycine usually helps people fall asleep, so if you try this option, take it at night or it could make you very drowsy. About 1 to 2 grams taken once at bedtime. You can certainly take more if you like the effects, and you're doctor says it's fine. I mean, it is known to calm aggression and improve anxiety and focus (now don't go putting it into your husband's coffee!)

Glycine may reduce cravings for sugar. If you like the effects and the "Ahhhh" you get from this, but you find that it's too sedating, take small doses two or three times a day and a heavier dose at night. Glycine may be helpful for children with attention deficit. As far as reducing those pain-causing compounds tied to headache, yes it does that too. It reduces IL-6, and TNFα. It happens to increase a good one, IL-10 which fights inflammation for you.[18,19]

Arnica Cream.

Arnica montana has been used for centuries, it should be applied to your skin to soothe muscle aches, reduce inflammation and relax muscles. It's commonly used by athletes with strains, sprains and bruises. Think of this if you hurt yourself in Runner's Lunge. Arnica or arnica-containing salves should be in any natural medicine cabinet. It's hard to believe but these gorgeous little Spanish flowers are powerful, they can slow down firing of the NFκB pathway (a good thing) and thus they halt production[20] of inflammation-causing chemicals like IL-1β and TNFα. I've written a special chapter for docs and nerds like me in case you want to learn more about those pain-causing chemicals, it's Chapter 12 "Reduce Pain-Causing Cytokines."

Now, if we were going shopping together, I'd suggest you buy a formulation that included arnica and other potent naturally-derived ingredients. My favorite product that fits the bill is Traumeel® made by HEEL. It's great for a wide range of aches and pains, joint pain, muscle tension and sprains and strains. The reviews for this product are very high so it must be doing something great for you. Traumeel® comes tablet, cream and gels. Unlike many other topical tension-relieving creams, this one is fragrance-free and non-greasy so it won't chase your spouse out of the room (due to any strong odor).

Taking arnica by mouth is not recommended unless you have an actual oral formulation intended for that use. In that case, it's safe and enormously helpful for anxiety and chronic stress or shock. If after someone has an accident and doesn't want to be touched saying "I'm fine, I don't need a doctor" and clearly they do, this is a good time to offer arnica. It is fabulous for restoring composure and releasing tension.

Botox Therapy

Since your head pain may be referred from myofascial trigger points, it stands to reason that Botox might work, since Botox paralyzes small muscle groups. Researchers set out to determine if it could help and their results were published in *Headache* in 2009. It was a small randomized, double-blind, placebo controlled study consisting of 23 volunteers.[2]

They injected botulinum toxin A (brand name Botox) into patients who had headaches pretty much every day of the month (average of 27 days per month). Headache intensity over the 12 week period did not change much for the treated group, however, the Botox treated group enjoyed reductions in headache frequency at the first part of the study. Unfortunately, these effects dissipated by week 12. From this, I gather that injecting Botox into trigger points may work for some people, but not all. It's not a lasting cure, just temporary. Considering the price, and the lackluster results, I'd skip it.

Get Rid Of . . .

Uncomfortable mattresses and pillows

Shoes that cause uncomfortable postures

Emotional conflict

Mental stress

Things on your To-Do list that you haven't done in 3 months

Things on your To-Do list that are not your responsibility (stop saying yes, when you mean no!)

Uncomfortable chairs

Headache Busting Yoga Pose

Tension headaches are caused by tight muscles and yoga relaxes those. Among yoga pros, it's well known that "Child's Pose" can help tension headaches. I do this all the time, sometimes when I wake up in the morning, I'll do this under the sheets just because the stretch feels good to me. You just sit on your shins, putting your forehead on the ground below your heart. This releases a tight low back. Extend the hands forward, or if you have shoulder issues, lay them by your sides so your hands are near your feet. This helps release tension, especially if you can breathe rhythmically, deeply, in and out, and try to quiet your mind. If you have trouble with that, just keep saying to yourself "I am inhaling" on every inhale, and "I am exhaling that's all I need to know" on the exhale. Or say whatever you want that brings you into the moment, and out of that misunderstanding you had with whomever. Direct the breath toward your back and feel it all stretch and expand.

I'm a Pharmacist, Let's Talk Medicine

If I was going to evaluate strictly medications for a person with chronic tension headaches my choice for you would be a combination of one NSAID and one tricyclic medication. Let's begin with NSAIDS. These drugs work by reducing pain-causing cytokines so they can be taken at the onset of your headache or during it. They don't help much with trigger point release, or free radical damage seen in tension type of headaches. The gold standard, often prescribed by doctors is ibuprofen 800mg taken 2 or 3 times a day, or as needed. Ibuprofen is sold over-the-counter in lower dosages, 200mg per pill.

NSAIDs or Non-steroidal Anti-inflammatory Drugs

Ibuprofen (Advil, Motrin, others)

Naproxen (Aleve, others)

Ketoprofen (Orudis KT)

Follow label directions on the package you buy. Try to take the lowest effective dose of any medication.

Caution: They may take up to an hour to kick in, assuming they are going to even work (some people get relief, others don't respond). NSAIDs are harmful to the stomach and esophagus. One more caution for you, in case you have already suffered a heart attack - using NSAIDs is not advised, I recommend you use acetaminophen or some of the preventive supplements in my Script section. Why? Because studies suggest that NSAIDS increase your risk for another heart attack, regardless of how long it has been since you had the first.[21]

Tricyclic Antidepressants

Examples: Amitriptyline (Elavil)
            Amoxapine (Ascendin)
            Desipramine (Norpramin)
            Doxepin (Sinequan)
            Imipramine (Tofranil, Tofranil PM)
            Maprotiline (Ludiomil)
            Nortriptyline (Pamelor)
            Protriptyline (Vivactil)
            Trimipramine (Surmontil)

I'm not a big fan of taking antidepressants for tension headaches however I am aware that a meta-analysis finds that they are effective for this condition so far be it from me to pooh-pooh a potential treatment option that could help you. According to the report,[22] researchers conclude: "Tricyclic antidepressants are effective in preventing migraine and tension-type headaches and are more effective than selective serotonin reuptake inhibitors, although with greater adverse effects. The effectiveness of tricyclics seems to increase over time."

The reason I'm not a fan of this therapy is just because of the side effects. You see, as a pharmacist, I am accustomed to evaluating risks vs. benefits. (This makes me think of the movie with Ben Stiller and

Jennifer Aniston, *Along Came Polly* where he evaluated every little detail of their relationship, it was very funny, he was a risk assessment analyst . . .) well anyway, tricyclic antidepressants are drug muggers[23] of CoQ10 which you need for proper muscle health. So you have to evaluate the risk of running short of CoQ10 (which may cause muscle cramps, memory loss, arrhythmias, fatigue) versus the benefits of taking medicine. If you decide to take the medicine, no problemo, just take the CoQ10 okay? Ask your doctor if 100mg daily helps offset the drug mugging effect, because you may need a little less, or a little more and I can't figure that out from here.

Additionally, these medications have side effects that make them a poor choice for seniors, as they may increase incidence of falls (think hip fracture). Side effect profile for Tricyclics (which are "anticholinergic" drugs) causes a drying effect on the body, so you may experience uncomfortable dry mouth, very dry eyes, blurry vision, urinary retention, constipation (see what I mean when I say "dry") as well as heartbeat irregularities, disorientation, confusion, lightheadedness, reduced sex drive (in men, problems with orgasm), and changes in appetite (usually increased).

I'm not trying to talk you out of these drugs, heavens no, if they are what bring you the most relief by all means, you have my blessings. I just want you to know what you're getting into if you are thinking about taking them (and have not yet begun) so that you can consider some of the other treatments listed in this chapter.

Dosage: Follow directions prescribed by your physician, as the dosage varies based upon which particular tri-cyclic you take. Side effects are dose-dependent so sometimes just backing off on your dosage will alleviate uncomfortable side effects.

Caution: They may take weeks to begin working, assuming they are going to even work (some people get relief, others don't respond). The combination of tricyclics with alcohol is not recommended. Get up slowly from a sitting or lying down position so you don't get lightheaded.

Opiate Analgesics

Medicines like hydrocodone, oxycodone, morphine, dilaudid, codeine and others. I don't recommend these for tension headaches, they do not work nearly as well as the anti-inflammatory drugs, or the tricyclic antidepressants. The risk to benefit with this class of narcotics is not good enough for me to comfortably recommend these, I doubt they will help.

Pacify Your Pain Right Now

Acetaminophen	500 - 1,000mg	every 4 to 6 hours	Max. 4000mg/day
Aspirin	325 - 1,000mg	every 4 to 6 hours	Max. 4000mg/day
Ibuprofen	200 - 800mg	every 4 to 8 hours	Max. 2400mg/day
Naproxen	220 - 550mg	every 12 hours	Max. 1100mg/day

Be Careful Combining Headache Medications

Your local pharmacist and primary physician play a key role in maintaining your safety, especially when it comes to combining medications and avoiding drug interactions. Certain combinations of medications used for headaches can cause excessive drowsiness or faintness. An example of this would be the combination of a tri-cyclic antidepressant (nortriptyline) and an opiate analgesic (ie hydrocodone). This combination can also cause severe constipation.

The combination of NSAIDs (ibuprofen) with one-a-day aspirin is not recommended. The risk of gastric bleeding goes up with this combination. The Food & Drug Administration's website posts a useful article entitled *"Information for Healthcare Professionals: Concomitant Use of Ibuprofen and Aspirin"* which you can read about if you have concerns about drug safety with this drug combination.[24]

TENS Transcutaneous electrical nerve stimulation

Picture a little device, about the size of a cell phone (or smaller) that sends electrical pulses through your skin to treat and eliminate pain. It transmits electrical pulses through your skin to stimulate your body to produce higher amounts of endorphins, your body's own natural painkiller. Don't let the word "electrical" scare you, it doesn't hurt, but it could tingle. You can change the settings so you feel less tingly sensations, I've tried this myself and it's safe and effective.

TENS units give effective pain relief with no side effects and can be used whenever you need it! I love that the portability of these little devices and think a TENS unit is a very effective complement or

ive to oral analgesics when your pain sets in. I recommend this
you based on anecdotal reports from my readers telling me
as well on findings from a study that found it to be effective
with CTTH (chronic tension type headaches).[25]
a TENS unit, you will need a prescription from a doctor, any
ing medical doctors, chiropractors, obstetricians, pediatricians,
or anyone. With your prescription in hand, you can either go
anding pharmacy (or call ahead) to see if they have a unit in
can buy one online from an Internet retailer. You mail or fax
ption and they ship you your TENS unit. I encourage you to
s as some devices are easier to use than others. Some have
s if your hands are big, some have bigger displays.

Make sure you know about the contraindications, your physician
should know, and of course you can research on your own. For example,
TENS units are not recommended for pregnant women or pacemaker
patients, also I don't recommend you place the electrodes on your face,
spine or neck. For tension headaches, the trapezius muscles are probably
ideal locations, but again ask your doctor what is right for you and then
double check with the company you buy your TENS unit from. One
more thing, TENS treatments are often 30 minute sessions but it will
differ for each person, and possibly the pre-set settings you have on
your personal unit. Don't go to sleep with these things on!

Weirdest Pain Relief Yet!

Imagine lying down on a table with a vessel above your head that keeps
pouring oil onto your forehead, very slowly in a continuous stream for
an hour and a half. The sound of this makes me want to blurt out every
secret of homeland security. It's called the shirodhara technique and it
is far from tortuous, in fact, it can be soothing and invigorating to your
senses and mind. Shirodhara is an Ayurvedic technique performed in
India for more than 5,000 years. Shirodhara means flowing of oil like
a thread (dhara) onto the head "shiro." The oil that is gently poured
upon you is a special medicinal oil but I've read that it can be milk or
even buttermilk. Cotton pads are placed upon your eyes to prevent oil
from splashing into them. The session is designed to calm your nerves
and help you recover from mental exhaustion. I read one site that said
Shirodhara "gives strength to the neck and head" and that alone is
helpful for tension headaches.

Think Outside the Doc Box

Light is a key to health. The use of light in the form of Light Emitting Diodes (LEDs) gained attention after NASA used it to promote plant growth in space. NASA research led to discoveries that both Red and Near Infrared (NIR) light is able to trigger healing in the body. It's an option that is "beyond the doc box" backed up by research that substantiates the healing power of LED light. The unit I like is the LightWorks by Sota. It's a hand-held unit with a choice of additional frequencies as well as the option to add other colors to the Red and Near Infrared paddles. More information on the use of light for health can be found at www.mylighttherapy.com.

Tea for Pain Relief: Lemon Balm Tea

One of the hidden treasures in the botanical world is lemon balm, Melissa *officinalis*. It reduces tension, anxiety and depression. It is a muscle relaxer. Sipping warm tea is soothing to your soul. Melissa *officinalis* can suppress pro-inflammatory cytokines[26] such as TNFα and IL-1β, something pain sufferers should make their goal. You can try lemon balm tea tabs, or buy dried herb in bulk to make your own, about 1 teaspoon per cup of hot boiled water. Let it steep (not boil) for 10 minutes then strain. Effects may be felt after one delicious cup. Sweeten your tea with natural sugars, maple syrup, coconut nectar, brown rice syrup or stevia, *but nothing artificial*.

Biofeedback Works

Back in the late 1990's, I got certified as a neurobiofeedback therapist. Neurobiofeedback is a technique that trains the brain to regulate and control bodily functions, and these changes show up on an EEG or electroencephalogram. The training helps improve temperature control, anxiety, pain levels, emotional symptoms and much more.

Back then I was still a gung ho pharmacist too. I never did anything with my certification because I couldn't bear to step away from my customers at the pharmacy, or those beloved metabolic pathways, nerd extraordinaire that I am. I've always remembered how wonderfully this modality worked to reduce blood pressure, ease stress, control heart rhythm, and improve pelvic floor muscle response (for incontinence). Could it help with headaches though?

After researching the literature, it's a resounding yes! I even found a meta-analysis that investigated the short and long term efficacy of biofeedback for tension headaches. According to an analysis of 74 studies, biofeedback was more effective than headache monitoring, placebo, and even relaxation therapies. The way that it impacted headaches the most is by reducing the frequency of attacks, but it also helped reduce symptoms of anxiety, depression and muscle tension. If you do biofeedback, you may be able to reduce the dosage of your medication. While adults benefit from biofeedback, it does appear that children and adolescents get the most value.[27, 28]

Know the Difference

The onset of any neurological symptom would be a clue that your head pain was beyond a tension headache. Time is of the essences. For example, a severe headache, often described as "the worst headache of my life" could be a warning sign of a cerebral aneurysm that is about to rupture, days or weeks after the headache first happens (sometimes sooner). Symptoms could include seizure-like activity, complete or partial loss of vision, weakness, double vision, eye pain or a stiff neck. If your headache is ever accompanied with eyelid drooping, sleepiness, stupor, difficulty moving a part of your body or numbness, I want you to immediately go to the Emergency Room or call 9-1-1 for an ambulance. If you have a long history of headaches that move around your head every few minutes to hours this could be tied to Lyme disease or Babesiosis which are tick-borne illnesses, discussed in Chapter 6.

Drug Muggers that Deplete CoQ10

Some medications rob your body of CoQ10 and this could affect your muscle health, since CoQ10 is food for your myocytes or muscle cells. As you have learned, the health of your muscles plays a direct role in tension headaches. Without enough CoQ10, your muscle cells starve to death and you become more prone to muscle tension. Recall from chapter 2 that CoQ10 deficiency also plays a role in migraines. Finally, a CoQ10 deficiency is tied to higher levels of IL-6, a pain causing chemical implicated in tension headaches. For a more comprehensive list of medications that zap CoQ10 from you refer to my *Drug Muggers* book.[23]

Antacids & Acid blockers
Atenolol
Cholesterol reducing medications
HCTZ (hydrochlorothiazide)
Hormone Replacement Therapy
Most medications for diabetes
Metoprolol
Oral contraceptives
Tricyclic antidepressants (doxepin, nortriptyline)

Quit Coffee or Drink More?

Tension headaches respond to different things. Many people find that drinking a cup of coffee, which is very stimulating helps reduce or eliminate the pain. This may occur due to the caffeine which constricts blood vessels. Caffeine enhances the pain relieving effect of analgesics, that's why you find caffeine in non-prescription pain-relieving formulas. I'm not a fan of caffeine for people with headaches. I received a very good question from Denise, a reader of my syndicated column "Dear Pharmacist" which I send out free in my newsletter (sign up www.DearPharmacist.com). Denise sent me this:

Dear Suzy

Is it better for me to take combinations containing caffeine, aspirin and acetaminophen as in the combo drug Excedrin? Or is it better to just take regular acetaminophen with caffeine as in "Tylenol Ultra Relief- Tough on Headaches" formula?"

I'll tell you the same answer I emailed to Denise. I think it's better to address the root cause of headaches versus relying on medications but if it's only once in a while, then I'd take the single agent, as in just acetaminophen (with the caffeine), not the two drugs such as aspirin combined with acetaminophen (with the caffeine). Excedrin is a good example of this, overseas, you may find it as Anadin Extra. By the way, acetaminophen is also known as "paracetamol" in many countries, and further, it is abbreviated as "APAP" sometimes. I'm basing my opinion to Denise, and you, on three very good reasons:

1) If you take just acetaminophen (with the caffeine) it's one drug (acetaminophen) so that exposes to only one set of side effects . . . those related to acetaminophen. If you take a combination

of two drugs (acetaminophen and aspirin) the combination exposes you to twice the amount of side effects because you expose yourself to two sets of side effects, those from acetaminophen and those from aspirin. Make sense?

Aspirin is known to thin blood, and cause easy bruising while irritating the stomach lining. Acetaminophen may harm the liver if you take too much. So you are opening yourself up potentially to both stomach *and* liver damage if you use a combination of these drugs with every dose of the combination pill.

2) Aspirin is a drug mugger of vitamin C. Acetaminophen is a drug mugger of glutathione. When you take the combination of these, you have to supplement with more nutrients. That costs you more money in term so replenishing what the drug mugger stole.[23]

3) A report analyzed 6 different trials, all conducted under similar protocols to see whether a caffeine-containing two analgesic combinations (like aspirin and acetaminophen) was better than acetaminophen alone, or placebo.[29] If you look this study up, you will see acetaminophen abbreviated as APAP, which is very common in pharmaceutical speak. Anyway, the patients all self-medicated themselves during episodes of tension headaches. In all 6 studies, the caffeine-containing analgesics performed significantly better than 1,000mg APAP, and better than placebo (well, we kind of expected that). They pooled the data and concluded that analgesic benefits were virtually the same whether you took aspirin and acetaminophen, or acetaminophen alone (both with caffeine) but *"The combinations [meaning aspirin AND acetaminophen] produced more stomach discomfort, nervousness, and dizziness than acetaminophen or placebo."*

Do all the studies agree? Of course not, why would medicine be that easy? In 2010, a study published in the *European Journal of Neurology* concluded the fixed combinations including the two drugs (with caffeine) was better than either drug alone (with caffeine).[30] They also said there's *"no evidence for higher prevalence of undesirable side-effects of combination analgesics in comparison to monotherapy."*

Really, you don't get more side effects from taking both drugs as compared to one? I've been a pharmacist for more than 2 decades, something's wrong with that picture. I simply don't buy it, and I don't suggest you do either.

And guys, get this, a recent study suggests that four or more cups of coffee might reduce the risk of prostate cancer recurrence.[31] Hmm, that's fodder for another book, right now, I'm focused on your head and some people do find relief with four cups of coffee, some find it with just half a cup every day.

On the other hand, some people are triggered by caffeine in coffee. For those of you, something calming maybe better. But don't stop cold-turkey, please realize that going off coffee (caffeine) is going to cause a rebound headache. Caffeine withdrawal is a very common cause of headaches. I know you know what I mean, if you are just 2 hours late for your usual cup of Joe, the pain begins, and only drinking your cup of coffee will soothe the beast. So if you want to see what life is like without coffee, wean off slowly.

Try Ice and Heat

Because tension headaches are often tied to knotted up muscles, try a hot compress on your forehead, or the back of your neck. The heat instantly relaxes the muscles in this area. Put a few drops of lavender essential oil on the compress for added benefit. You could jump into a hot shower. (Warn your spouse that you may exit in 2 hours looking like a prune) as the shower trick works wonders for most people and you just don't want to get out! The heat and moisture can be very enjoyable.

Now if heat makes you cringe, and it does for some, then try applying a cold pack to your temples, or to the back of your neck for 5 to 10 minutes.

Your Plan of Action: A Dozen Ways to Minimize the Pain

If you feel a tension headache coming on, here are some ideas. For the supplement or medication ideas, you need to get permission from your practitioner:

1) Stop working if you can. Stress is a huge contributor to tension headaches. Get off Facebook, who cares that someone just unfriended you or tagged you in an unflattering photo. Let it go, it isn't worth the stress and the pain in your head that you'll feel for the next hour! Whatever you are working on can wait, you need to come first right now.

2) Get at least 30 feet away from any charging electrical device like your computer, iPad or phone, especially if it's been on your ear for a long conversation. The stress of working and the electromagnetic radiation doesn't make a headache better. It's either neutral or bad.

3) Drink a full glass of water.

4) Try a hot shower. If you prefer, take a hot bath with a full 3 to 4 pound bag of Epsom salts which is a way to get magnesium in through your skin. Epsom is magnesium and that mineral is a potent muscle relaxer, just what you need right now!

5) Try a mini massager on trapezius muscles, which may be referring pain. Of course, if you have quick access to get a real massage, I'd go for that.

6) Take 5 deep breathes, breathing in about the same length of time as you breathe out. Relax your shoulders, and let them fall to their natural place (I'm betting you keep them up high, guarding your head a bit). Let them go down.

7) Unclench your teeth, this is a common cause for tension headaches.

8) Make tea. Lemonbalm is my pick for you, however it is very relaxing, and somewhat sedating if you make it strong enough. As an alternative, ginger tea may help because it is a strong anti-inflammatory and helps with nausea. It has natural blood thinning properties, so if you take anti-coagulant drugs, don't combine.

9) Put a TENS unit on.

10) Turn on your Lightworks by Sota. For me, I use the red paddle for 5 minutes on each side of my forehead.

11) Turn on Heart Math program, this is a type of biofeedback training that you can do at home. www.heartmath.com for devices that you can buy.

12) Ask someone to get behind you, and with the palms of their hands to gently compress and traction your temporal region (basically squeeze and pull up on the temples). Hold for 10

seconds and release, then again. And combine that with a little forehead and temple massage. If nothing else, it should feels good but of course if there's any pain or worsening of your symptoms you need to stop immediately. If you like this, make sure you unclench your teeth and relax your jaw.

Sip Relief

Headaches sometimes occur as a result of dehydration. Drinking fresh water or tea (about 6 to 8 glasses per day) may make the difference for you because detoxification is the name of the game. We're exposed to toxins all day long, getting them out is important. If nothing else, adequate hydration dilutes the poisons in your body and helps you eliminate them in your urine. You know you're dehydrated if your lips are dry or cracked. Another sign that you need to drink more is concentrated urine that is deep yellow or has a strong odor.

Chapter 4

Cluster Headaches

Sometimes cluster headaches are termed "alarm clock" headaches because they wake you up at pretty much the same time each night. I've also heard them called "hypnic" headaches. Call them whatever you want, they're excruciating. And they occur in cycles, hence the name "cluster."

One headache can last a few minutes, or a few hours, more often happening between 1 and 2 am. This could cause serious sleep dread. No matter what time of day or night you get these headaches, please know reprieve should come in-between the episodes. The seasons matter, with spring and fall the most common start for a cluster headache cycle in both men and women. Some of you have these cluster headaches *chronically!* These are knife-like, burning, horrendous bouts of head pain, like a hot poker or an ice-pick right into your brain, or your eye and almost always one-sided.

My husband Sam used to get these occasionally and wake up in the middle of the night. I'd see him lunging out of our bed, practically throwing himself into a wall because of the shock of it. You wake up to the sensation of getting stabbed in the head! He is completely cured of this and trigeminal neuralgia now. So hold on to hope! A complete cure is absolutely possible.

Where Do Clusters Come From?

There are many theories about why cluster headaches occur, but no fully determined medical cause. It could be a compromised area in your brain, perhaps from prior blunt trauma to the head, say a football injury in high school, a concussion from a car accident, or whiplash. It may not be easy to figure out. Whether or not we know the exact cause of your headaches is irrelevant to me. I'm still going to point out ways to help you reduce frequency and duration, and possibly even get rid of them altogether.

This chapter is going to give you lots of information, some of which will ruffle the feathers of many doctor you've been to. *You realize I'm going to get some lip from the conventional medical community don't you? Once you've been helped, could you please give my book a 5-star review on Amazon? It'll help pay me back for the grief I get from conventional docs.*

I specialize in "far-out" ideas and I'm proud of my detective abilities. I'm not sure why I'm this way, maybe seeing first-hand the horror of chronic pain when I was a nursing home consultant, and also up close with sweet Sam.

The pain and sleep deprivation caused by cluster headaches are unfathomable. They are called "the suicide headache" by some. Poor response to conventional treatment is your clue something "far out" may be going on.

The underlying cause for cluster headaches could be different for every person reading this. So let's begin our journey, because no matter the cause, even if you don't yet have a diagnosis, I still have tricks up my sleeve to help you.

Man Versus Women

One very interesting survey was done and it examined the differences between men and women when it comes to cluster headaches. This was published in 2012, in the *Journal of Neurological Sciences*.[29]

Statistically-speaking:
Women who get cluster headaches are more likely to experience depression or asthma.

Women are more likely to respond to inhaled lidocaine than to injected triptans.

Women develop cluster headache at an earlier age than men.

Women are more apt to have a family history of headaches or Parkinson's disease

Aura duration is shorter in women.

Women are much more likely to have sensory, language or brainstem auras.

Women's cluster pain is more likely to radiate into the jaw, cheek and ear.

Women more likely to have nausea.

Women have more attacks per day and higher pain intensity.

Women less responsive to triptans and nasal spray than men, but statistically more responsive to inhaled lidocaine.

Women are less likely to be diagnosed at the first doctor's visit compared to men.

Women's cluster headaches are not influenced by menses or menopause

Half of women surveyed said their headaches improved with pregnancy.

Women are much more likely to lose their job compared to men.

Anatomy of a Cluster Headache

Cluster headaches may involve demyelination or some other defect in the trigeminal nerve in your face. Myelin is a protective substance that surrounds every nerve in your body, much like the electrical cord that protects the interior wiring on electrical appliances. Demyelination is a process that involves damage to that protective coating. It leaves those sensitive nerve wires exposed.

New research suggests that our natural myelin production is ramped up during sleep. Clusters occur during the time you are supposed to be asleep, so sleep deprivation contributes to more pain. It's a vicious cycle. If you're not sleeping, myelin production goes down, and myelin is what protects you from pain. Myelin is comparable to your body's skin, which also protects you from outside influences.

Demyelination means a stripping away of the protective layer of your trigeminal nerve, leaving it exposed. The painful syndrome called "Trigeminal Neuralgia" is fully discussed in Chapter 5, so I urge you to read that chapter next if you have cluster headaches since the same exact cranial nerve (cranial nerve V) is involved. If you have a demyelination process going on, you could have both of these conditions, meaning trigeminal neuralgia bouts during the day, and cluster headaches at night!

Your goal would then be to figure out what is causing the demyelination. It could be related to insomnia. Remember, poor sleep contributes to poor myelin production, according to emerging research. Also, sometimes demyelination is caused by gluten, found in barley, rye, spelt, and wheat-based products, such as bread, pasta, bagels, and muffins. Demyelination can occur for other reasons too, but I point out the gluten connection because it may apply to you. Within months of going gluten free, or even grain free, your headaches and pain may retreat. It really can be that easy.

Sometimes, cluster headaches are the result of swollen blood vessels around the brain, which puts pressure on your delicate trigeminal nerve. Anti-inflammatory medication can be beneficial here. Recent MRI studies suggest that this swelling around the brain has to do with structural changes that occur deep inside, in the hypothalamus. Your hypothalamus regulates your biological clock (circadian rhythm). This explanation makes sense to me, because it explains why cluster headaches tend to be seasonal, and why they occur around the same time each night when melatonin levels are supposed to be high (and they're not). All this research, and still the true underlying cause for clusters remains elusive.

While scientists are trying to figure out why these headaches appear, one thing is clear. You're still suffering, and I'm here to help you. As a Functional Medicine practitioner, I've always got my mind wrapped around complex studies that have something to do with metabolic pathways that drive pain. Forgive me momentarily while I lapse into some chemistry for you. I'm just trying to help. I know for a fact that with cluster headaches several imbalances with chemicals that cause pain (cytokines) occur.

For example, we know that in folks who get cluster headaches the cytokine IL-1β is at a high level all the time, and the cytokine IL-2 is significantly higher than it should be in between headache attacks during the active cluster headache period.[1,2]

If you want to know more details about those cytokines, read Chapter 12 "Reduce Pain-Causing Cytokines." If you can reduce them (and you can), you're another step closer to living headache free.

Table 1 Most Common Pain Sites Clusters

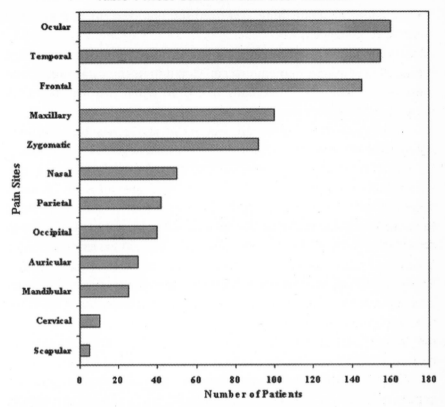

Now, I know that you want all the information you can get about how to end this pain. Before we discuss my Script for Clusters that can help over the long haul, I want to tell you about the number one pain reliever for clusters. And it's not a pharmaceutical or a nutritional supplement. It's O2, as in oxygen.

Most Important: Breathe Baby Breathe!

Pure oxygen is usually the only thing that can stop a cluster headache attack, but you have to breathe it in almost immediately.

Triggers for Clusters

There is some evidence that cluster headaches might be triggered by the following:

Alcohol
Chocolate
Heat
Perfume
Infection
Disrupted sleep patterns
Melatonin deficiency
Smoking

Normally, taking deep breaths are nice and helpful for most headaches; however, for clusters I think you need the real deal, as in a portable home tank of oxygen.

Oxygen inhalation can successfully abort a cluster headache. I'm talking here about a treatment that can stop it in its tracks. However; the treatment needs to be immediate, like right when you wake up with the pain. It has little effect once the pain has reached its peak.

Scientists at the *Taiwan Headache Society* characterize cluster headache as "severe and excruciating pain which develops within a short time," and recommend emergency treatment. Yeah, I'm sure you can attest to that! They determined that high-flow oxygen inhalation appears to be most effective for the people they saw. It's interesting to see what other countries do. According to this article, the Taiwanese recommend intranasal triptans as first line pharmaceutical agents (examples include Imitrex or its generic sumatriptan and Zomig or its generic zolmitriptan). As a second line drug for acute attacks, the oral triptans are recommended. As for prevention, verapamil is their choice, and then second line agents included lithium, melatonin, valproic acid, topiramate and gabapentin. Corticosteroids (hydrocortisone, prednisone) were named but only for use within two weeks of the cycle.[3]

Do you think you need to take the triptan with the oxygen? If you said no, you're correct. This was shown in one large, randomized, double-blind study (the best kind of study) that was published in the *Journal of the American Medical Association (JAMA)* in 2009.[4] This study showed that oxygen alone can render people pain-free in about 15 minutes!

You can get an oxygen tank delivered to your home by asking your physician to order it for you. I know this for a fact, we've had one in and out of our home several times. The doctor phones the pulmonary company, and places the order for you. Then the

Feel Better at Sea Level?

Some people have a genetic predisposition that causes more headaches at high altitudes. You might be able to tell, if you fly to sea level and you feel better, breathe better, get fewer headaches, but then you fly home to the mountains, and the nonsense begins again in your head. You can take a saliva test to see if you have this predisposition. The "ACE D" and "AGT 235M" alleles were found to be significantly associated with both acute and chronic mountain sickness.[46]

www.23andMe.com

company calls you, set up a time to come to your home and drop it off for you. You could go to sleep with it too, the nasal cannula just rests in your nostrils and you breathe it in. Insurance often covers this, but check with your carrier to make sure. It is worth a try, and might be a great rescue aid for those 2 am alarm clock headaches! There are other ideas to help you relieve pain in Appendix IV, "Facebook Friends Helping Friends."

Before I leave the section on oxygen, I need you to consider undiagnosed sleep apnea as a cause for your clusters. With sleep apnea, you temporarily stop breathing while asleep. Most people with apnea are loud snorers. This creates periods of hypoxia (low oxygen to the brain), and this triggers clusters. To treat apnea, you just need a CPAP mask that delivers oxygen to you while you sleep. You might not look so sexy in the breathing contraption, but nowadays the masks are fairly small and comfortable. The CPAP literally breathes life (in the form of oxygen) into you while you sleep. It should reduce your attacks, if not cure them. Get a "sleep study," done to find out whether you have apnea.

Suzy's "Script" for Cluster Headache Relief

Before you take any of the following supplements, you must ask your doctor(s) if they are right for you. My intention here is to educate you about possibilities and options. Do not misconstrue my ideas for medical advice. I have no idea what is right for every individual reading this so take my list to your practitioner(s) to ask if they're right for you with your medical history. Dosages are also just basic guidelines, some people tolerate different dosages than what is stated here:

Lithium orotate
Melatonin
Skullcap extract
Licorice Root
Taurine
Diamine oxidase

How This Helps You Become Headache Free

Lithium.
Lithium is a natural over-the-counter supplement that may reduce feelings of anger and actually cause cheerfulness. People think of

lithium as a prescription drug useful for bipolar disorder, but lithium (even the natural, over-the-counter version I'm suggesting) is essential for every human being, just in small amounts. We all use it in our body; it is quite abundant.

Research suggests this mineral may reverse early Alzheimer's, improve spatial memory, and reduce symptoms of Ménière's disease, an inner ear disorder that affects balance and hearing. Plus, get this, it was shown in 2006 to help prevent cluster headaches.[1] Low lithium levels are associated with seizures, and you can have seizures even if you don't have any mood problems. Sometimes this mineral can help with encephalopathies, a category of brain diseases.

Prescription versions come in exponentially higher dosages (300mg, taken 3 times a day, for example). If you need that much, you could ask your physician.[2]

The 5-mg dose I'm suggesting should involve minimal side effects. In fact, it may help with memory. But everyone is different, and I'm not sure how you'll respond. You know you're getting too much lithium if you notice any of the following side effects: tremor, nausea, heart palpitations, weakness, excess urination, or confusion.

Side effects usually don't occur at all with small doses, as lithium is natural to our body. Keeping steady salt levels (i.e. the amount of sodium you get from your diet) will help to reduce the side effect called hyponatremia (which means that you have too little salt in your body). This is commonly associated with excessive lithium.

Melatonin.

Your body makes the hormone melatonin on its own. The pineal gland in your brain produces the hormone, which acts as your body's clock. When taken in supplement form, melatonin may be helpful, especially as a preventative. It won't help stop clusters that are already underway. One theory is that taking melatonin helps reset your circadian rhythm.

In studies, melatonin reduced pain intensity by blocking the nociceptive sense. "Nociceptive" refers to pain from the stimulation of nerve cells, which is different from damage or disease in the nerves themselves. In other words, melatonin acts a little bit like a mild tranquilizer to the brain, slowing down the firing of overactive cells.

One particular melatonin study I read about still has me thinking. Published in the journal *Current Neuropharmacology* in June 2012, the study was based on other studies that took place in India.[3] The authors mention that people experience different intensity levels of pain in the daytime and at night, and that the intensity of pain perception is lower at night, when it's dark. That's when our natural levels of melatonin are high, presumably so we can sleep. So researchers have discovered that the hormone melatonin is an anti-nociceptive substance, meaning that it helps the brain feel less intensity of pain. So far, it appears that melatonin affects sensation in the spinal cord, and up towards the shoulders and neck.[4] And, equally fascinating is the fact that that melatonin is involved with receptors the same way narcotic and central nervous system medications might be.[5] Melatonin has been used to treat both migraines and cluster headaches, as well as fibromyalgia and irritable bowel syndrome.[6] But here's what really surprised me: Researchers have actually administered melatonin during surgeries, and found that melatonin helped control pain both before and after the surgery![7] That's one powerful hormone!

I read one study that said people with chronic cluster headaches, or people who have episodic cluster headaches for whom prescription medication does not work, do not appear to benefit from adding melatonin to their "usual treatment regimens."[8] I disagree with that.

People who get cluster headaches are often low in melatonin, and I think it's worth a try. In fact, there's a chemical basis for why melatonin is so crucial. My theory is that it has to do with poor methylation. Methylation is a detoxification process in your body, and things like medications, foods, and genetic problems interfere with that process. If you are a poor methylator, you cannot effectively convert serotonin to melatonin, leaving you in a state of melatonin deficiency. And we know that melatonin deficiency is tied to cluster headaches in some folks.

There isn't a direct study to prove me correct, so my comments are based upon my understanding of the chemistry of metabolic pathways. You either have this important pathway functioning smoothly, or you don't. I am sure that many people who get cluster headaches are dealing with raging pain because they are poor methylators. To read about tips to override methylation defects, see Chapter 8 "Detoxification Matters." For anyone who gets cluster headaches, this is a must read. I looked on Internet forums where people talk about their experiences, and I found this from someone who used melatonin to relieve pain from cluster headaches: *"After 39 years I am headache free!"*

The dosage varies for melatonin. I would normally recommend 0.3mg to 1.0mg for a headache-free person with insomnia. After all it is a potent hormone. With cluster headaches though, the dosage is much higher, something like 3mg to 10mg nightly. I want you to ask your doctor what's right for you.

Consider the following 1996 study in which people with cluster headaches took 10mg melatonin nightly.[9] Half of those treated noticed a decline in headache frequency by day 3 or 5, and "and they experienced no further attacks until melatonin was discontinued." Not one individual in the placebo group felt any better!

As for pro-inflammatory cytokines (the pain-causing chemicals associated with cluster headaches), melatonin is a master at reducing these. I talk about these chemicals in greater detail in Chapter 12, "Reduce Pain-Causing Cytokines" so you can check that out if you are really into this kind of science. For simplicity, in this section, I'll just tell you that melatonin inhibits the activation of the pain-causing pathway NFκB. Melatonin is also known to reduce levels of pain-causing interleukins, such as IL-6, and IL-1β , as well as TNFα. As if that's not enough, melatonin reduces levels of IFNγ.

Now I know that all those letters probably don't mean much to you unless you're a scientist or a science nerd. So I'll translate into plain English: Wow! It's just a fabulous thing to suppress all those pain-causing chemicals with one single hormone.

And don't forget that melatonin also helps you sleep. So you're getting a lot of action from this one hormone.

Caution: Of course, melatonin does cause drowsiness. Yes, and that's the point of taking melatonin. It's your natural sleep hormone taken in pill form! Some people have also reported a few side effects such as vivid dreams, daytime fatigue, altered taste sensation, nausea, stomach pain, and possibly diarrhea. It may not be right for everyone, I've had people with rheumatoid arthritis tell me they flared up after taking melatonin.

Skullcap *(Scutellaria latiflora).*

The herb skullcap, a gorgeous flower found in damp woodlands, is one of the best pain-relieving nervines (which means it tends to soothe

nervous excitement) in the plant world. It also has mild aphrodisiac properties and antibacterial components. In particular, it is soothing and restorative to the nervous system. I've selected this herb in part because people with cluster headaches have a touchy nerve, the trigeminal nerve among others. Skullcap is also helpful for withdrawal from narcotics. In addition to all that, this herb has pain-relieving analgesic qualities. In short, skullcap gives your brain a deep sigh of relief. Skullcap also reduces MMP, one of those pain-causing chemicals (cytokines) implicated in headaches. So that's another reason I've recommended it for you. Anything that reduces MMP can help with cancer, so by that token, skullcap must also have some anti-cancer benefits. But more than that, skullcap is a powerful reducer of numerous cytokines. It is known to shut down the NFKβ pathway, so that you don't have that outpouring of nasty pain chemicals. It can suppress production of IL-1β, TNFα, IL-2, IL-6, and COX2.[10] It blocks the VEGF pathway too, something important to patients who have a history of cancer.[11] OK, OK… I'm getting into all those science letters again. The point is simple: Although Skullcap may sound ominous, it actually puts a warm fuzzy cap on your skull so that you can finally catch a break! Try skullcap and see if it helps you, especially in combination with the other supplements in my Script.

Caution: Skullcap causes drowsiness, so combining it with medications that also cause drowsiness is not a wonderful idea, even if the herb is very gentle. Taking skullcap and melatonin together should be OK, though. I recommend that you avoid consuming alcohol at the same time as skullcap. Skullcap has a mild diuretic (water pill) effect, so if you are also taking lithium for your headaches (or for bipolar disorder) be very careful. The change in water balance in your body could increase the amount of lithium in your system, leading to more side effects.

Licorice root *(Glycyrrhiza glabra).*
Your adrenal glands take a beating with all the stress in your life. Licorice root helps your adrenal glands produce the hormones cortisol and adrenalin if you are exhausted. So licorice root improves cortisol imbalances. It increases the circulating levels of cortisol already there by *reducing its breakdown,* not by making extra cortisol.

Cortisol imbalances, particularly when the hormone dips low in the middle of the night, have been closely linked to cluster headaches.[12] Studies have shown that people who suffer from cluster headaches usually have lower levels of cortisol than people who don't suffer from cluster headaches. So when licorice is on board, it may help prevent those dips, and thus lower your risk for a cluster episode. That's my thinking, and the reason I've recommended it; however, you should ask your doctor what's right for you.

You can brew a cup of licorice tea every day for a very gentle effect, or you can take supplements. Licorice root is strongly flavored. I think it's delicious myself. If you like, you can add a small piece of cinnamon, some peppermint leaves, or honey to the tea.

Caution: While absolutely safe when used properly, licorice root can magnify the effects of many drugs and cause fluid retention, which can raise blood pressure. So use this herb only with your doctor's consent. The DGL version of licorice root will not work for what we are trying to do here. Read Chapter 9 "The Adrenal Hormone Connection" to learn more about cortisol and other adaptogens that might work if you can't take licorice.

Taurine.

The amino acid taurine is the most abundant in your heart. It is often used in supplement form to help normalize heart rhythm in people with cardiac palpitations. I love taurine, and think it is one of the most impressive amino acids we have when it comes to feeding the body at a cellular level.

Taurine puts your brain at ease, by activating (yes, activating) an inhibitory neurotransmitter called Gamma Amino Butyric Acid (GABA). When you activate GABA, you put your brain at ease. Some people are so relaxed from taurine, it helps them sleep, but that depends on the dose. In fact, GABA is extremely plentiful when you are sleeping. I can't tell you why manufacturers put GABA in energy drinks. It does not give you energy. *Au contraire.*

Drugs that are used to treat cluster headaches (valproic acid, gabapentin) raise levels of GABA. But you don't need to take the drug to get this benefit. You can buy taurine at health food stores, and taurine helps you naturally produce GABA.[13] If increasing GABA helps, then it makes sense to consider taking taurine, even though there have been no direct scientific studies examining taurine as a treatment for cluster headaches. Taurine also reduces the damaging effects of the neurotoxin glutamate.[45] In and of itself that is enough reason for me to recommend it for you. As an aside, it supports pancreatic health and is helpful for those with diabetes.

I think taking taurine can be helpful for you unless you have a genetic snp (pronounced "snip") that prevents you from utilizing it properly. That discussion is too complex for this book, but the snp involved may be a "CBS enzyme" upregulation. Genetic tests like those through 23andMe.com can determine if you have this snp. You be able to tell if it was a problem for you (without genetic testing) because your mind would become sluggish and thinking slowed down from it. Side effects of taurine are usually minimal, but do jot down in your headache diary the times when you take it, so you can track any effects. If you feel really slowed down from it, then I'd stop.

Caution: Taurine can lower your blood pressure, so be careful if you're also taking drugs that lower your blood pressure. The two together will work really well, too well actually, and you may feel faint if your pressure drops too much. Ask your doctor if reducing your medication dosage is okay. Hopefully, your doc would allow that, rather than stop the taurine, which has heart benefits galore.

Sometimes people report itching, nausea, dizziness, drowsiness, or headache, while taking taurine. You can always lower your dosage if necessary. As I always tell you, take the lowest possible dose possible, while still reaping the benefits of what any drug or supplement has to offer.

Squash Histamine with Diamine oxidase or DAO

Cluster headaches are also called "the histamine headache" because they may be tied to high levels of histamine (which your body produces). It's a chemical that is released from your mast cells in response to an allergic reaction, causing itching, sneezing and wheezing. It causes a dilation of your blood vessels, and that's not necessarily a good thing if you're prone to headaches, because it produces more pressure in the brain. Histamine occurs naturally in certain foods, see my list coming up in the next section. This connection of histamine as a chemical mediator of migraines and cluster headaches has long been known so I hope your pain specialist has told you this by now. We never knew how prevalent it was though, until recently.

I got my hands on a study that showed a remarkably tight connection to migraines and DAO. What is DAO? It's one of the enzymes that allow histamine to break down. DAO stands for diamine-oxidase. What if you didn't have a lot of DAO in your body? You'd have higher levels of histamine! The objective of the study,[44] published in the October issue of *Journal of the Neurological Sciences*. Scientists tested 137 people that suffered migraine attacks 4 to 14 times per month. The test was basically to give them a DAO supplement (or placebo) three times daily for one month and see if their headaches got any better, and if they needed as much medication as they normally took. Not a surprise, the folks taking DAO supplements experienced fewer hours of pain, and significantly reduced need for migraine medicine. Researchers found that natural DAO activity in the body was reduced in 119 of 137 patients meaning 87% of them had reduced DAO activity. That's why taking DAO supplements helped them so much. You can test yourself for DAO activity. You can also buy supplements of DAO without a prescription, these are sold online and at health food stores. I recommend DAO supplements for people with cluster and/or migraine headaches along with a low-histamine diet.

Dosage: 1 or 2 capsules (20,000 to 40,000 HDU) daily, usually before eating a meal that is high in histamine. Sometimes you will find brands that are 10,000 HDU and those are often taken as 1 capsule with each meal. There isn't a hard fast rule with dosing as long as you stick to what I've outlined here, or what your physician recommends (or the label directions for the brand you buy).

Get Rid Of . . .

 * Alcohol
   Artificial sweeteners packets (aspartame, sucralose, etc)
   Bright lights
   Deli meats (that contains nitrites)
   Diet soda (mainly because of the artificial sweeteners)
   Dried fruit (that contains sulfites)
   Foods allergens: dairy, gluten, soy, corn, eggs
   Gluten
   GMO foods
   Heat (hot baths, hot weather)
   High altitude (trekking, flying)
   Histamine-rich foods
   MSG
 * Nitroglycerin
   Perfume
   Pollen, dust mites, anything that creates histamine
   Smoking

 * *Vasodilators such as nitroglycerin, alcohol, and carbon dioxide may trigger a headache during a cluster period.*

Histamine-Rich Foods

I'd avoid or at least minimize histamine-rich foods and take a DAO supplement for at least 6 week trial. The supplement called "Diamine Oxidase" or DAO can help you if you are intolerant to some of the foods above, or if they trigger headaches.

Alcoholic beverages, especially beer and wine.

Anchovies

Avocados

Cheeses, especially aged or fermented cheese (parmesan, blue, Roquefort)

Cider and home-made root beer

Coffee or black tea

Dried fruits, such as apricots, dates, prunes, figs, and raisins

Eggplant

Fermented foods, pickled or smoked meats, sauerkraut

Ketchup, barbecue sauce, pickles, pickled beets, relish, olives (it's
    the vinegar)
Mackerel
Mayonnaise (if it contains vinegar)
Mushrooms
Processed meats (sausage, bratwurst, hot dogs, salami, etc.)
Sardines
Smoked fish (herring, sardines)
Sour cream, sour milk, buttermilk, yogurt
Soured breads, pumpernickel, sourdough, coffee cake
Soy sauce
Spinach
Sunflower seeds, or sunflower butter
Tomatoes
Red wine vinegar or balsamic vinegar
Salad dressing
Yogurt

Histamine-Releasing Foods

*These cause your body to produce more histamine. You may feel better
off them.*

Alcohol	Papayas
Bananas	* Pineapples
Chocolate	Shellfish
Eggs	Strawberries
Fish	Tomatoes
Milk	

* Even though you see pineapples as a histamine-releasing food, you
sometimes see one of its extracts "bromelain" sold as a dietary supplement
that works as a natural antihistamine. Fine by me, I like bromelain for people
with allergies; you'll just have to see if it's right for you, by seeing if you get
a flare.

Gluten and Headaches

Gluten attacks the brain and causes release of pro-inflammatory, pain-
causing chemicals known as cytokines. I recommend reducing or
eliminating gluten from your diet as a measure of safety for your brain.

If this is going to help you, you may notice in the first month. Even if you don't notice any difference, I recommend eliminating all gluten for at least three months. If you don't find any reduction in the frequency of headaches by then, it's okay to re-implement gluten if you must. But if you've found some relief, just stay on the diet. There are a bazillion great gluten-free products out there now, making it a lot easier to go gluten-free. Rice flour is a great gluten-free substitute for wheat flour, and it tastes just as good if you bake with it. You won't even notice the difference.

> ### Feverfew: Don't Go There!
>
> The herb feverfew *(Tanacetum parthenium)* is a preventive for migraines. It's helpful for those who have already tried prescription meds for migraines with no positive results.[10, 11] When it comes to cluster headaches, I do not recommend feverfew. This herb is a vasodilator, and you do not want that.

I'm a Pharmacist, Let's Talk Medicine

Medicines that help reduce the incidence or severity of cluster are not foolproof, nor are they without side effects. Nevertheless, they can be a Godsend. Treatment approaches involve a two-fold process: 1) Immediate pain relievers 2) Preventative drugs.

Because cluster attacks come on so suddenly, I think pain relievers are basically not effective because they take 20 to 30 minutes to get past your stomach and into your intestines, where they are absorbed. At least that's the case with oral analgesics. You can still try them, because they may be useful at preventing your cluster from reaching its normal peak. Taking long-term analgesics out of fear that you might get a cluster headache is not the ultimate solution. This can complicate matters because these pain-killers are addictive, sedating, and constipating. With clusters, you really have to look at things like oxygen and melatonin as treatments.

Immediate Pain Relievers

A variety of drugs are designed to relieve headache pain. You can buy them over-the-counter or with a prescription. It depends on the type of medication. Let's look first at the pain-relievers that you can buy over-the-counter: The most popular over-the-counter (OTC) medications are ibuprofen (Advil, Motrin, others), naproxen (Aleve, others), and ketoprofen (Orudis KT) all of which belong to the NSAID class (pronounced "N-said"). NSAID stands for non-steroidal anti-inflammatory drugs. Acetaminophen (Tylenol, others) is another pain-relieving drug sold over-the-counter. You can also find medications sold at pharmacies nationwide that combine these ingredients along with some caffeine (Excedrin Migraine).

Dosage: Follow label directions on the package you buy.

Caution: All of these medications may take up to an hour to kick in, assuming they are going to even work. This category of drugs is simply not effective at aborting clusters.

Always try to take the lowest effective dose of any medication.

Medications containing acetaminophen can harm the liver if taken in excess, or long term, or in combination with wine and alcohol. Be very careful not to combine different products that contain acetaminophen because the maximum daily dosage is 4,000mg. Taking a multi-tasking cold formulas along with your pain-relieving drug, for example, could easily take you over that amount.

Preventative Drugs

Triptans

Examples: Zolmitriptan (Zomig)
Sumatriptan (Imitrex)
Naratriptan (Amerge)
Almotriptan (Axert) and others...

Triptan drugs are often prescribed to prevent cluster attacks or reduce pain. They can be taken orally, but don't overuse them. Follow your doctor's directions. Some triptans are available in injectable form, so that they enter the system quickly and can be tried for a cluster.

If you do use a triptan, don't combine it with any other triptan drugs, ergotamine drugs, or serotonin agonists (drugs or supplements that produce more serotonin in the body). Like all triptan drugs, Zomig requires a prescription. Certain people should not take triptans: Anyone with uncontrolled high blood pressure, ischemic heart disease, or vascular disease. I've written a great deal more about triptans in Chapter 2, "Migraine Headaches." I suggest you read that if you're thinking of using any of the tripans. Thank goodness we have triptans because the older alternatives that were our only choices back when I graduated in 1989 were rarely effective and riddled with problems.

Let's talk about some of those older drugs, in case you rely on them, first up methysergide and after that, methergine.

Methysergide

This drug has been discontinued in the United States due to bad side effects, such as retroperitoneal, cardiac, and pleuropulmonary fibrosis. It was useful for some people because it constricts blood vessels and reduces inflammation. Even if it's sold in your country, I don't recommend taking it because of the serious side effects.

Methergine

Known generically as Methylergonovine maleate, this drug is a close relative of methysergide (see above). It's one of the active metabolites of methysergide, meaning it's capable of causing similar side effects as that drug. Why am I including drugs here that have potential for harm? Because the side effects don't happen to everyone who uses the drug. And let's face it, all drugs have potential for harm, all of them.

Methergine reduces cluster headache frequency by more than 50% in 19 of 20 people according to a pilot study.[30] You never want to take this drug if you have high blood pressure or while pregnant. In fact, just like methysergide, methergine should be approached with extreme caution (or avoided) in people with vascular disease, liver damage, kidney compromise, or coronary heart disease. This drug is closely related to LSD, no joke! It can cause hallucinations if you take too much.[31] Depending on which manufacturer you get, the inactive ingredients include talc, parabens, several artificial colors, synthetic black iron oxide and gelatin in case you are sensitive to any of those.

Pregabalin (Lyrica)

This prescription drug is relatively new (in pharmaceutical years), and it soothes nerve pain, but it causes a lot of drowsiness and dizziness. It comes as an easy-to-swallow capsule in varying dosages. It helps to reduce the chemical Substance P.[35] Why would you want to reduce Substance P? Pretend the "P" stands for pain, because this is a pain chemical.

I definitely think pregabalin is worth a try, and recommend you ask your doctor if it is a safe option for you. I have to warn you that some people have to discontinue pregabalin because of the adverse side effects, such as wobbliness, abnormal gait, daytime fatigue, trouble concentrating, weight gain, chest pain, and visual problems. Some of these side effects are dose dependent (so take the lowest effective dose); some of them go away over time too.

When you begin taking this drug, you must start with a low dosage and gradually increase it over the first few days. You may not need the maximum dose, which is 100mg taken TID (pharmacy speak for three times a day). You'll just have to see how much you need based upon the pain relief you get. I always recommend starting out slowly with any medicine to see how you react. If you decide to stop taking pregabalin, you don't want to stop suddenly. Taper off gradually over a minimum of 1 week, preferably 2 or 3 weeks.

Corticosteroids

Examples: Prednisone, methylprednisone, hydrocortisone
Corticosteroid drugs, called "steroids" for short, are transitional drugs, not really intended for long term. They just stabilize you after an attack until you can get on an anticonvulsant medication, calcium channel blocker, or another medication. You usually see them dosed in a pack. The dose is higher on day one, then tapers down over a week. Doctors prescribe steroids because they reduce pro-inflammatory pain-causing cytokines. These drugs are extremely effective, but long-term use can lead to immune suppression, psychosis (or mental and cognitive changes), and other serious side effects.

Butorphanol Nasal Spray (Stadol)

This prescription drug comes as an injection, but the form used for cluster headaches is nasal spray, so that's what I'm going to talk about here. Stadol and its generic forms come as a liquid solution that you spray into your nose. It works pretty fast if it's going to work at all, usually within an hour or two. If you sneeze right after administration, do not take another dose, as this will give you a potential overdose. This drug is an analgesic, and it's not used that much. The side effects really mess people up, making them feel almost like a zombie, drowsy but unable to sleep, with a bad taste in their throat. The only reason I mention the drug at all is because once in a while I hear it helps someone, and my book is all about options. I like to give you options. It may be something that helps you. So look it up, talk to your doctor, and make your own decision as to whether this is right for you. Besides drowsiness (which you can almost expect with this one), other side effects include unusual dreams, gastrointestinal side effects (nausea, vomiting, stomach pain, constipation), flushing, sweating, cold clammy skin, pounding or erratic heartbeats, neuropathies in hands/feet, confusion, uncontrollable shaking, tinnitus, blurred vision, unpleasant taste, dry mouth or difficulty urinating, and sudden emotions, which could be a sense of euphoria, or floating, or hostility, or sadness. As with any nasal spray, you could experience irritation in the nostrils, nasal congestion, or nosebleed.

Dosage: Usually 1 spray in 1 nostril only delivers 1mg of medication based upon the concentrations of the drug currently on the market. If you experience no pain relief within 60 - 90 minutes, an additional 1mg dose (1 spray) may be given. Sometimes, depending on the severity of the pain, your doctor may suggest an initial dose of 2mg (which means 1 spray in each nostril). The initial dose sequence outlined above may be repeated in 3 - 4 hours as required after the second dose of the sequence.

Depending on the severity of the pain, doctors may suggest an initial dose of 2mg (1 spray in each nostril) for patients who will be able to remain lying down in the event drowsiness or dizziness occurs. In such individuals single additional 2mg doses should not be given for another 3-4 hours.

Caution: This nasal spray can be habit forming. If you use the spray routinely, it becomes problematic when you want to stop. You should not suddenly stop this drug, as you may experience withdrawal symptoms, such as agitation, chills, sweats, confusion, hallucinations, the shakes, and diarrhea. It's better to wean yourself off the drug gradually, not suddenly stop. Also, if you have an allergy to preservatives, this one contains benzethonium chloride. It's not normally a problem for most folks; however, I'm aware that people with headaches have sensitivities to many different things.

Intranasal Lidocaine Solution

I really like this prescription option, especially for women, because statistics show women respond to it well. Men may benefit too, but men have other options they respond to, such as injectable triptans (which don't appear to work so well for women).

Lidocaine is a popular anesthetic that comes in all sorts of forms, including cream, patch, and viscous liquid. For cluster headaches, I recommend the intranasal form, which requires a prescription and is made by a compounding pharmacy. I've seen it made in 4% and 5% solutions. We've known about the benefits of this treatment since 1995, so I hope your doctor has mentioned it to you. I'm sharing it here just in case. This is a good option. How good? In a study published in *Cephalalgia* about 14 years ago, intranasal lidocaine was shown to reduce pain after just five minutes, and all nine of nine treated patients were pain free after 35 minutes![34] I think I heard you just say, "Dang!" Back in 1995, thirty men were enrolled in a study and given a solution of 4% lidocaine intranasally during a cluster attack. They got four sprays, and 27% of the men reported moderate relief. Another 27% reported mild relief, and 46% reported no relief. In summary, half the participants found some benefit. (Hey, some is better than none when you're dealing with excruciating clusters). So about half found no relief in this particular study. The best part is that side effects were minimal. Because of the ease of administration and the 50/50 odds, I say give this one a try.[28]

When All Else Fails

Boy, do I ever dislike including an option like this, but my book is about options. For chronic cluster headache sufferers who do not respond well to medications or treatments, surgery may be an option. The procedure may involve damaging (deadening) the trigeminal nerve with radiofrequency, which blocks the pathway that transmits the pain. My problem with this option is that cluster headaches may be due to an infection or a nutrient deficiency, so this option doesn't always work. Not to mention it's invasive! Promise that you'll only go this route when you've tried everything else in my book, and read every chapter,

Be Careful With Yourself

I know you're in pain but before you take anything at all, including herbal remedies, you must ask your prescribing clinician to make sure there won't be any interactions. For example, if you are taking a prescription SSRI (selective serotonin reuptake inhibitor for depression or fibromyalgia, you should not be taking other drugs that raise serotonin, like triptans or St. John's Wort or MAO inhibitors.

And know that I am not in any way "prescribing" anything for you or providing medical advice. I trust you are going to ask your doctor about what is right for you. This goes for all my "Scripts" in every chapter. OK? OK then.

because you may find a clinical pearl that solves your brain pain without surgery. There's something else on the horizon. In April 7, 2013, a scientific paper was published in the *Journal of Oral and Maxillofacial Surgery* that describes a minimally-invasive procedure that brings permanent relief to people with cluster headaches.[12] Before you get too excited, this procedure, which entails cauterizing the maxillary artery (the side of your face) was only done on five patients. In 4 out 5 patients, the "cluster attacks ceased immediately following surgery." Wow, that is amazing. I'm super excited about this procedure being performed on a larger group of patients. I can't recommend it just yet, not until it's studied further.

Anticonvulsant Medications

> *Examples: Valproic acid*
> *Divalproex (Depakene, Depokote)*
> *Topiramate (Topamax)*
> *Gabapentin (Neurontin)*

These medications help calm down the firing of neurons in the brain, which may help prevent the clusters from occurring. These drugs work by increasing GABA, a naturally occurring brain chemical that slows things down and helps you relax and sleep.[14] The dosage varies. That's why I have not listed it here. If you take any of these drugs, you'll start with a low dose, increase the amount gradually, and then stop increasing the dosage when you reach optimal function. That amount differs for everyone. These drugs do not raise or affect levels of the hormone melatonin.

Caution: Side effects are more common with valproic acid (older one) as compared to gabapentin. With continued use, the side effects tend to lessen. Side effects of valproic acid vary, but may include tinnitus, nausea, vomiting, visual disturbances (blurred, double, eye pain, poorer eyesight), drowsiness, odd movements, higher risk of PCOS (polycystic ovary syndrome), and liver damage.

Side effects of topiramate (Topamax) vary, but may include visual disturbances, neuropathy (burning, prickly tingling, or numb sensations), clumsiness, confusion, dizziness, drowsiness, unusual eye movements (this is not common), memory problems, nervousness, and menstrual changes. Side effects of gabapentin (Neurontin) vary, but may include visual disturbances, loss of coordination, dizziness or drowsiness, tremor, unusual eye movements, and liver problems. A small number of people may experienced changes in thoughts, such as more depression or ideas about suicide. If you notice this while on an anticonvulsant drug, please call your doctor to find a different type of medicine. It's not common, but like I said, if you start to think about harming yourself, get on a different type of medication. There are plenty to choose from.

Calcium Channel Blockers

Examples: Amlodipine (Norvasc)
Verapamil (Calan, Verelan, Covera)
Nifedipine (Procardia)
Nicardipine (Cardene)

These medications are generally used to reduce blood pressure and help with certain heart rhythm problems. For some people, they work very well to prevent cluster headaches during the actual cluster cycle, but they can also be used daily to prevent clusters. Constipation, fatigue, and swollen ankles are rather common with this type of medicine and so is orthostatic hypotension (low blood pressure upon standing). Verapamil is one of the first line agents used in cluster headaches, so I want to focus on this drug. In one double-blind, randomized clinical trial[32] researchers gave verapamil to 15 people. Twelve of the 15 experienced improvement — a reduction in the frequency of attacks — within just two weeks. In another double-blind study, published in *Headache*, researchers compared verapamil to another drug (lithium) and half of those tested noted improvement during the first week of treatment. So of the calcium channel blockers, you have my blessings to try verapamil first.[33] The dosage is usually between 120 to 160mg taken three times daily by mouth.

Ergotamine

Examples: Ergotamine (Ergomar)
Caffeine/Ergotamine (Cafergot, Wigraine)
Dihydroergotamine or DHE 45 injections

This medication is sometimes used for people with migraines. You can buy some brands like Ergot as a sublingual (under the tongue) tablet or rectal suppository. This drug squeezes off blood vessels that would otherwise swell and cause a headache from the increased blood flow.

You should never combine this drug with a triptan, which is another drug used for migraines. The combination is dangerous. Ergotamines can also be dangerous for the heart, so approach with caution and only with your physician's approval.

The Jury Is Out on Nitric Oxide

Many people, especially men, take supplements containing the amino acid arginine. These supplements work by increasing levels of nitric oxide or "NO" a substance which opens up blood flow to the brain and other parts of the body (ahem). Men take these sex-boosting supplements for erectile dysfunction, but the same types of ingredients show up in supplements for cardiac health. If you take a supplement containing arginine, your headache status may improve. That's because low nitric oxide can trigger headaches. But there's a point where it could be come too much for you, and your levels of nitric oxide rise to such a point that you get backlash. I went straight to the expert on NO, my good friend Nathan Bryan, Ph D a scientist and researcher of nitric oxide. Dr. Bryan said, "The jury is still out, regarding the role of NO in migraines. Most migraines are caused by cerebral vasospasms due to an imbalance in vasoactive substances (it's the imbalance between vasoconstrictors vs vasodilators). If you restore the balance, then the migraine will subside and even prevent recurrence. The only condition in which inhibition of NOS was thought to be effective is in sepsis but all trials using NOS inhibitors in sepsis have led to higher mortality than placebo. Incidentally, we have many chronic migraines sufferers who take nitric oxide-producing supplements and see significantly fewer occurrences of migraines or less severe bouts." To learn more about Dr. Bryan's formulas visit his site, www.neogenesis.com.

So an arginine supplement may, or may not trigger more headaches. Like Dr. Bryan said, the jury is still out. Have you noticed more frequent headaches while on an arginine supplement? That is the real question for you. Gauge usage of your supplement based upon the answer to that.

What About Misdiagnosed Cluster Headaches?

I have a different perspective on illness than many health care practitioners. Truth be told, I'm not the most trusting sort when I see people quickly labeled with a diagnosis and treatment, only to watch the treatment fail.

Could Brushing Your Teeth Contribute to Headaches?

Your pineal gland which is deep inside your brain gets damaged by fluoride.[27] Over time, this damage interferes with your ability to make melatonin. I always recommend switching to a fluoride-free toothpaste if you have cluster headaches, migraines or insomnia.

If you have the disorder you were diagnosed with, and that's a great big "if," then you should respond to the treatment for that disorder. Time and time again I hear of people being misdiagnosed. I've seen this happen in my own family. Take my mom, who was told she had diabetes. I found out that what she actually had was a simple case of hyperglycemia (high blood sugar levels), induced by her statin cholesterol medicine. When she went off that drug, and took a few herbs mentioned in my *Diabetes Without Drugs* book, her "diabetes" disappeared.

A friend of mine was told she had rheumatoid arthritis, but failed to respond to her medicine. As it turned out, I asked her to investigate the possibility of Bartonella infection. She tested herself for this. Her test

Chiropractor to the Rescue

I love one of these guys (my husband Sam) so I'm all about chiropractic. For me though, chiropractic treatment has to be gentle, as in the "Activator" method. I don't like the sudden jerky movements. I asked the good "Dr. Cohen" if I should just recommend the Activator method since it's gentle, and that was his primary method of treatment, and he said, *"No, there are a many adjustment methods and they all have merit, depending on the specific problem in the spine. When it comes to headaches, I've seen people get better from a variety of different techniques and you can't argue with success. So if someone has a preference about their adjustment technique, and it works for them keep it up for a few weeks. Be picky about your doctor because, if it's going to work at all, you should start to see results within a few weeks. If they want you to come several times a week for months on end, and you're not getting positive results, I'd question that."*

Chiropractors can make minor adjustments, giving you a big payoff. There are as many techniques as there are nuances of headache pain.

was negative, but that's only because labs can only test for 2 strains of Bartonella, and there are dozens more. Regardless, her doctor prescribed antibiotics (Rifampin and minocycline) to target a possible infection. She recovered over a period of 6 months, after years of suffering. These drugs are not for everyone, but they did work for my friend.

So I pose the question to you: Do you really have cluster headaches? If your symptoms are unresponsive to the classic medications used to treat this condition, and you've gone off dairy and gluten and you still suffer, maybe you too have an infection. You might want to consider this possibility if you've had other symptoms besides headaches. Such symptoms include other neuropathies or joint pain, fatigue, or assorted symptoms that come and go from day to day. That is the hallmark for infection. It feels almost as if bugs are crawling inside of you, annoying one organ after another. (Well, and they are!)

Brain Pain and Lyme Disease

Lyme disease, usually contracted from a tick bite that you don't even feel, causes symptoms that include tremendous headaches that can move around your head and face, even behind your eye, making your eyeball hurt! The Lyme spirochetes are more active in the spring and the fall, and they love to infect the brain and the eyes. Look what else they cause when they are active:

Heat sensations like hot water is pouring on you
Burning scalp sensation
Eye and eyeball pain
Difficulty concentrating
Buzzing, ringing, ear pain, sound sensitivity
Blurry vision, visual snow, floaters, light sensitivity
Painful headaches similar to clusters
Vertigo
Neuropathy in the head, face or extremities

See yourself in that? If you do, then you may have been misdiagnosed with cluster headaches, and you'll probably not respond well to any of the treatments in this section because you need antibiotics instead. The infecting organism of Lyme is *Borrelia burgdorferi* and there are co-infections too; Lyme doesn't travel alone. When the pathogens get into your brain, it causes neuroborreliosis, dubbed "neurolyme" and the horrible headaches and brain fog begin.

The discussion of Lyme disease is in Chapter 6, and testing is in Appendix I. The big deal is this, *you probably never even saw a tick*, or felt it bite you. So don't be too quick to rule out this infectious disease. It's a myth that you will always feel it, or get the characteristic rash from a tick bite. Ticks are tiny, silent creatures, causing one to be miserable and sick and misdiagnosed with a fibromyalgia, chronic fatigue syndrome or some kind of autoimmune disorder almost every single time. They cause many years of suffering, many years before the infection is detected. I'm giving you a head start here. Many people get Lyme from a pet, or from a walk in the park, or a picnic.

Put Down the Phone!

There are forces that we cannot see, but they affect our brain. EMFs, or electromagnetic forces around us, are an invisible field produced by electrically charged objects. EMFs can break down the blood-brain barrier, a microscopically thin sheath that wraps and protects your brain from toxins in your blood stream.

I recommend that you turn off your cell phone at night if you keep in on your bedside table, and reduce EMFs as best you can during the day. There are entire websites and books on the subject of EMFs. Some experts feel that invisible EMFs are the scourge of our time, and the cause for most, if not all disease. So please, learn more about this important topic on your own. And do your best to sleep as far away as possible from EMF radiation. Attached as you are to your cell phone, it does have EMF radiation. I wouldn't talk on it for very long, or sleep with it turned on, resting on your nightstand, because it's next to your head all night long! Turn off your phone, give your brain a mini vacation.

Think Outside the Doc Box

Try a cup of gold. California poppy is a stunning orange flower that blankets the hillsides of California every spring. Someone figured out that compounds it contains can relieve pain. Botanists know this beauty as *Eschscholzia californica,* and it goes by other names, including "a cup of gold" or "California Sunlight" or "Golden Poppy." It's a natural pain reliever, and that's why I've included it in my book.

California poppy is frequently used for insomnia, nervousness, agitation, liver problems, and bed-wetting in children. I think this is tremendously helpful for people with anxiety, especially when taken with magnesium at bedtime. Of course, no matter how wonderful I think something is, you need to ask your own physician whether it's right for you. I can't possibly know what's right for you. I'm just giving you options to discuss with your own doc, shining a beacon of hope to help you end the nightmare of clusters and the sleep dread and anxiety that go with it!

Poppy is a calming herb. It slows down your CNS (central nervous system). That is the point of it. However, that means you should be very careful combining it with anything else that causes CNS depression, including benzodiazepine drugs, such as Valium, Xanax, Ativan, alcohol, pain-killers, Benadryl, and headache drugs. I do not think that poppy is going to stop the headaches entirely, though I hope I'm wrong. I'm recommending it here because you won't hear about poppy from your doctor, and I think it is a great natural sedative and nervous system relaxer. Many people with chronic headaches are afraid of getting addicted to pain meds like Oxycontin, MS Contin, Hydrocodone, Oxycodone, and others. Before

Tea for Pain Relief

The herb passionflower (passiflora) has nothing to do with passionate sex like you might think. Ok, fine, maybe it was just me that thought that. Anyhow, it is known to help with headaches, and it calms the nerves and reduces the anxiety and restlessness often associated with cluster headaches. Studies support passiflora's role in generalized anxiety disorder, insomnia and depression.[26, 41,42,43]

This herb helps with panic attacks and narcotic withdrawal. You can buy prepared passionflower tea at any health food store. All by itself, it is relaxing, but if you can add lemonbalm, lavender or chamomile it would be fantastic. The ratio I would use is like this:

1/2 cup dried passionflower
1/4 cup dried lemonbalm
2 tsps. dried lavender (it's strong)
1/2 cup dried chamomile

Put this all in a glass jar and shake well. When you're ready to make tea, add 1 tablespoon of the mixed herbs to 1 cup of hot water and let it steep (not boil) for about 2 to 5 minutes. Sweeten if desired with Manuka honey or coconut nectar.

starting those, try California poppy. This herb may be just the ticket to mitigate pain, reduce anxiety, and help you sleep through the night. When you are shopping for California poppy at your natural health food store, or online, you will see liquid herbal extracts. You can try those. Just look for a brand that is alcohol-free because alcohol is sometimes a trigger for clusters. I'd love it if you can find one grown organically too. If you'd like a gentler option, you can brew some tea at home. I found both an organic (alcohol-free) liquid extract and the dried herb to make tea on Amazon from a company called Hawaii Pharm.

Have a Baby?

Women report their headaches dramatically improve when pregnant. Gives new meaning to that "bundle of joy." Yes, yes! And let me count all the ways!

Drug Muggers that Deplete Melatonin

Some medications rob your body of melatonin, and this could affect your headache status. Remember, melatonin deficiency is sometimes implicated in cluster headaches. Even though melatonin supplements are sold over-the-counter, I want you to ask your doctor about the right dose for you. The following medications are known to deplete melatonin, so if you take any of these, it's particularly important to add a melatonin supplement at nighttime:

Alcohol

Nicotine

Sleep medications like Lunesta, Ambien, Sonata

Benzodiazepines like temazepam, diazepam, lorazepam

SSRI antidepressant drugs (fluoxetine, sertraline, etc)

Octeotride (Sandostatin)

Any drug that mugs vitamin B1, B6, niacin, calcium or magnesium (all needed to make melatonin)

That last one, "any drug that mugs vitamin B1, B6, niacin, calcium or magnesium" is a big category. Listing all those drugs would entail about 50 more pages to this book, so please refer to my other book, Drug Muggers, available on Amazon. If you're taking a drug mugger of any of those vitamins or minerals, you're goal should be to replenish those nutrients. In fact, it wouldn't hurt for you to take a multivitamin that contains these nutrients if you take any medication at all. It helps fill a nutritional gap. If you do this, make it high-quality version.

Know the Difference

There's a condition that mimics cluster headaches called "orbital myositis," a painful inflammation of the muscles that control the eyes. There are several differences, the primary difference is that orbital myositis has a shorter duration as compared to clusters.

Weirdest Pain Relief Yet!

Psilocybin, the active ingredient in "magic mushrooms" is getting attention in the cluster community. Some benefit has been seen in case studies but before you get the thumbs up from me, I want to see more research. Back in 2006, scientists interviewed people who experience cluster headaches[36] who were taking psilocybin or LSD. Of the 26 people who took psilocybin (magic mushroom) during an attack, 22 of them (85%) found it aborted the attack. The LSD worked too! In that group, 7 of 8 users (88%) reported termination of at least one cluster attack. Here are more details directly from the article published[36] in the journal *Neurology: "Twenty-two of 26 psilocybin users reported that psilocybin aborted attacks; 25 of 48 psilocybin users and 7 of 8 LSD users reported cluster period termination; 18 of 19 psilocybin users and 4 of 5 LSD users reported remission period extension."*

Cannabis & Clusters

Marijuana increases melatonin. If you have cluster headaches, that's helpful. The downside, other than the obvious, is that marijuana may cause gynecomastia in men (swollen breasts) and psychoactive effects. Unless you can get pure or high CBD which have reduced psychoactive effects then you really have to think about it. The THC causes all the psychoactive effects. This herb is decriminalized in many states nowadays. Medical marijuana (cannabis) is available in many forms today, including lozenge, capsules, edibles, and the well-known "joint" form, but your doctor has to prescribe it.

Taken together, this means that some folks who get cluster headaches have found a way to help themselves using natural plant extracts, albeit illicit ones! I'm not recommending this treatment to you, but I've included it here since I think it's the weirdest pain relief yet! How can mind-bending drugs have such a beneficial impact on this pain syndrome?

Fresh News: Headaches and BDNF

You make a protein called "neurotrophin" in your brain that helps you grow new brain cells or "neurons" from stem cells during a process termed "neurogenesis." So the protein, neurotrophin, stimulates and offers the 'call to action' for stem cells to morph into brain cells. We want that! And scientists have told us for years that after birth, we can't grow neurons anymore. Feh! You want neurotrophin protein hanging around, especially as you get older, because it helps you remember things and keeps your mind working well.

So what's the name of the specific fabulous protein responsible for this? It's called "Brain-Derived Neurotropic Factor" or BDNF for short. You may be reading about it for the first time here, and that's okay, I am often ahead of the game.

Scientists bring up BDNF in lectures while talking about "neuronal plasticity." That is how our brain interacts with the environment, how we think, how well we remember, how intense we feel pain and much more. We know that BDNF is a critical factor for healthy neurons, and we're finding out now that BDNF plays an essential role in controlling pain signaling.

Since I'm here to help you stop the brain pain, that fact (BDNF is involved in pain signaling) caught my attention. You know the old saying, "too much of a good thing. . . ." I did some research, and guess what? Levels of BDNF are *significantly increased* during migraine and cluster headache attacks! This is some seriously cutting edge stuff. Under normal circumstances I'd want lots of BDNF in your brain, even if you have headaches yet this research implies it's bad.

As I've explained, BDNF are proteins made in the brain and central nervous system that support the endurance of existing neurons and encourage their growth.

Based upon the results of a clinical trial published in August 2012, in *Journal Headache Pain*,[37] it's safe to say that BDNF goes up both in people who get clusters, as well as in those who get migraines. Dr. M. Fischer and his team of researchers enrolled 106 people into three groups, based upon whether they had migraines, clusters, or tension headaches. There was also a placebo group. In both the migraine and cluster headache groups, blood samples were taken during the actual headache episode, and again after the headaches. One blood sample was taken from the participants in the tension headache and placebo groups. None of the participants reported taking any pain medications, including non-steroidal anti-inflammatory drugs (NSAIDS), triptans, or opiates in the 48-hour period prior to the blood sample collection.

After the data was collected and analyzed, researchers concluded that BDNF was substantially elevated in individuals with migraine and cluster headaches during the attacks, compared to tension headache sufferers and those in control groups.

Interestingly, the BDNF decreased in concentrations after the headaches subsided, so it's going up during the attacks and then coming down, but only in the migraine sufferers, not in those with clusters. With clusters, the BDNF is high during and after the attacks.

This suggests that excess BDNF causes an inflammatory cascade in the brain that is somehow tied to migraine and cluster headaches. The scientists are saying that BDNF expression is increased, but it begs the question. Is it increased because of the attack, as in some effort to rescue you? After all, BDNF is neuroprotective under normal circumstances. That is what I think, and I'm just thinking out loud with you, but I suspect the increase in BDNF is meant to be your body's attempt at controlling inflammation and protecting or repairing your neurons during the headache. BDNF is reduced in people with depression, BDNF is in and of itself an 'antidepressant.' Cortisol (as in stress) lowers BDNF, and here's a fun fact (though I'm not advocating you take any of these drugs), Prozac, Zoloft and Risperdal happen to raise BDNF to some extent, accounting for the mood lifting benefits of these drugs.

The other side of the BDNF story could sound like this: Somehow BDNF goes rogue, like other cytokines do in excess, and its raging levels go out of control to actually trigger an attack. It's just too preliminary to tell.

What we do know is that exercise increases BDNF and exercise as well as overexertion are triggers for some of you. It's just fascinating to me that we normally seek to raise BDNF, because it helps us think better and remember more things yet it is implicated in headaches. Avoiding high sugar is imperative because a high-sugar diet is the fastest way to lose your precious BDNF. But as it pertains to brain pain, I'm saying the very things we use to raise BDNF could backfire on headache sufferers.

So what's the bottom-line here? We are not sure if BDNF goes up and triggers the headache, or if it's there to try and rescue your neurons. Here's my advice based on what we know today:

Watch your response to exercise. If you note a headache on the days you exercise, back off and do something less strenuous.

Reconsider Alpha Lipoic Acid. This supplement raises BDNF, so if you recently started taking it for neuropathy, and now you have more headaches, then stop it.[38]

Reconsider resveratrol. This supplement raises BDNF. So if you're taking it, try going off it and see if your headaches subside. On that note, avoid red wine (a known trigger for migraines) because it contains some resveratrol.[39]

Reconsider vitamin D. This nutrient, especially when combined with progesterone hormone, is known to raise BDNF. This may explain why some migraineurs do poorly after taking vitamin D for a few months.

Another study published in March 2013, in *Frontiers of Neurology* took a closer look at all of this. Working off the fact that we have a growing body of evidence implicating BDNF and other cytokines tied to migraines, they set out to compare the levels of TNFα and BDNF in people with episodic migraine headaches.

Drs. D. Pinchuk and O. Pinchuk and 2 other scientists examined the blood samples of 9 patients during a migraine attack, and during a headache-free period. As it turns out, this study concluded the very same thing that the first study on BDNF did. That is, BDNF serum levels goes up significantly during the migraine attack, and drop back to normal in the pain-free period. The scientists stated, *"This is the first report showing that BDNF serum levels increase during migraine attack. This reinforces the view that BDNF may be implicated in the physiopathology of migraine."* As for TNFα there was no significant difference in serum levels during this particular study.

Your Plan of Action: A dozen Ways to Minimize the Pain

If you feel a cluster attack coming on, try any of the tips below. Naturally, you'll want to make sure all of this is alright with your practitioner(s):

1. Breathe pure oxygen. Medical grade oxygen is the best cluster

buster I know of. You want oxygen flowing at approximately 8 to 10 LPM (liters per minute) via mask or cannula. Continue this treatment for up to 15 minutes.

2. Spray away pain. Spray it away. Use intranasal lidocaine, which requires a prescription.

3. Take one dose of your lithium. Lithium, you want either the prescription version (which is dosed at 600 to 900mg total per day, given in divided doses), or a fraction of that dose, taken in the form of natural lithium orotate, sold at health food stores. That is usually 5 to 10mg at bedtime. Lithium is something you stay on with your doctor's supervision and routine blood testing. It is not a rescue remedy because it does not work fast. It requires physician supervision, even the over-the-counter form because if you get too much, it can cause heart palpitations. Drink plenty of water, you never want to become dehydrated on lithium.

4. Go for cold! Choose either a cold compress or an ice pack if that is soothing. Put it right where it hurts.

5. Apply heat. Take a washcloth and dampen it with water, then microwave for 15 to 30 seconds. It will be very hot. Cool it to your comfort level and apply to your head where it hurts. You can also use a heat pack with calming lavender chamomile beads inside!

6. Try both hot and cold. Alternate ice packs with a heading pad. Do each for one minute. Keep going back and forth between the two.

7. Sleep. Take a high-quality melatonin supplement before bedtime.

8. Triptans anyone? I'm not in love with this option but every now and then I hear someone finds it effective so it's an option. Zomig nasal spray (only at onset, it doesn't help much if you've peaked). Read Chapter 2 "Migraine Headaches" for some cautions and contraindications.

9. Breathe better while you sleep. Talk to your doctor about a CPAP mask, a device that delivers oxygen to individuals with sleep apnea.

10. Take supplements. Taurine supplements, and GABA may reduce levels of glutamate, an excitotoxin that causes

headaches. So will theanine, found in green tea (which has a small amount of caffeine). Theanine is also sold as a supplement.

11. Relax with scent. Put lavender essential oil in an aromatherapy diffuser and let it fill the room with relaxing fragrance at night.
12. Kill Germs. Take about 5 to 30 drops nightly for a minimum of 3 months. This is a broad-spectrum antimicrobial which kills a lot of different pathogens. If there's an infection causing brain inflammation and triggering your headaches this could solve the problem, gently, naturally.

It's all natural and available at www.nutramedix.com. Some people wonder if a herpes related virus could be driving the headaches. In this case I recommend the prescription drug Valcyte taken twice daily for a week; if it's going to work for you, you'll notice effects within a week or perhaps two at the most. It should not be a forever drug, you take it and then you're done taking it until the next cycle (if it ever comes back). This helped two of my friends get well, however, there isn't hard data to prove it; talk to your doctor to see if Valcyte is right for you.

Chapter 5

Trigeminal Neuralgia

Can you imagine feeling as if someone plugged your face into a socket? That's what trigeminal neuralgia, often abbreviated to "TN" feels like. It is one of the hardest syndromes to diagnose and treat.[15] That's why I included this chapter, I'm all about options. Hopefully, you will find the answer to your prayers within these pages. I want you to stop living in fear of your next attack, stop hoarding pain medications (and thinking about taking a handful!). Please.

If searching on the web, or in medical books you will also see the term "tic douloureux" as well as hemifacial cranial pain, and atypical facial pain or AFP. AFP is like having TN but it goes on almost all the time, it's not episodic like TN which comes in waves and sudden outbursts. There are no rest periods with AFP, it is constant and unrelenting. It's much worse to have AFP as compared to TN because the shocks and stabbing pain are constant. When you think of AFP think head banging, screaming, rocking, cursing, crying, making deals with God, deep depression, suicidal thoughts . . . that's the kind of pain I'm talking about. It's cruel.

TN is more common than AFP. TN and AFP are commonly referred to as the "suicide disease" which just saddens me to the core. I've seen it first hand, because my wonderful husband, Sam, dealt with AFP for over 1 year!

Sam is cured, he gets one 'facial pain' attack per year, at best, and it's because he did heavy lifting, or sneezed a lot for a day or two. It goes away completely now. It's an absolute miracle, he has no facial pain. I'll help you too, it doesn't matter how long you've had it, I can help. If you have a loved one that is complaining about TN, take them seriously. Just because you don't see their pain doesn't mean they don't have it. Right now they need your support and care, not judgment. I never for a minute doubted Sam's pain, and I don't want you to discount it for someone you love either.

Statistics vary, but there are about an additional 150 people per million who suffer with this condition annually. Some estimate that there are anywhere from 10,000 to 25,000 new cases every year. I think it's higher, though, because it is frequently misdiagnosed as something else. According to *The Dana Foundation,* 60 % of people with the disorder are women, and if your parents or grandparents were prone to TN, you may develop it at an earlier age.[16]

Signs & Symptoms of Trigeminal Neuralgia

Shocks like electrical sensations in the face or head

Pain may radiate into head, jaw or teeth

Drowsiness or dizziness

Depression, secondary to chronic pain and fear

Made worse by chewing, touching or exposure to cold

Recurrent pain every few seconds or hours

Anatomy of Trigeminal Neuralgia Pain

Trigeminal neuralgia or TN causes lightning bolt shocks of pain in the head that just come out of nowhere, often starting near the ear and moving around your head, teeth, jaw and eyes. The pain is usually one-sided but it can be bilateral too, or it can start out on one side and then spread to other areas in your jaw, teeth, eye region and head. Many patients develop the pain in one area of their head, then over the years the pain travels through other areas. This is happening because different branches of the nerve become involved.

TN is a facial pain disorder but I've read that some people get shocks down into their fingers. Those shocks can't be coming from the trigeminal nerve (as that only wraps around your head) so it supports my theory that TN is a systemic (whole body) disorder, related to some bigger disease or problem that damages the trigeminal nerve. Maybe it's an undiagnosed food sensitivity that is attacking your nerves, a virus or bacteria causing infection. Even nutritional deficiencies cause you to lose the protective myelin sheath.

There is a reason or reasons that TN happens to people and if you can figure out what is driving it, you can fix it or minimize it. I don't know why some neurologists call it an "idiopathic" syndrome. According to Merriam-Webster dictionary,[32] idiopathic means *"arising spontaneously or from an obscure or unknown cause."* If the the cause is "unknown" how are you supposed to get proper treatment? I don't buy it! Don't accept the "idiopathic" diagnosis, stop at the first 4 letters "idio." Trust me, whether it has been uncovered today or not, there IS and HAS TO BE some underlying pathology (a "path" that causes disease or illness) for your pain.

Pain doesn't just happen randomly, something triggers it. Perhaps your trigeminal nerve is getting squeezed or compressed by a nearby artery or from inflammation or ischemia (sometimes the result of vasculitis). Or it may be from an infection, as there are organisms known to attack the trigeminal nerve. It's kind of like saying to you, there's no known cause for your illness, you're stuck with this. Garbage! Sam was told this also, and nothing was further from the truth.

Kim's Story

Kim came to my pharmacy one night and confided in me she had "idiopathic" trigeminal neuralgia and since there was no cause for the condition (and her surgery didn't work), that she would need morphine the rest of her life. She was surprised I even knew what that meant, so she kept talking. She already wrote her suicide note and had it hidden in a drawer for when she was ready. She was my customer at the local pharmacy I worked. (She had no idea that I was dealing with this very same issue at home). There are no accidents.

I told her to do some blood tests, specifically a test to evaluate B12. As it turned out, she had a severe vitamin B12 deficiency. I also suggested she eliminate all gluten from her diet. Then I suggested she try rubbing capsaicin cream on her face in between the TN attacks since she had hours of relief in between. And I recommended some massage therapy, once a week just to get away for an hour and decompress. She did everything. She corrected the B12 deficiency with injectable methylcobalamin (not cyanocabalamin) about 500 mcg every week and after a few months she came back to tell me (all teary eyed) that she felt 80% better and was taking half her medication dose, and no more pain pills! She couldn't believe how many thousands of dollars she'd spent on doctors, surgery, 4 different MRI scans, missed work and opportunities to be with her children.

Herpes types of germs like one called Human herpesvirus 6 or

HHV-6 as well as Lyme organisma (Borrelia burgdorferi and coinfections) are known to invade your central nervous system, take up residence there forever and essentially try to destroy your cranial nerves.[12] Lyme organisms always deplete thiamine (vitamin B1) which plays a protective role with your nerves. Neuroborreliosis (Lyme disease) can cause symptoms of trigeminal neuralgia.[38] One of its hallmarks is intense, lancinating, radiating pain, especially at night (caused by the Lyme spirochete)! I know right? Shocker. As it turned out, my husband had undiagnosed Lyme disease, and it was one of the Lyme germs that attacked him, and caused horrendous facial pain 24/7.

When I learned that I almost fell out of my chair. How many of you have been bit by a tick, possibly one toted into the house by your pet cat or dog. Physicians can medicate you all they want, but if the underlying infection is not treated, your progress is very slow. More about infections in Chapter 6, "Lyme Headaches."

You Have Some Nerve! In Fact, You Have 12...

You have 12 different nerves that come out of your brain and help you to enjoy life. They are named by roman numerals, as in the following:

Cranial nerve I	Olfactory nerve	Smell
Cranial nerve II	Optic nerve	So you can see
Cranial nerve III	Oculomotor nerve	Eye movement, pupil constriction
Cranial nerve IV	Trochlear nerve	Eye movement
Cranial nerve V	Trigeminal nerve	Somatosensory information & chewing
Cranial nerve VI	Abducens	Helps you roll your eyes
Cranial nerve VII	Facial	Make facial expressions
Cranial nerve VIII	Acoustic	Helps you hear and balance yourself
Cranial nerve IX	Glossopharyngeal	Helps you taste and move your tongue
Cranial nerve X	Vagus	Speak; this nerve wanders all over the body
Cranial XI	Accessory	Helps you move and shrug shoulders
Cranial XII	Hypoglossal	Helps you speak and swallow

More About Your Nerves

You have two two trigeminal nerves, one on each side of your face. These trigeminal nerves sit above your ear. Since the trigeminal nerve is cranial nerve number five (Roman numeral V) you will often see it in the literature. Each nerve has three branches on each side of the head. For that reason you will sometimes see V1, V2 and V3 in the literature. These branches (when affected) are what cause the spreading of the pain to other areas of your head. V1 goes to your forehead, eye and sinus area, V2 goes to your cheek, and V3 around your jaw.

Cytokines: Love 'Em or Hate 'Em

Pain is driven by pro-inflammatory cytokines (which are pain-causing chemicals) that your cells make in response to injury or infection. Those cytokines are 'spit out' by your immune system as the result of activation of NFκB, a metabolic pathway that, when 'angered' starts pumping out nasty chemicals. The resulting ouch is all you ever see or feel.

Shutting down NFκB for a bit will reduce the level of cytokines and that helps to reduce pain so I always have this in mind when I research the best ways to get you more comfortable. And in fact, I found studies showing that certain cytokines are elevated in people with TN. For example, recent studies have "shown that cytokines IL-1β, IL-6 and TNFα play a very important role in the origin and development or "pathogenesis" of the immune response within the trigeminal nerves.[17] One demonstrated that some pro-inflammatory cytokines (IL-1β and TNFα) are capable of sensitizing nociceptive neurons (the ones that allow you to experience pain). When produced in excess, these cytokines give you a heightened

> **Triggers for Trigeminal Neuralgia**
>
> Touching your face
> Dental work
> Chewing
> Kissing
> Hugging (if your face hits another)
> Talking
> Brushing teeth
> Brushing or combing hair
> Cold breeze
> Shaving your face
> Showering (water hits your face)
> Injury or trauma to head or neck
> Whiplash or Traumatic Brain Injury
> Applying capsaicin at the wrong time

sense of pain. Therefore, you can have an effect on the "inflammatory response," and release of these cytokine by reducing those compounds.

Another study, published in 2012, showed, for the first time that the presence IL-1β can promote an increased sense of pain around the fibrous membranes that surround the central nervous system or the "meninges" that is different from what IL-6 does![18] These pain chemicals travel together, and apparently hurt us in different mechanisms. Not to worry, there are ways to squash them. Curcumin, astaxanthin, resveratrol, fish oil, saffron and green tea are thought to reduce IL-6, so those are all considerations. More in Chapter 12 "Reducing Pain-Causing Cytokines."

Suzy's "Script" for Trigeminal Neuralgia Pain Relief

Before you take any of the following supplements, you must ask your doctor(s) if they are right for you. My intention here is to educate you about possibilities and options. Do not misconstrue my ideas for medical advice. I have no idea what is right for every individual reading this so take my list to your practitioner(s) to ask if they're right for you with your medical history. Dosages are also just basic guidelines, some people tolerate different dosages than what is stated here:

Takuna

Meadowsweet extract

Methylcobalamin

R lipoic acid

Biotin

Jamaican dogwood

How This Helps You Become Headache Free

Cecropia strigosa or "Takuna"

You may not have heard of it but it's a 100% natural herb that has antibiotic, antifungal and strong antiviral properties. Cecropia strigosa is sold by the brand "Takuna" and it does not require prescription. I never see it at retail outlets. You can buy it online, or by phone from the makers.

It comes from a tree found throughout South America. It has powerful antiviral properties. Is it known to cure or even relieve TN pain? No, it's not proven; hardly any studies are done on natural plant-derived antibiotics. My rationale for this herb is to help reduce viral load in your nervous system should this be the underlying cause of your pain. I feel it is worth a try. Think this out with me. We know how devastating the herpes virus can be on the nervous system, in some people it's disabling, think of Shingles or post-herpetic neuralgia.

Those lesions and the terrible nerve pain is caused by a herpes virus called "Varicella" zoster. Those pathogens know precisely how to destroy a nerve and cause terrible nerve pain. They can lay dormant, and attack you at will. The herpes virus called HSV-1 or Herpes Simplex Virus infects the mouth and lips, then the virus hides in the trigeminal ganglia.[12] The cold sores come and go while the virus hides in the trigeminal nerve. Does that sound like TN to you, how the pain comes and goes? With HSV-2, the virus hides in the sacral ganglia and affects the genital regions. Have I convinced you that herpes types of viruses cause tremendous pain in the nervous system. There's already speculation in the medical community about the connection of herpes viruses to trigeminal neuralgia, so I'm not alone. My recommendation to address a herpes virus, just in case it's affecting your trigeminal nerve should make sense to you now, especially when the side effects are slim to none with an herbal antimicrobial that is very gentle and mild on the system.

Nutramedix brand uses a proprietary extraction process that makes this extremely effective. Follow the label for dosing instructions. If it says 30 drops per day, then titrate up starting with 5 drops daily, then 5 drops twice daily for a few days, then 10 drops in the morning, 5 at night, and so forth.

Since Takuna is particularly good at lowering viral load it can be used for any herpes related virus. It's not as strong as Acyclovir, the drug or Valcyte another drug, but it is an option you can try yourself at home (if you buy it online, do get your doctor's blessings). Anti-viral drugs and herbs would be helpful for mild cases of viral hepatitis (sexually transmitted), herpes zoster (Shingles), EBV (Epstein Barr virus), CMV (Cytomegalovirus) and mild symptoms of viral encephalitis/meningitis. Naturally, do not delay seeking medical attention if you have serious infections, this is considered a remedy to do in addition to what a physician tells you to do (known as "adjunctive" remedies).

Meadowsweet

Known botanically as "Filipendula ulmaria" and dubbed "Queen of Pride of the Meadow." My opinion is that this herb is terrific for pain syndromes, such as trigeminal neuralgia and even rheumatoid arthritis. It suppresses IL-1β which you learned is elevated in TN.[39]

Meadowsweet is a natural pain-killer due to its active ingredient salicylic acid, the principle ingredient in household aspirin. Aspirin was created from meadowsweet in the olden days. Why not just take aspirin? The digestive upset and irritation to your gut lining is a concern for me (and it should be for you too). Meadowsweet is a gentle herb but it has anti-inflammatory compounds, humans have known about it for centuries. The pretty little white and yellow flowers (and leaves) of the fragrant meadowsweet plant are used to make herbal medicines. The flowers smell delightful, and interestingly, the leaves smell a bit like almonds.

Since it has a slight blood-thinning effect like that of aspirin, I'd be careful with this (get permission) if you take blood-thinners or are prone to bleeding. If you have migraines, this may not be right for you because some migraineurs get affected by higher blood flow into the brain, and blood thinners do that. I recommend the liquid herbal extract by Herb Pharm because you can easily gauge your dosage since it's a dropper formula. There are other brands of course, choose what you like.

Methylcobalamin

Methylcobalamin is the more technical name of natural vitamin B12, a water-soluble B vitamin that is commonly associated with energy and mental well-being. B12 is vital for you to make healthy red blood cells, and protect your nervous system. The reason it is in my "script" to help TN sufferers is plain and simple, it helps your body to heal injured myelin, the coating that wraps around your cranial nerve V (trigeminal nerve). Because vitamin B12 plays a role in myelin production, it is crucial for people battling neuropathies, especially TN or any type of facial pain.

While no one has made the definitive discovery of exactly how methycobalamin (Vitamin B12) helps, one study in the journal *Neuroscience* showed that B12 hastened recovery of nerves, specifically within a bicep muscle of a laboratory rat.[19]

But does it affect your body's production of cytokines? Yes, in fact, methylcobalamin, was shown a long time ago (1992) to reduce production of the pro-inflammatory cytokine IFNγ (interferon gamma) by about 50%, isn't that remarkable?![20] If you have trigeminal neuralgia, levels of IFNγ are elevated so B12 comes to the rescue.

One more reason I recommend B12 for you is that animal studies have shown a deficiency of this valuable nutrient will cause an increase in TNFα production, which leads to more pain when it's pumped out in excess. Improving levels of methylcobalamin, or methyl B12 as it is sometimes called, brings down TNFα, thus putting out the fire a little bit.

The most common supplemental form of vitamin B12 is called cyanocobalamin; it's also the most affordable to produce. But the most effective form is methylcobalamin, because that's what the human body recognizes. So if you supplement with B12, please read the label; you want "methylcobalamin" for the optimal effect. I recommend it as a sublingual lozenge or spray (as your stomach may not be able to utilize it well). You can buy all sorts of good brands of sublingual or lozenge methyl B12 at any health food store, and the beauty of that is you get it fast.

Now, if you want to get a superior brand, I'd buy it online from Dr. Ben Lynch's site, www.SeekingHealth.com. Why? Because his product called "Active B12" is exactly that, superior! It contains two of the most active forms of B12 in your body. First one, as you most likely know is methylcobalamin. The other one, adenosylcobalamin, is used by your mitochondria giving you energy. This blend in "Active B12" is good for people with methylation defects (see Chapter 8 "Detoxification Matters") which is common among persons with migraines and painful neuralgias. Did you know that there is a common genetic snp (mutation) which limits the conversion of methylcobalamin to adenosylcobalamin? This is why Dr. Lynch formulated "Active B12" using both forms. Use coupon code "Headache Free" for 15% off purchases at *seekinghealth.com*

Caution: You can also get injections of vitamin B12. The typical solution for intramuscular injection sold by prescription at the pharmacy is "cyanocobalamin" so to get the methylcobalamin that I recommend, your physician (or nurse practitioner) must call it in that way to a compounding pharmacy. If there isn't one local to you, many compounding pharmacies will ship it to you. I don't recommend cyanocobalamin shots (or oral supplements) because it is unnatural.

R-lipoic acid

This antioxidant squashes free radicals that attack your myelin sheath and 'fray' your nerve wiring. You make lipoic acid naturally, in your body, but you can buy supplements. Every cell in your body uses lipoic acid, especially the nerve and brain cells. It's used for energy and neuralgias very commonly. There are two kinds, alpha lipoic acid, and R lipoic acid. These are isomers, similar to how your left hand is to your right hand, mirror images. Lipoic acid protects you from oxidative stress, and soothes your nervous system. It can also dramatically lower your blood sugar. Lipoic acid is able to pass readily into the brain and reach all parts of a nerve cell.

Natural "R lipoic acid" is a little harder to find than "alpha" lipoic acid, which is also okay to use. I'm recommending the R isomer of this antioxidant because it is body-ready, it is active. So try to find the "R" version because it works faster and better, at a lower dose and it's natural. You take half of the "R" version as compared to alpha. In other words, 200mg alpha lipoic acid equals 100mg R lipoic acid. The alpha lipoic acid that you commonly find at health food stores is not dangerous, it's less active, and your body has to spin a couple of antioxidant cartwheels to convert it to an active usable form.

Lipoic acid is a well-known nerve soother. It has been studied for people with multiple sclerosis, which is where the body experiences a demyelination of the nervous system.[33, 34] Lipoic acid is commonly used for diabetic neuropathy so it makes sense to me to include this natural nutrient if you have TN since that is a neuralgia of the face.

Caution: Too much alpha or "R" lipoic acid will deplete you of biotin, so lipoic acid is a 'drug mugger' of biotin, you will need some of that nutrient to compensate. More on biotin right now.

Biotin

Biotin belongs to the B complex family. Generally speaking all the B vitamins are needed to help the nervous system function properly. Biotin is found in many cosmetic-aimed supplements to help with hair and nail growth. Biotin is made from your intestinal bacteria but most people don't have enough of those good bacteria. By taking probiotics, you can naturally cause your body to produce more biotin. Will it be enough to restore what the lipoic acid is taking out of you? Probably not, but I always recommend probiotics since they support our immune system and help reduce pro-inflammatory cytokines. Severe biotin deficiency is unusual unless you have Celiac or Crohn's disease, or irritable bowel syndrome.

Milder deficiencies are very possible though, and if you have it, it will cause cracking in the corners of your mouth, hair loss, scaly skin, a painful, swollen tongue or dry eyes. A biotin deficiency may lower your appetite and cause depression and insomnia. If this sounds like you, biotin supplements may be just what you need. Dosages vary, often 2 - 10,000 mcg per day. As an added benefit of biotin, it could help with hair and nail growth.

Caution: Always put back what medication stole, so if you're taking one or more anticonvulsants, you need biotin. Lipoic acid reduces your body's warehouse of biotin, so this is to restore what lipoic acid takes out. I call lipoic acid a "drug mugger" of biotin, although it's not a "drug" that is just my term for compounds that rob your body of nutrients. See my book, *Drug Muggers* to learn about side effects that result from depletion, which are almost always diagnosed as new diseases.

Jamaican Dogwood (Piscidia erythrina)

Jamaica is best known for picturesque beaches with the sparkling blue waters. But more than the beauty of the little island (and the beautiful people who enjoy reggae music), we have the dogwood tree. Jamaican dogwood (also common in Florida) is part of my "script" for treating facial pain. It's just an option, I'm never sure what will work for you, and what will work for another. In the Carribean, it's common for doctors to use extracts from this plant for anxiety, insomnia, cramps, migraines (possibly cluster headaches) and pain in general.

Piscidia contains many natural compounds (isoflavones, tannins, resins, glycosides and others) that account for its anti-anxiety and pain-relieving properties. Piscidia is a strong antispasmodic too. You can buy it as a liquid herbal extract or as a tea. The tea is gentler (i.e. weaker in action) and it is caffeine-free. If you take a supplement, get one from a very reputable maker so you can be sure they are using the correct parts of the plant. Use the wrong part and it's toxic! I feel comfortable recommending the herbal liquid extracts by Herb Pharm called "Jamaican Dogwood" because it's never fumigated or irradiated; and there's another one made by Gaia Herbs that combines Feverfew with it, called "Feverfew Jamaican Dogwood Supreme." Feverfew is another well-studied herb that reduces incidence of headache.

Caution: As with any herb, an allergic reaction is possible. Only the root bark should be used. If it's not made properly, Jamaica dogwood can be toxic (like any herb). Also don't take too much, an overdose may cause numbness, tremors, salivation, hallucinations and sweating. This stuff works, respect it, use the lowest effective dose. Make sure it's right for you by asking your physician. Pregnant or nursing women should avoid dietary supplements unless your obstetrician orders it. Jamaican dogwood may help with painful menstruation.

Kava Kava (*Piper methysticum*).

This is an incredible herb because it has pain-relieving qualities and it calms the nerves. When it comes to cytokines, the "kavalactones" in kava reduce TNFα.[21] It's remarkably helpful to reduce muscle contractions that your neck and shoulder probably have. I know you 'guard' yourself a little, which is why you may raise your shoulders toward your ear, or hunch over, or hold tightness in traps. I understand. Kava may help. It may boost mood, and help with fungal infections (a benefit that is superb for people with candida, athletes foot, ringworm or tinea). Do not drink this with alcohol, or take while pregnant or nursing. Ask your doctor if it's right for you, there are many interactions.

Get Rid Of . . .

Foods containing MSG
All artificial sweeteners
Gluten, preferably all grains
Cold foods like ice cream
Icy drinks or smoothies
Linens that aren't soft
Toothbrushes that are too big
Nicotine (affects blood vessel contraction)
Electronic pollution
Artificial dyes and colors
Cell phones, limit use, don't sleep with them near your head
Cordless phones- don't talk on them more than 15 minutes
Don't keep your head near clock radios or microwave ovens

Instant Skin Soothers for Facial Pain

Lidoderm patches. These require a prescription and contain lidocaine 5%, which numbs the area. Some people really think these help, reducing pain sensations for a few hours. It really depends on the amount of pain you feel. You can cut them with scissors making one 10 cm X 14 cm patch go a little further than one application. (Cut it in half, make it work for 2 applications).

No Scream Cream. This is a brand of cream that numbs your skin after applying it. It takes about 20 to 30 minutes to take full effect and it works great. I found out about it when I went to the salon who does my waxing and whined like a baby that it hurt too much. Why I don't opt for a razor, I cannot tell you, but my caring cerologist, Krista told me about a secret weapon, "No Scream Cream." Yes! I can attest to that! This brand says "Relax and Wax" on the label also. Nevermind that this is a numbing cream sold without prescription for Brazilian's and bikini waxes (and eyebrows), it just so happens to numb the skin and that is why I'm suggesting it to you. It's not an instant numb, it takes 10 - 30 minutes. It costs about $20 online.

Geranium oil. Those gorgeous blooms of geranium in your garden can bring more relief to a TN sufferer than you thought possible. Essential oil of geranium (not germanium) is helpful for neuralgia. You put about a few drops on your fingertips and gently massage it to your scalp and face (wherever it hurts). You can use a cotton ball too. It's included there because studies show it can help relieve pain from "shingles" (aka herpes zoster virus). You can buy essential oil of geranium at many health food stores, or online.

Neuragen PN. A topical ointment sold at pharmacies and online. Some studies suggest it might be helpful for shingles neuralgia, diabetic or HIV neuropathy or trigeminal neuralgia. It's a homeopathic blend of St. John's wort extract, as well as eucalyptus, bergamot, lavender and geranium. You apply it to your skin and it goes to work quickly to instantly soothe and calm the pain.

Prescription Relief from a Topical Pain Gel

A long time ago, someone created relief you could apply to your skin and these are my secret weapons for you. When my sweet husband Sam was dealing with constant facial pain he tried a prescription gel, which immediately went to the top of his list for relief.

This topical prescription gel which was compounded for him by a pharmacist named Sam Pratt, who over the course of one single meeting became my good friend! He is seriously a nice guy, and his pharmacy can create all kinds of safe and effective compounded medications. Sam's pharmacy makes two different formulas that I know of, one is called "Pratt Gel" and the other is "Sam's Magic Gel."

Whichever you choose, they will get applied to your skin and they both contain a strong anti-inflammatory and a topical nerve soother which quiets overly rambunctious nerve firing. Put together, this combination may feel soothing to your face over time, which feels like it's on fire! Yes, you can buy a tube of relief! Applications offer a cumulative effect, it isn't instant for everyone. Both the creams require prescription, they are never sold at health food stores. Let's start with Pratt Gel.

1) **Pratt Gel:** To give credit where credit is due, this formula was originally created by a pharmacist named George Roentsch from Keene New Hampshire. George liked to tinker with his formulas so when Sam Pratt, a colleague of his at the time, saw how amazing this base was, he labeled it Proprietary Roentsch Anhydrous Trans-Tissue or "PRATT" gel. This was easy for Pharmacist Sam Pratt to remember because Pratt is his last name. This base was used as a vehicle for the combination of Naproxen 5% and Gabapentin 5% mixed thoroughly into an anhydrous gel (anhydrous just means there's no water in the mixture). The final compound has a strong affinity for the lipophilic structure of the nerves which is amazing because (and maybe you have to be a pharmacist to appreciate this), it's a clear gel that dissolves in water but it's a carrier for ingredients that dissolve in lipids or fatty tissues (like nerves).

2) **Sam's Magic Gel:** This one is made with Ketoprofen 10% and Gabapentin 5% and mixed into an anhydrous gel. This does not completely relieve the pain on contact, but over time, perhaps hours or a day, you'll notice a reduction in pain. It's either naproxen in the Pratt Gel, or ketoprofen in Sam's Magic Gel but both contain gabapentin, the nerve soother. There is not a whole lot of difference between these 2 gels, it's just the anti-inflammatory portion that changes, but both are offered because some people note a difference. It uses the same base as Pratt gel, so it penetrates the nerves just as well.

These come in a tube or a little tub, for easy dispensing at home. It will last a long time, several months if you use it as directed. The directions for using transdermal pain gels are pretty simple. You rub about a pea size amount of gel in front of, AND behind your earlobe, down the back of your jaw and around your face and temples (or other focal points of pain).

Careful, more is not better, this is a drug you know. Over time, like a few days to weeks, the pain should be lessened. Some people find relief even quicker. It may make you a little drowsy if you're super sensitive. Your doctor can call this into a compounding pharmacy, he'll have to have the exact recipe though, and preferred instructions.

I think you're better off calling in "Pratt Gel" or "Sam's Magic Gel" to the man himself, Dr. Sam Pratt. His pharmacy is reputable, and local in the Orlando area however they will ship to states where they are currently registered, or they can refer you to an accredited pharmacy in your area as some states prohibit pharmacies from shipping medications across state lines. As for your insurance, both of these medications are compounded, so I don't know what your plan covers. Pharmacy Specialists will be happy to let you know if your insurance will cover the gel. Call 407-260-7002 or 800-224-7711 or email Juan@MakeRx.com.

Astaxanthin: Get On My Nerves ASAP!

You may have read about the many marvelous properties of astaxanthin for your eyes in Chapter 7 "Mystery Headaches Solved." It also appears to support nerve health.[13] In particular, one article noted the antioxidant action and "anti-inflammatory protection" of astaxanthin and canthaxanthin. They appear to have potent abilities in fighting against neurodegenerative disorders. This means the compounds may protect you against the degeneration of the neurons in your brain. I recommend the brand "BioAstin by Nutrex-Hawaii" and take 12mg of this myself, every day. If you happen to buy BioAstin off their website www.Nutrex-Hawaii.com, use coupon code "suzy" to receive 25% off your purchase.

I'm a Pharmacist, Let's Talk Medicine

A variety of drugs are designed to relieve headache pain, and you can buy some over-the-counter, and others with a prescription. It depends on the type of medication. I'm not a doctor, but if I were picking the pain-reliever for you that I thought would do the best job, it would be one of the anti-inflammatory drugs. They work much better for people than narcotics (such as oxycodone, or hydrocodone) and they are not addictive either. But most of all, they address the inflammation that might be occurring and pushing against your trigeminal nerve. Narcotics won't do that. It's okay to combine both of them, an anti-inflammatory drug along with a narcotic pain reliever.

Some experts feel that anticonvulsant drugs are best for TN, and that is true, a drug like Lyrica may be in order for you, if only temporarily. I don't recommend steroids like prednisone or hydrocortisone though. You may have been offered those, but I have to say the long-term side effects are just not worth it. These drugs have the ability to suppress your adrenal function, and to trash your ability to fight infection. I think you're better off with anti-inflammatories, analgesics and anti-convulsant (aka anti-seizure) medications, as opposed to steroids. As you try different medications, you have courage and keep going.

Listen to me, they call trigeminal neuralgia the "suicide disease" so I want you to take whatever you need right now, until you uncover the true underlying cause of your pain, then you can get off your medicine slowly, as you start to see more time pass in between your attacks, and the severity of them lessen. It can happen for you. For now though, let's see what medicines are available and how to stay as safe as possible on them.

Over-the-Counter Pain Relieving Medications

The most popular medications sold over-the-counter (so you can get them in a hurry) are ibuprofen and naproxen, which belong to the NSAID class, pronounced "N-said") and it stands for nonsteroidal anti-inflammatory drugs. Follow label directions on the package you buy.[15] For ibuprofen it is about 400mg taken 3 times daily. This may not be strong enough. The prescription version of this drug comes in an 800mg dose, and it is dosed three times daily with a little snack or juice/milk, for a maximum dosage of 2,400mg per day. The 800mg dosage form requires prescription, whereas the smaller tablets (lower dose of 200mg per tablet) are sold at pharmacies nationwide.

Although NSAIDs are effective for a person with TN, at least in my professional opinion, they may take up to an hour to kick in and minutes matter when you are in pain. So you might have to take these during the day, or around the clock, prophylactically. If you know your attacks happen around midnight, take your medication around 10 or 11pm so it's on-board when midnight rolls around.

NSAIDs are harmful to the stomach and esophagus and have a knack for attacking the gastrointestinal (GI) lining and in sensitive individuals; they can cause ulcers, stomach or intestinal bleeding. To avoid this side effect, a compounding pharmacist can make you a suppository form, but your physician will have to phone that prescription in and it could take a few days to fill. If you take the oral medications, I suggest a little marshmallow root herb taken as an extract or infusion. You can watch me on Youtube.com make a marshmallow infusion, it's easy. Or you can take something like DGL, a dietary supplement which coats and protect your stomach from the harsh effects of NSAIDS.

Another idea is to take acetaminophen, this is better for people with an existing ulcer because ibuprofen is a no-no if you have an ulcer. Medications containing acetaminophen can harm the liver if taken in excess, or long term, or in combination with wine and alcohol. Acetaminophen is a drug mugger of glutathione. For acetaminophen, be very careful not to combine different products that contain it (for example, multi-tasking cold formulas with a sleep aid) because the maximum daily dosage is 4,000mg.[14] You must ask your doctor what is right for you. One more caution for you, in case you have already suffered a heart attack. Using NSAIDs are not advised, I recommend you use acetaminophen or some of the preventive supplements in my Script section. Why? Because studies suggest it increases your risk for another heart attack, regardless of how long it's been since you had the first.[16]

Anticonvulsants

Examples: Carbamazepine (Tegretol, Carbatrol)
Gabapentin (Neurontin)
Phenytoin (Dilantin)
Oxcarbazepine (Trileptal)
Pregabalin (Lyrica)
Clonazepam (Klonopin)

Neurologists prescribe medications from the anticonvulsant categories because they calm down excessive nerve firing. These medications don't work fast to reduce pain like a pain reliever would, you have to think of them as prophylactic. Carbamazepine is the most commonly prescribed drug for TN, or it's long-acting version called Carbatrol. This is more than likely the first drug that a doctor will prescribe for you, upon diagnosis, it is that common. Dizziness or drowsiness, and unsteady gait are the most frequently reported side effects when you first begin using it.

This has good effects for many people, but not all. One problem with carbamazepine is the blood abnormalities that occur such as aplastic anemia and agranulocytosis. Reduced platelet and white blood cell counts may occur too. But the limiting factor is the serious, potentially fatal dermatologic reactions such as "toxic epidermal necrolysis" and "Stevens-Johnson syndrome" which occur in 1 to 6 people per 10,000 new uses in caucasian populations. The risk is estimated to be about 10 times higher in Asian countries. It is most frequently reported in people who have the HLA-B gene, on 1502 allele. That might sound weird to you, so if you want to know if you have this gene, you have to do a saliva test from 23andMe.com. If you have the gene, I would not recommend carbamazepine for you.

Lyrica's another frequently prescribed medication, and works well in combination with Klonopin (clonazepam), a benzodiazepine sedative that is similar to another drug you might know called Valium. With continued use, perhaps a few weeks, you will find that anti-convulsant drugs, regardless of their category, slow down the electrical firing in your brain and therefore reduce the frequency or severity of TN pain. Some lucky folks get a complete remission, and this combination did help my honey for awhile so I think it's worth a try for you. See your physician routinely for lab work, especially if you take medications. Some of the anticonvulsant medications that I've listed above are drug muggers of B vitamins.

Antispasmodic Agents or Muscle Relaxers
Baclofen (Gablofen, Lioresal)
Tizanidine (Zanaflex)
Muscle-relaxing agents may be used alone or in combination with anticonvulsants. Side effects may include dry mouth, blurry vision, dizziness, confusion, nausea and drowsiness. You really want to be careful driving on these agents, I would avoid it until you are completely sure of your dosage, and how the drug affects you. Most people take these before bed, if that gives you an indication of how drowsy you will feel.

I interviewed some TN patients, and several said the pain began again, post-surgically within two months, for others, it took a year. But it came back. I haven't met anyone (yet) that had surgery and remained cured for more than 18 months. This leads me to suspect there's some other underlying pathology that continues to take place, despite the surgical procedures, perhaps an infection, demyelination or gluten sensitivity among other causes that surgery can't fix. Microvascular decompression and Gamma knife radiosurgery are the two main procedures which you can look up on your own. There are other procedures you can read about such as "glycerol injection," "balloon compression" and "radiofrequency thermal lesioning." I won't pretend to know all about these options as it is out of my expertise. I just want you to know about a few more options so you can have a conversation with your doctors.

Surgery

The surgeons' goals is to stop the blood vessel from compressing or damaging the trigeminal nerve.

We do know that aging is a risk factor for TN, and neurosurgeons frequently see elderly folks develop the condition. I read an article in the *Journal of Neurosurgery* (Jan 2011) that evaluated the safety of microvascular decompression (MVD) in 36 elderly patients and 53 non-elderly patients. The authors stated, "the majority of elderly patients with TN can safely undergo MVD."

Acupuncture Might Be an Answer to Your Prayers...

I know your face sometimes feels like there's already a thousand needles burning into it, but don't rule out acupuncture too quickly. I found an excellent scientific paper about a 66 year-old woman who had TN for 25 years.[17] She had been through the mill as you can imagine and had tried different prescription medications over the years. She had a nerve block and underwent a radiofrequency rhizotomy (of the infraorbital branch) of the trigeminal nerve.

Sadly, after enduring all of these procedures, the expenses, hospitalizations, the medications (and their side effects) she still rated her pain as "10" for the "worst pain imaginable." She went to an acupuncturist who did 3 treatments a week, each session lasting about 45 minutes. After her fourth treatment, she said she was almost pain free. After 14 sessions (her 6th week . . . and keep in mind she had been suffering for 25 years) she was completely pain free! She remained pain free even after 6th months. Isn't that amazing?!

Can you be this lucky? Since I'm a fan of acupuncture, I suggest you try it. If you don't like your treatment, or your doctor, go to another one. I've been to five different acupuncturists and experienced five different styles as a result. I only liked two of those doctors and their respective methods. Why do I tell you this? Because you should not give up if you don't like your first session, or your first doctor. Some of them are truly gifted, you have to find a practitioner who is right for you. For me, I simply don't like it when they have "to find your chi" and start digging around with each needle until they're 4 inches in. They're not actually doing that, but that's how it feels to me. I start to sweat. I simply do not want to feel pain when I'm on the table so whether it is right or wrong, it's my personal opinion. I prefer acupuncturists who are gentle, who put the needles in completely painlessly. That's just me. Chinese medicine and acupuncture varies according to how and where your practitioner was trained.

I spoke to one of my favorite acupuncturists, and TCM practitioner Jason Blalock, LAc from *Good Earth Acupuncture* in Boulder, Colorado. He is very gentle and mindful when "poking me" as I call it. Because I think he's brilliant, I asked him how to help you with trigeminal neuralgia pain. Jason said you should be treated on an individual basis since the causes for TN vary. He explained, "You have to evaluate the patient as a whole, not just target your treatment on a few square inches of their face, although that may be helpful also. Certain herbs may work for one patient, but not another. A popular herb called Xi Xin (Herba Asari), which should be certified aristolic acid free, is generally helpful in many patterns of trigeminal neurlagia, however this herb is almost always combined into a bigger formula that addresses aspects of the underlying cause."

Jason, who is the coauthor of *Qin Bo-Weis, 56 Treatment Methods: Writing Precise Prescriptions* says to ask your TCM practitioner if this 'pain decoction' would be right for your particular needs:

Rhizoma Praeparata Typhonii (Zhi Bai Fu Zi)
Radix Chuanxiong (Chuan Xiong)
Radix Angelicae Dahuricae (Bai Zhi)
Scorpio (Quan Xie)
Bombyx Batryticatus (Jiang Can)

These herbs, in combination with acupuncture may be just the trick to help you get out of pain, even if you have been suffering for many years. Practitioners who would like a copy of Jason's book, a clinical reference for TCM practitioners can find it on Amazon.com.

Weirdest Pain Relief Yet!
Got Pain? Need Weed?

In states where it is has been decriminalized, marijuana is prescribed by authorized medical doctors to manage disabling pain such as TN in their patients. Cannabis is sometimes called "medical marijuana" and often used for facial neuralgias or neuropathic pain, such as that related to post-herpetic neuralgia. I've put it in my "weird" section because most people think that marijuana does little more than make you high, but that is a myth. One of my fans read a column I wrote about it, and emailed me to thank me for keeping him from putting a gun to his head.

There is Nothing "normal" about TN!

The *"TN may be part of the normal aging process..."* that is what I read at the website of the *National Institute of Neurological Disorders and Strokes.*[18] That makes me mad because the "normal" aging process does not include lightning bolt pain in your face. If a white-coat professional tells you this is part of your "normal aging process" RUN! It means they don't know squat.

The chemical reason that marijuana can relieve pain is because the herbal ingredients stimulate receptors in the brain and may abort an attack within minutes. A study found that vaporized, low THC cannabis (which is the type of marijuana that has low amounts of psychoactive compounds so it's less likely to cause that 'stoned' feeling) is associated with a significant reduction in pain. This was based upon clinical data from a double-blind, placebo-controlled crossover trial (yes TIGHT study) published in *The Journal of Pain*, in January 2013.[19] Researchers in this study reported, *"Both the low and medium doses proved to be salutary analgesics for the heterogeneous collection of neuropathic pain conditions studied. Both active study medications provided statistically significant 30% reductions in pain intensity when compared to placebo."*

They concluded: *"Both the 1.29% and 3.53% vaporized THC study medications produced equal antinociception at every time point. ...*

[T]he use of low doses could potentially be prescribed by physicians interested in helping patients use cannabis effectively while minimizing cognitive and psychological side effects. Viewed with this in mind, the present study adds to a growing body of literature supporting the use of cannabis for the treatment of neuropathic pain. It provides additional evidence of the efficacy of vaporized cannabis as well as establishes low-dose cannabis (1.29%) as having a favorable risk-benefit ratio."

Previous clinical trials have indicated that inhaled cannabis can safely and effectively relieve neuropathy, a hard-to-treat nerve condition often associated with cancer, HIV, spinal cord injury, diabetes, multiple sclerosis, and other conditions. Separate trial data further indicates that inhaled "cannabis augments the analgesic effect of opioids" and therefore *"may allow for opioid treatment at lower doses with fewer side effects."*

The literature has many references that point to the therapeutic potential of marijuana, cannabis and other cannabinoids (which include any of a group of closely related compounds that include cannabinol and the active constituents of cannabis), and I have cited a couple in the reference section of my book.[20, 21]

In states where cannabis has not been decriminalized, your pain doctor could write a prescription for the drug "Marinol" sold in pharmacies, but it is terribly hard to find. The FDA approved it to treat nausea and vomiting that is associated with chemotherapy. The pharmacies simply don't stock this. Marinol is not exactly marijuana, it's a slightly modified version that is different enough to get a patent by a pharmaceutical company. It has a similar effect on the body to the natural herb, and it's completely legal. Let me say it here up front, as much as I prefer natural herbs to synthetic drugs, I am absolutely not advocating that you take or grow anything illegal so please follow the laws in your state.

Tea for Pain Relief
Catnip (Nepeta cataria) the herb that cats love...

Apparently, a chemical in the plants produces a slightly intoxicating effect in cats, somewhat akin to the effect of marijuana on humans. That's why cats are always rolling around in gardens where catnip grows. The two plants (marijuana and catnip) are distantly related but don't get too excited (or worried), you are not going to get any kind of marijuana-like high from catnip tea.

I recommend this catnip because it is a "nervine" it's soothing to your nervous system, it is a strong anti-inflammatory, and it's known to reduce sensations of pain by increasing your pain threshold. I use dried herb which I buy in bulk at my local apothecary, Rebecca's in Boulder, Colorado. I use 1 teaspoonful herb steeped in 1 cup water for about 15 minutes. There are prepared commercial brands that you can just dip into hot water like normal tea bags. Drink 1 cup at night, you'll probably want to sweeten this one. Avoid if you're allergic to mint.

Think Outside the Doc Box

Hot chili peppers could ease the burning, stabbing type of pain in your face.[22]

While this may sound counter-intuitive, the application of capsaicin cream (derived from chili peppers) to your skin could help you, so don't dismiss it too quickly. It must be applied in-between attacks, never when you are having an attack as it will cause even more pain and burning. The reason this works for some people is because it numbs nerve endings, by depleting substance P, a compound that transmits pain. Chili peppers aren't taking your pain away, they're just making you feel less of it. It's a great fake-out that I recommend for people with TN because over time, it can lessen the sensation of pain.

When you apply the skin cream, it binds to pain receptors in the skin, causing an initial excitation of the neurons so you feel hot and prickly all over, maybe even itchy. Under normal circumstances, this is followed by a period of reduced sensitivity (as in relief). With repeated applications, your skin becomes desensitized. This could work for you, but it may not so I hate to sit here and promise. The facts are such that in neuropathic conditions (looking at six trials for a total of 656 patients), topical capsaicin (0.075% strength) worked better than placebo. After eight weeks, 60% of participants reported less pain.[23, 24]

Here's what you do if you want to try it. Wait for a time when you are free of pain, and not having an attack. Apply capsaicin cream to your face/head where it hurts. You should use the lowest possible strength when you do this, just to be sure it doesn't burn you. While there may be a warming sensation, it should be tolerable and okay, you do not want it to feel uncomfortably hot. Whenever the 'hot' sensation is gone, reapply it. While this differs from person to person, it is usually about 4 to 6 hours later. You just keep doing that (unless you get a TN attack, then do not apply).

After a week or perhaps two, the nerve endings should be numb. Please be careful when applying it. Perhaps use a roll-on form of it. If you use your bare hands, definitely avoid your eye area and wash hands well. These types of creams are sold over-the-counter at pharmacies nationwide, under such brand names as "Zostrix" for example, and many store-brand generics. Many chiropractors offer a similar type of pain-relieving gel called Sombra. There are various brands sold online too, just make sure the active ingredient in yours is capsaicin. While doing the hot chili pepper cream, it's important to continue searching for the cause of your TN pain, as this just temporarily numbs the pain.

The procession of nerve damage (or infection) continues. In January 2007, I sent my column to newspapers like normal for syndication. at the time, I was trying to help everyone I could with trigeminal neuralgia because I saw first hand what a catastrophe it brings to a family's life. Remember, Sam did not have episodes which are indicative of TN, he actually had nonstop facial pain, very severe, which is termed "Atypical Facial Pain" or AFP. So I was studying and writing about what I learned, as I kept his secret safe. I received this note from Marilyn who found relief with the chili pepper cream.

Dear Suzy,

You have incredibly changed my life. In 2006, I had two surgeries designed to relieve the pain of trigeminal neuralgia. By September 06, my neurosurgeon told me that there was no treatment or relief for the type of pain I was experiencing. He was wrong! Since using the capsaicin you recommended in your column, hours of pain have been reduced to minutes. I am now living an almost normal life. I owe you an enormous debt of gratitude. Thank you, thank you, thank you.

Marilyn, in Gainesville Florida

Your Pasta Could Cause Nerve Damage

If you have facial neuralgias, it could be related to a process called demyelination, a big word for what happens when nerve cells (neurons) lose their outer coating – their 'insulation.' This is what happens to people with multiple sclerosis. When neurons "demyelinate" a lot of weird nervous system problems result, such as sensations of hot water pouring down your leg, or someone pulling one of your toes and the feeling that ants are biting you. Sometimes numbness can occur. Did you realize that the protein in wheat, barley and rye contain gluten and that gluten can cause nerve damage?[25]

This study concludes *"Gluten sensitivity may be aetiologically linked to a substantial number of idiopathic axonal neuropathies."* The part that caught me was that they found gluten was linked to "idiopathic" (meaning from an unknown cause) neuropathies and if you recall, I said that I didn't believe anything is "idiopathic." I know there's a cause for this condition, and there you have it, straight out of the researchers mouths to our ears, maybe it's gluten!

Gluten is known to stimulate your body to release pro-inflammatory cytokines like IL-8 and TNFα as well as IFNγ (interferon gamma).[26, 27] I'm proposing the possibility that you have demyelination happening to your trigeminal nerve. That could absolutely cause TN in a person who is sensitive to gluten and it doesn't matter if you have Celiac disease or not. You don't have to have irritable bowel syndrome to have your nerves fried by gluten. You can test yourself, see Labs in Appendix I. If you can't afford testing, you certainly have nothing to lose by eliminating gluten (if not all grains, and that would be my choice for you).

Removing an offending food additive such as gluten will do 3 huge things:
1. It will allow your nerves to catch a break, perhaps remyelinate because they are not being attacked
2. Reduce pain-causing cytokines like IL-8 and TNFα as well as IFNγ
3. Reduce intake of fungi which will parasitize you and trigger migraines. Fungi survive in grains, they hate steak and eggs! Wheat, rye, barley (beer too), become contaminated with fungus and so avoiding gluten (which is found in all those grains) reduces your toxic load.

What else would you like to know, going gluten-free doesn't hurt you, and reduces pain all over the body. Wouldn't any of us give up biscuits in a heartbeat if it offered the remotest possibility of living pain free?

. Let's say you actually have the autoimmune condition called Celiac disease as opposed to just gluten sensitivity, (although both are caused by eating wheat, barley and rye containing foods). If you have Celiac (whether or not you've not been diagnosed correctly is not the issue right this second), then you have that particularly nasty cytokine IL-17 which I discussed in Chapter 12 "Reduce Pain-Causing Cytokines." I found a study[28] that ties it all up, "gliadin may induce the activation of IL-17-producing T cells and that IL-17 expression in the CD mucosa correlates with gluten intake." Gliadin is a part of the gluten molecule, and here it is clearly implicated in IL-17, the neurologically damaging cytokine.

Corn gluten causes the same villous atrophy in your gut that wheat gluten does. And then there is the subject of molecular mimicry, where your body attacks your own tissue instead of gluten. For example, it attacks cartilage in your joints because it resembles the gluten protein causing autoimmune disease, in this case rheumatoid arthritis. Cross-reactivity is different than molecular mimicry. Your body attacks itself because it confuses gluten with other food proteins. For example, dairy's protein "casein" causes strong cross-reactivity in people sensitive to gluten. You may be strictly gluten free, but because you are so reactive to gluten, your body attacks the casein too, in whatever organ it has landed on. Basically your immune system has been fighting like a soldier, and it's used to fighting, and shooting the invader. After years of being in attack mode, your immune system (the soldier) is just shooting whatever comes near, without discerning anymore. You might say it has blinders on after awhile. This explains why some people who go gluten-free complain about it, and say they notice nothing. It's likely because they need to also cut out the cross-reactive food proteins and substances. The worse offenders in this case are lectins, legumes, seeds, corn and dairy. Seeds can be very bad for some of you. If you're very sensitivie, just consume clean meats, seafood and fruits and vegetables for 30 days. See how you do, you'll probably feel so good you'll stick with it forever.

I've known for years there was a connection and heated debates with practitioners who didn't believe me. If you read my syndicated column, which you can get for free by signing up for my newsletter (www.DearPharmacist.com) you knew about the gluten-neuropathy connection at least 7 years ago! It's really common sense if you think about it.

Testing for Celiac can be done through Cyrex Labs.[30] Doctors are so used to testing for alpha gliadins, that's been the standard for many years. I'm saying you could be highly allergic to the gamma form of gluten, and not to the alpha form that old tests look at. What if you're okay with both alpha and gamma, but highly sensitive to the omega part of gluten, or other components like "wheat germ agluttinin." If you are using old standard tests that 99% of physicians today still use (can I scream out loud now?) then you would be incorrectly told that you're okay when in fact your body may be on fire from the allergy and you will continue to live in pain because you were tested incorrectly. Read more about Cyrex Labs in Appendix I.

Gluten is A Food Additive

Gluten is not what it used to be! It's genetically modified, and it's a food additive. It is pro-inflammatory. It's pretty much just 'glue' in your food. I know I don't need to hammer you too much because you are suffering with a potentially disable nerve disorder, so you're probably willing to do anything right about now. So do this: Change your mind. When you think of gluten, think of it as you would MSG, food colorings and artificial sweeteners . . . by that I mean, it's not needed in your food, it's added. It can attack the nervous system, in fact, it has a strong affinity for nerves, and can very well cause neuralgia, in the face or elsewhere.

It may take up to a year to get optimal relief (if you're not cheating) but you should notice some positive changes within 3 to 6 months. Stick with it! I found this post on a forum by a person who had been dealing with trigeminal neuralgia: "One blog stated that a gluten free diet could help. I tried it and it worked, thank god. If you have trouble with acid reflux, feel bloated and feel tired after you eat, you may be sensitive to gluten. Try getting rid of the bread and all gluten in your diet. I saw results in 48 hours."

If I could have it my way, I'd urge you to eat a completely grain free diet. Popular diets include the "Paleo diet" and "Phase One" diet. Grain free is my preference, and what Sam ultimately did to get well. The reason is that all grains seem to be pro-inflammatory in some people, and they sometimes contain fungal contaminants.

You don't need to get tested, you could just clean out your kitchen and start eating this way immediately. You could lean into it gently, slowly, like refrain from eating pasta from now on. And then after a 2 weeks, cut out the muffins and cakes. And if you're still doing okay, have bread only on Fridays and Wednesdays. Then cut that out, and after awhile, cut out hamburger buns. One day you'll notice how much weight you've lost because that is an incredible, inevitable side effect. I can promise you that. Then you'll notice more energy and better digestion. And then it won't matter anymore, you'll want to give up your Eggo's!

Know the Difference between TMJ and TN

Cool packs or warm packs? Yes! Apply whichever feels better. Some people like the warmth because it relaxes the muscles while others prefer the cool because it reduces the 'burn' sensation. You can alternate too.

The pain condition referred to as "TMJ" syndrome which stands for temporomandibular joint syndrome is more of a mechanical or structural issue, where as TN has more to do with nerve damage, irritation, demyelination and/or compression. The pain is much more severe and debilitating with TN than it is with TMJ. The two conditions affect the same region of the face and head. It's usually not that difficult for your dentist and neurologist to sort out these conditions. If you've ever had TN, you will never get confused because the pain is much more intense and acute.

Drug Muggers that deplete B12

When your body starves for B12, you lose the myelin sheath and your nerves short circuit. This can cause neuropathy, fatigue and depression. B12 deficiency is tied some pain-causing cytokines such as IL-8, TNFα and IFNγ (interferon gamma).

There are hundreds of drug muggers of B12 and they're not all drugs: Processed foods, sugar, the condition of celiac, Crohn's, gastric bypass, and being a vegetarian or vegan. Here are other drug muggers of B12:

Antacids & Acid Blockers
Diabetes Medications (Actos, Glyburide, Metformin)
Hormone Replacement Therapy (HRT)
Potassium medications
Birth control pills
Haloperidol
Breast cancer drugs (Tamoxifen, Arimidex)
Levodopa/carbidopa
A vegan diet, it lacks B12
H. pylori infection, associated with reflux and ulcers
Poor probiotic status

Try Hot Towels

This can bring almost instant relief, at least minimizing the pain. I recall staying up hours at a time, in the middle of the night, night after night using hot towels on Sam. (Yes, I crashed my adrenals but I love this guy, and he pulled through 100%). Anyway, you'll need a dish towel, some Epsom salts and a few drops of lavender essential oil. If you only have hot water, it is okay. It would be awesome if you had someone to help you do this during an attack (so you could just lie down). Run the hand towel under hot water and gently place the towel on your face or head (wherever it hurts). If it feels good, very gently apply a little pressure to the area and hold it. This tip may work for you, or may not. It's a bit of an experiment. I used to 'pump' the area by alternating the hot towels with cool ones, changing every other towel. I think the changing sensations on his skin helped distract from the pain. I would also give it a rest, and apply St. John's wort essential oil (or another one, geranium essential oil) and let that sit on his face for 10 minutes, and then I'd start the towels up again. Remember, he had AFP, atypical facial pain, so the trigeminal neuralgia pain was almost constant, around the clock.

The hot towel applications were very helpful. Of course, you may need to let it cool a few seconds, you want the temperature to feel nice on your skin, not burn it. It's ideal to wear dishwashing gloves because these towels get hot. You can even microwave it for a few seconds, just check it for hot spots.

For added benefits, you could take your towel and soak it a concentrated solution of epsom salts and water: Use 2 cups of Epsom salts and 10 drops of Lavender essential oil to a sink full of water. Soak the towel and wring it out, then microwave for a few seconds. Place that on your face or head. You (or your loved one) will have to keep doing this 5 to 10 times over the course of 15 minutes but it may take the edge off with each application.

Doing it once doesn't usually work because the towel cools off quickly as you will see when you try. So if you enjoy the treatments, keep doing the process a few times until you have enough relief. Inhaling essential oil of lavender would be a wonderful treat as well, it is very relaxing. One more option is to buy a microwavable hot pack which lasts a little bit longer. I've seen nice ones made with flax seeds sold in salons, at the mall and Etsy.com. Whatever you use, breathe deeply and try not to clench your teeth. Just hold on, breathe deeply, this trick can reduce the intensity of an attack.

Estrogen is Essential

Teasing out the estrogen scenario is difficult, and it's clear that estrogen levels matter because the highest incidence of migraines is among women between the ages of 20 and 40. One study (done in rats) concluded estrogen *excess*, specifically "estradiol" causes nerve sensitization, which means your nerves are more reactive and touchy.[35] The researchers go so far as to say that estrogen status and chronic inflammation enhance your pain perception through a common pathway.

Another study (done in mice) says that estrogen *deficiency* is implicated.[36] I wish I could lock up these researchers in a room and say, *"C'mon people, make up your mind, you're not getting outta here until you decide if it's high or low estrogen!"*

Well, I can't do that, so let me make this simple for you. First of all, we can't automatically deduce that rodents react the same way as humans, and both these contradictory studies were done in 4 legged critters. The next thing I deduce is that estrogen levels matter, and it should be balanced with progesterone. You do not want your estrogen to fall too low beneath your "normal" levels, and you do not want them to be higher than normal either. Please read Chapter 10 "Estrogen, Progesterone and More."

Dive But Not Underwater

Hyperbaric oxygen therapy is an excellent way to reduce facial neuralgia pain. It may sound extreme but neuropathic pain is sometime unrelenting and extreme. It may take a few "dives" but this could offer long-term relief. Insurance probably won't cover it for a diagnosis of TN, but if you have extra cash, look into HBOT. This is getting more common place around the country, and there's some research that suggests it helps.[37] This study suggests that a reduction in pain medication may be possible, after approximately 10 consecutive treatments and "long-lasting analgesic effects" were clear based upon the treatment.

Hairdos and Don'ts

Don't put your hair in a ponytail. No hair clips, claws or braids. Some people have such a heightened sensitivity on their scalp that this triggers an attack.

Your Plan of Action: A Dozen Ways to Minimize the Pain

If you feel facial sensitivity or get an attack of TN, or you deal with these chronically, here are some options:

1) If the attack is associated allergies (because sneezing can bring this on), take an antihistamine such as loratadine (Claritin).
2) Make a comfortably hot, wet towel and place it on the area of pain.
3) Take an anti-inflammatory such as ibuprofen, no more than 800mg per dose
4) Apply a topical ointment like Neuragen or Traumeel® sold at pharmacies
5) Apply Pratt Gel or Sam's Magic Gel, discussed earlier in this chapter.
6) Try gently tractioning your head, your partner can help, sometimes just the position of your head makes a difference, even turning it left or right.
7) Deep tissue massage (but be very gentle) on the back of neck, near the base of the skull.
8) Capsaicin but ONLY in between attacks and very low dose, this is chili pepper cream, do not apply during an attack. Ever.

9) Eliminate gluten, and preferably grains which are pro-inflammatory in the body.

10) Apply St. John's wort oil, topically, to the area of your face where the nerve pain is. This is a known nerve soother. It may help on contact for some of you.

11) Apply essential oil of geranium directly to the facial nerve pain, it is sometimes soothing, on contact. You don't have to dilute that one.

12) Take anything from my script section that your doctor has approved.

Living With TN

There's an online site run by people like you, who have trigeminal neuralgia and other facial pain disorders. This site allows you to get on the discussion group and forums, conduct a live chat, read success stories, watch videos and peruse articles. www.LivingWithTN.org

Chapter 6

Lyme Headaches

Do you have symptoms that come and go? Are you on a medication merry-go-round? Have you been to 10 or 20 doctors without relief? Maybe you've been misdiagnosed with fibromyalgia, chronic fatigue syndrome or idiopathic migraines and you really have Lyme disease. It's caused by *Borrelia burgdorferi*, and Lyme is the number one vector borne epidemic worldwide.

Lyme disease causes headaches of all types, it can leave you feeling very tired. Sometimes that is the only symptom. For others, it will disable them. Lyme disease mimics symptoms of other diseases such as multiple sclerosis, autism, Rheumatoid arthritis, Parkinson's, ALS, Alzheimer's, fibromyalgia, Chronic Fatigue Syndrome and epilepsy so it's hard to pin down. Bummer, because if you're diagnosed incorrectly, precious antimicrobials needed to kill Lyme bugs are never taken, leading to potentially catastrophic problems. I'm not being melodramatic, ask any Lyme sufferer! No two patients have the same symptoms, which come and go.

Lyme is transmitted by ticks, but also possibly by fleas, biting flies and mosquitos. It's transmitted inutero, from mother to child, and possibly by sexual relations. Tick born infections can also be transmitted from blood transfusions. This is scary, Lyme has been found to persist in stored blood, and Ehrlichia and Babesia (two co-infections) have been reported in patients receiving blood transfusions.

Ticks are a common vector, and they are often brought into your home as they hitch a ride on your pet cat or dog. They often infect pets, but many times, because pet lovers take such good care of their animals and use tick and flea spray, and collars, the ticks are repelled from your pet and jump onto you. Once a tick latches on to you, and spits its saliva out, it injects you with more than the Lyme germ. So you can get headaches from the causative agent of Lyme, *Borrelia burgdorferi*, as well as its co-infection pathogens like Babesia, Erhlichia, Anaplasma and Bartonella.

Sadly, most of you don't even know if you were bit by a tick, they are tiny, the size of the period at the end of this sentence and you may not feel the bite. If you have moving headaches, or migraines and you live on pain medications or triptans, or you have trigeminal neuralgia or clusters, the underlying cause may be one thing, Lyme disease! From my experience, headaches are a huge chunk of the Lyme pie.

How do I know? I helped my husband Sam deal with (and conquer) every kind of headache in this book for many years, and every one of them was tied to Lyme! I assume many of you reading this chapter have different types of headaches or "brain pain" or brain "buzzing" or vibrations in your head, or heat sensations, moving headaches, eye pain, and facial pain . . . is that you? To me, it's Lyme until proven otherwise.

Doctors almost always fail to recognize Lyme unless you get a skin rash, and know that you've been bitten by a tick (even then it is sometimes dismissed). That's disgraceful but I hear it all the time. My editors have asked me repeatedly why I wanted to include this chapter when it's so controversial. *Why not?* Who else is going to tell you this when the controversy surrounding Lyme is latched on tighter than a tick. Here's a question that I received from a reader.

Dear Suzy

I have headaches of an "unknown etiology" and take all sorts of medications. Nothing works and my brain scans are normal. Could it be Lyme disease even if I never saw a tick bite, or felt one? I never got the bullseye rash. I do take routine walks in the park with my dogs. My only other symptom I have is occasional days where I feel fatigue (but not every day).

Monique

Answer: Yes it could be Lyme. Test yourself. Here's my thinking:

Your pets are a red flag (they bring ticks into your home).

The fact that you take regular walks in a park.

The fact that doctors haven't yet been able to pinpoint the cause for your headaches, so you have this "unknown etiology."

The fact that your brain scans are normal (that is often the case with infections because germs don't show up on MRIs).

The fact that you sometimes have fatigue, another common symptom of Lyme.

The fact that none of your medicine helps, I bet none of them are an antibiotic. Pain relievers don't kill germs. Neither do triptan drugs. When you have Lyme, the goal should be opening up your detox pathways, eating highly nutritious foods and taking supportive immune-boosting supplements and killing Lyme germs (in that order). No triptan migraine drug is going to do any of that, so maybe that is why you remain unresponsive to treatment.

Now, and this is VERY important. Don't assume there has to be a tick bite, followed by a bullseye rash. Some people carry Lyme even though they're asymptomatic and well. Oh, and it can remain dormant for months to years. Some people get a tick bite in camp at age 14, and don't get symptoms until 35.

Lyme Headaches Can Vary

Lyme disease can cause headaches anywhere in your head. If they are more frontal, I would suspect Lyme's co-infecting parasite called Babesia. It's actually a protozoal infection termed "Babesiosis" but you can be infected with either *Babesia duncani* or *Babesia microtii*. This is not technically Lyme disease anymore, but it's transmitted the same way, and from the same tick. Ticks have all sorts of germs when they bite you. So if you're unlucky enough to get bit by one that infects you with a Babesia parasite, your head will suffer quite a bit! Lyme headaches tend to hurt towards the back of your head, whereas Babesia headaches tend to be more frontal. If you feel like your brain or your head is smoldering or hot, this could be either Lyme or Babesia. And then there's Bartonella, another co-infection of Lyme.

Many Lymies have all 3 infections (Borrelia, Bartonella and Babesia) so your head pain changes constantly, you may also have facial pain, as in trigeminal neuralgia.

Even with a good lab, those with Lyme will only have a positive test 80% of the time. Ultimately Lyme may just have to be diagnosed based on your clinical presentation of symptoms. Are you the poster child for Lyme? Is it possible that you got a tick bite, even if you don't remember one? For example, do you take walks, lay in the grass, have pets that go outdoors, work at a job where animals are allowed, and so forth. The big shocker to people (and some physicians) is that only half of those with Lyme disease ever remember their tick bite, the other half just get sick and have no idea why. Not every one gets the famous bullseye rash (and it's not always a bullseye either), so that complicates diagnosing Lyme. Only 30 to 50% of those with chronic Lyme have a bulls-eye rash, and sometimes it doesn't even look like a bulls-eye.

Meet the Stealth Lyme Organisms

There is a lot of overlap with symptoms. For Lymies reading this, I realize your experience of symptoms is very individual, and it may be different than what I've outlined here. I'm starting with Babesia, then Borrelia followed by Bartonella. You'll notice that no matter what Lyme-related pathogen you read, headaches are part of the picture.

Babesia microtii

A parasite that can be transmitted along with the Lyme microbe. Testing can detect only one or two strains. This means you can have a negative test, but still be severely infected with a Babesia parasite.

Headaches or migraines
Pressure sensation "My head is in a vice!"
Vertigo
Racing heart or cardiac palpitations
Shortness of breath
Chronic fatigue
Crawling sensations in the head
Easily lost, even in familiar areas
Short term memory loss
Difficulty concentrating
Depression
Suicidal ideation
Anxiety or panic attacks
Bizarre dreams or nightmares
Deja vu
Memories or visions out of nowhere "I just saw myself at a playground, I couldn't remember that if you paid me!"
Sweats, can be drenching
Occasional fever or temperature fluctuations
Blurred vision, it may come and go

Sensations of heat or pain that come out of nowhere
GI problems, especially gastric motility.
Neuropathy (pain, burning or numbness)
Rubber band sensation on your head, your feet or ankles, or hands
Dysautonomia
Severe insomnia and fitful sleeping
Air hunger (feels like asthma attack)
Yawning attacks (an expression of 'air hunger')
Need to sigh
Brain fog
Cognitive problems, sometimes severe
Feeling of being drunk
Tinnitus
Spleen enlargement, left side abdominal pain

Borrelia Burgdorferi
Early symptoms
Red rash, sometimes bulls-eye
Flue like symptoms
Fatigue
Joint pain
Myalgias
Back ache
Stiff neck
Fever

Late symptoms (after 1 to 3 months)
Headaches
Neck pain sometimes called "nuchal" headaches
Anxiety
Bipolar disease
Depression
Light and sound sensitivity
Cranial neuritis
Neurological problems
Symptoms of meningitis
Stiff joints
Crepitus (joint noise)
Bells palsy (unilateral or bilateral)

Chronic fatigue or napping
Fibromyalgia pain
Low body temperature
Hashimoto's thyroiditis or Graves' disease
Memory loss
Thick blood

Bartonella Hensalae

Headache
Migraines
Ice-pick sensation in the eyes, or head
Seizures
Tender subcutaneous nodules
Morning fevers, mild
Pain in feet or heels (usually worse in morning)
Joint pain
Cognitive problems and brain fog
Mild splenomegaly (radiating pain under rib cage)
Occasional conjunctivitis
Blurred vision, may be intermittent
Sore throat
Restless legs syndrome
Mild liver impairment
Gallbladder pain
Stretch marks on abdomen
Stomach pain
Crawling sensations
Neuropathy- pain, burning or numbness
Bipolar disorder
Anxiety, irritability or unexplained rage
Cystitis or bladder burning
Rib or chest pain

> ## Get Rid Of . . .
> Alcohol
> Smoking
> Food allergens
> GMO foods
> Carpets
> Sugary foods
> Artificial ingredients
> Any source of ticks

Cats and Bartonella Infection

Don't play rough with kitty or let him lick your wounds because about 40 % of cats are a natural reservoir of *Bartonella henselae*. They may not show symptoms, but if they infect you by biting or scratching you, then you might show symptoms. It's called "Cat Scratch Fever." Growing up, my rather savage cat named "Sugar" attacked me all the time. I was lucky! If you're not, cat scratch disease can cause an infection at the site where you got bit or scratched, along with swollen lymph nodes, headaches, fatigue, low appetite and/or fever. It's almost impossible to eradicate and can cause life-long problems. Bartonella infections from your cat (or a bite from any vector for that matter) are known to cause anxiety, panic attacks, seizure disorder, encephalopathy, memory problems, brain fog, chronic fatigue, joint pain, rheumatoid-like pain and foot/heel pain and dozens of other symptoms.

Why So Much Lyme Controversy?

In a nutshell, the infectious disease doctors don't believe "chronic Lyme" exists, despite scientific studies in animals and humans that the germ lives

Where you live matters

In 2011, Delaware had the highest incidence, followed by Vermont, then New Hampshire, but Lyme disease is a global issue, so don't let any physician tell you that you can't get it because "Florida doesn't have ticks." Oh yes, it does! They're everywhere. Even the CDC says their numbers represent only about 10% of actual cases, which means about 500,000 people or more go undiagnosed every year, just in the United States.

well beyond 1 month of antibiotics. Those physicians belong to the *Infectious Disease Society of America*, or IDSA.

Not all physicians feel this way, and make assumptions . . . luckily.

The other group of medical doctors and practitioners who belong to the International Lyme and Associated Diseases Society or ILADS group, www.ilads.org believe that Lyme persists beyond a few weeks in some people.

Borrelia burgdorferi really is a stealth organism, it can morph into 3 different forms in your body, and it morphs all the time, this is a dynamic situation and provides rationale for different types of antibiotics, taken long term.

Lyme germs are smart and strong and can hide inside any organ of your body for years and do not usually die in 3 weeks. Have the 3 forms of *Borrelia burgdorferi* been proven to exist? You betcha! While the doctors are busy arguing about whether chronic lyme is real, and how long to treat, most Lymies are misdiagnosed. They bounce from doctor to doctor, suffer beyond belief and some die. Others want to.

Jarisch-Herxheimer Die-Off Reaction

This is what is more commonly referred to as a Herx reaction. It is your body's reaction to toxins (and dead bug parts) that are released when you kill pathogens in your body with herbal antimicrobials or prescribed antibiotics. The death of these harmful organisms causes poisons to be released, and then your body faces that. If you have trouble detoxifying poisons, for example you have a methylation defect (read Chapter 8 "Detoxification Matters") then your body will hang onto poisons more tenaciously. A herx reaction causes your body to pump out more pro-inflammatory cytokines, like IL-6, IL-8 and TNFα. Detoxifying the body can help speed clearance of the poison, but it doesn't prevent or stop a herx.

Killing Lyme germs can often cause elevated levels of quinolinic acid, ammonia, histamine, not to mention dead bug parts. This in turn causes release of pro-inflammatory cytokines. It's the cytokines that make you feel bad, not so much the germs. Ask your doctor if these are right for you:

Steroids- Never in a Lyme patient. I see these prescribed all the time, but I think they can make a Lymie lose their mind, feel disoriented, separated from their body, foggy and irritable. On top of that, steroids dampen your ability to fight Lyme, which is already dampened because Lyme germs have already hijacked your immune system! It's rare that I ever recommend steroids, they can worsen encephalopathy, which could be a life-threatening situation. You could get me to agree to these if the dose was extremely low, like 5mg hydrocortisone, or 1mg prednisone. If you take one, and you're alarmed now, you need to ask your doctor if they're right for you, don't stop taking them, especially, don't stop suddenly.

Curcumin- This is a strong natural anti-inflammatory considering it's a spice extracted from turmeric. It helps to reduce TNF alpha, a pro-inflammatory cytokine as well as other inflammatory compounds. This reduces quinolinic acid, often high in Lyme patients.

Astaxanthin- This protective antioxidant is a strong anti-inflammatory derived from purified algae. It penetrates the brain very easily (unlike curcumin) and so if there is any kind of neurological difficulty, this would be a consideration. This reduces TNF alpha, a pro-inflammatory cytokine, as well as other inflammatory compounds. It has well-documented research to support its ability to support joint and eye health. I personally take and recommend BioAstin Astaxanthin by Nutrex-Hawaii (www.Nutrex-Hawaii.com) Use coupon code "suzy" to get 25% off.

Cholestyramine (Questran)- A prescription drug normally used to reduce cholesterol from the GI tract that binds toxins and sweeps them out of your body. It can cause constipation. You should build up slowly on the dose. Ask your doctor if it's right for you.

Bentonite clay- Works in a similar way to cholestyramine, but clay does not require a prescription. Redmond makes a brand, and it it's sold at health food stores, please make sure your brand is the purified, edible sort. If you take too much it may cause constipation.

Benadryl or Claritin- Helps reduce histamine. I recommend using the children's liquid so you can gauge dosage. My experience is that Lymies are very sensitive to medications, and need less, rather than more. With the children's liquid, you can take very small doses. Side effects are drying, constipating, or sedating. As an alternative, you could take a natural anti-histamine, like quercetin.

Substance P Means Pain

Substance P is what transmits pain from your nerves to your brain. The

"P" actually stands for "peptide" but you can think of it as pain if you prefer. It has been detected in chronic lyme disease (especially neuroborreliosis), not a surprise as that condition can cause a condition of encephalopathy (brain swelling) and in fact, substance P is totally capable of doing that. Remember, substance P also increases an excitotoxin in your brain called glutamate (different than the amino acid supplement "glutamine" that body-builders take, or those with leaky gut). Anyway, the increased glutamate overstimulates your central nervous system causing very mild brain edema and cognitive deficits like brain fog, feeling drunk, lightheaded, confused, anxious, etc. So to hear that substance P is involved finally validates and lends proof for Lyme patients who deal with cognitive problems galore, who are dismissed so cavalierly by their physicians (or loved ones) being told, "You look well, we can find nothing in your blood, so it must be all in your head." Yeah, it is! Now you can tell them it totally is, it's due to the substance P and glutamate!

Substance P may also be released at the juncture where nerves connect to muscles, causing your muscles to be feel tight, sore or achy. Stretching helps discharge substance P, think yoga and Pilates.

Probiotics Are Necessary to Get Well

It's important to stay on your medicine if you're infected with Borellia, Bartonella, Babesia, certain species of Clostridium, E. Coli, MRSA, West Nile, Legionella, Morgellon's, Strep and others. Just FYI, that last bug eats flesh! It's harmful to your health to take antibiotics without also taking probiotics, and yet many of you have never been warned of the dangers. Once the antibiotic goes off like a shotgun in your gut, killing the pathogen as desired, but also the innocent bystanders (your beneficial bacteria), then any bad yeast, parasites, worms or dangerous organisms that the antibiotic missed become opportunistic and start growing.

People with Lyme disease notoriously take multiple antibiotics. These drugs harm your gastrointestinal tract. Your gut microbiome is partially responsible for production and breakdown of neuro-transmitters. If you are stressed, nervous, sad, overwhelmed or you cry easily, I suggest trying probiotics. It helps modulate serotonin and other brain neurotransmitters. Read more about the importance of beneficial bacteria as it pertains to thyroid, metabolism, allergies and autoimmune disorders in Chapter 7 "Mystery Headaches Solved."

Low Dose Naltrexone

One of the most inexpensive medications for immune boosting is LDN, short for low dose naltrexone. I'm a big fan of LDN. It's used most commonly to raise endorphin levels and normalize immune function, and it can be very helpful for Lyme patients. That's why I've included it in this chapter. There are several books written about this drug, which I've tried for the purposes of experimenting and writing to you. I had no problems taking it; but it may interfere with sleep. I took 3.0mg per night, but 4.5mg is the most often prescribed dose. This drug has to be compounded by a pharmacy, and has been used successfully for many years for numerous autoimmune diseases, including multiple sclerosis, lupus, rheumatoid arthritis, Crohn's disease and fibromyalgia. Several small studies have been conducted that confirm its efficacy. LDN is not traditionally used for migraines but I feel compelled to tell you about it because some of my readers have written to me to thank me for telling them about it. One woman said that she experienced "remarkable" relief after suffering with migraines for almost 3 years, and it also lifted her brain fog a little bit. Another woman said after using LDN, she was able to get off her medication (Topamax) without getting as many headaches. They're not completely resolved, but she is much better. If you want to read more about LDN, there are several books you should read, including:

* *Honest Medicine: Effective, Time-Tested, Inexpensive Treatments for Life-Threatening Diseases* by my friend Julia Schopick.

* *The Promise of Low Dose Naltrexone Therapy* by Elaine Moore and Samantha Wilkinson.

* *Up The Creek with a Paddle* by Mary Boyle Bradley.

LDN has to be made by a compounding pharmacy, in a special way. A list of compounding pharmacies that are known to compound LDN correctly may be found at http://lowdosenaltrexone.org/index.htm#pharmlist.

Triggers for Lyme Headaches

Unlike most other headaches, Lyme headaches don't really have a "trigger" in that it doesn't matter much what you eat or do, the headache is the result of the germ residing in your brain, or the neurotoxins that ensue. The goal for every sufferer is to eradicate the actual infection. Some people relapse due to:

Anxiety or emotional stress
Herxheimer or Herx die off reaction
Quinolinic acid, a neurotoxin
Ammonia, a neurotoxin
Acetylaldehyde from Candida yeast, a neurotoxin
Mycotoxins from yeast overgrowth
Methylation difficulties
Caffeine
Artificial sweetener
Toxins in non-organic foods

Worried About Flu Season?

There's a non-prescription homeopathic throat and nasal spray formulated to provide relief from cold and flu-like symptoms. It's called FluNada® and it is sprayed directly to your throat and nasal pathways, where most viruses enter the body. I like this product because it's natural, and the homeopathic blend is derived from eucalyptus, menthol and elderberry. It also has very solid laboratory testing data against both influenza and common cold viruses. www.flunada.com

---

Suzy's "Script" for Lyme Related Symptoms

If you go to 5 LLMDs in America, you'll get 5 totally different treatments and since I'm not a doctor, I'm not going to pretend to know what is right for you and your co-infections.

I'll happily weigh in on some supportive remedies here, because I think these might be useful for you, no matter what infection you have. The remedies below are not at all intended to treat Lyme. Before you take any of the following supplements, you must ask your doctor(s) if they are right for you. My intention here is to educate you about possibilities and options. Do not misconstrue my ideas for medical advice. I have no idea what is right for every individual reading this so take my list to your practitioner(s) to ask if they're right for you with your medical history. Dosages listed anywhere in this book are basic guidelines, some people tolerate different dosages than what is stated here:

Magnesium
Probiotics
HomocysteX Plus
Sarsaparilla
Proteolytic Enzymes

How This Helps You Become Headache Free

Magnesium

This mineral is depleted from the body because the Lyme organisms use it for their biofilms. You have to supplement yourself because magnesium deficiency is a very common cause for migraines and headaches.

Probiotics

These support your immune system, and you need all the help you can get to build your T cell immunity. Probiotics are immune modulators, they help you whether you are Th1 or Th2 dominant, meaning whether you have autoimmune disorders or if you are prone to infections and allergies. It means it helps all kinds of people. Your probiotic genome weighs more than your brain, so make it count. I recommend Dr. Ohhira's Probiotics, however there are many others, including high-quality brands sold through physician offices. You just want to make sure they are live and viable. For more on probiotics, refer to the end of Chapter 7 "Mystery Headaches Solved."

Methylcobalamin

Sometimes you will hear that herxing is a good thing, that it means your antibiotics are working. I don't buy that. If you're herxing, that means you have more toxins (or dead bug parts) in your body than you should and it's a bad thing. I see nothing good about it. It may mean that you have a genetic snp (pronounced "snip") such that you can't eliminate toxins well. It may mean that you're going too fast with your antibiotic therapy and you have to slow down. It may mean that you have not fully addressed your detoxification pathways properly and you need supportive supplements. One of my favorites is "HomocysteX Plus," which you can read about it in Chapter 8 "Detoxification Matters." It contains active B9 which is called "methylfolate" or sometimes "5-MTHF."

This is a much better form of what you call folic acid (which I no longer recommend). HomocysteX Plus has this special methylfolate, as well as natural vitamin B12, needed for cranial nerves, energy and clarity of mind. Vitamin B12 will nourish your nervous system, including your brain. It should help with fatigue, muscle cramps and myelin production for your cranial nerves (often attacked by Lyme germs). As you learned in the Chapter 5 on "Trigeminal Neuralgia," B12 can reduce production of the pro-inflammatory cytokine IFNγ (interferon gamma) by about 50% as well as TNFα, two compounds that are almost always high in Lyme patients. You can buy products anywhere you want, I'm only trying to help. You can find folic acid and B12 combinations at any health food store, but you can't find them with the active 5-MTHF, or the active methylcobalamin [it's usually cyanocobalamin] and that's why I recommend HomocysteX. I negotiated a discount with the maker because we are study buddies (nerds stick together you know), so if you want Dr. Lynch's "HomocysteX Plus" use "Headache Free" at his site to get a discount www.SeekingHealth.com.

Sarsparailla

Used to make root beer, this contains saponins which are strong anti-inflammatories and studies suggest it is a strong neuroprotectant; it helps restore brain receptor function, cognition and memory. Helpful for rheumatoid arthritis and gout too. I think it can help with neurologic manifestations of Lyme. We used to get this from a Chinese Medicine practitioner, and make tea out of it but it comes as a tincture and oral dietary supplement.

Proteolytic Enzymes

This dietary supplement helps you break down and digest proteins. In doing so, it suppresses inflammation throughout the body, you need that if you have Lyme disease. Bromelain is one enzyme derived from pineapple stems; papain comes papaya plants/fruits. These are sold at health food stores. Proteolytic enzymes modulate the immune system. Holistic physicians utilize this supplement in the treatment of cancer, hepatitis, viral and bacterial infections, suppressed immunity and inflammation. Some use it to control cholesterol.

What If You Don't Respond to Lyme Treatment?

I have seen time and time again, a person chase out Lyme *(Borrelia burgdorferi)* with antibiotics, get better for a little while and then crash. There are no studies to back me, but one reason you may still plagued with terrible symptoms is because of a Babesia infection. Until you eradicate that parasite, getting completely well will be tough. The

Babesia speaks so loud in your body that until that parasite is under control, it's hard to clear any other bugs. Without knowing which organism is causing your headache, it's hard to choose a treatment. Some of my friends have flown to Germany where medical ozone is commonly used on cancer patients and seriously infected individuals like Lyme, HIV and Hepatitis. Most have had positive experiences.

Medical Ozone?

Yes, I'm for ozone. Ozone was really a helpful tool for my husband. He had trouble tolerating all of the antibiotics prescribed for him, he tried them all, and all the antifungals, antivirals, antiparasites and others. After 1.5 years of weakening his body, we decided it was too much of a tightrope to kill the Lyme germs without killing him. Ozone is an indiscriminate treatment. It doesn't matter what infection you have, these "oxidative" therapies are going to hone in on them. It's not a direct kill, like an antibiotic. Ozone ends up producing more oxygen in the bloodstream, and Lyme 'and friends' can't stand that. Microbes are anaerobic, they die in the presence of oxygen. This is a very important topic, and it warrants a bigger discussion with your own lyme doctor. I do not know what's right for you. Ozone is not right for everyone.

EGCG from Green Tea

It contains many compounds, but the main one is EGCG which stands for "Epigallocatechin-3 gallate." This is a well-known antioxidant used for chronic infections and cancer because of it's strong antioxidant and anti-inflammatory effects. What you don't realize is that this compound is strong medicine and highlights the potential benefits of EGCG against Babesia parasite infection.

Both "in vitro" tests (meaning tests done outside of the human body) and "in vivo" (meaning in the body) were completed and when all the scientific literature is put together, green tea, or more specifically, EGCG inhibits growth of various species of Babesia. High quality supplements may be an option for some of you, if you cannot tolerate drugs. EGCG has activity against B. bigemina, B. bovis and B. microtii. I really like this natural option for killing babesia, especially if you are okay with a small amount of caffeine (present in green tea). Serendipitously, I got an email from one of my sweet fans on facebook, the day before I turned this manuscript confirming the benefits of green tea. I'm so grateful because I love to include real people, and their stories. The "study" that Nancy refers to was published in 2010, in *Parasitology* and it's entitled, "Inhibitory effects of EGCG from green tea on the growth of Babesia parasites."

Dear Suzy,

One morning I woke up, with yet another Babesia migraine! I had a cup of green tea and my migraine started to subside. So I googled, green tea and Babesia migraines. I found this recent study.

Sincerely,
Nancy F. from Colorado

Tea for Pain Relief
Sarsaparilla, the herb your brain loves...

A good tea for a Lyme headache is sarsaparilla tea. You can buy this from an herbal apothecary, or a Chinese Medicine doctor. I'd use about 1/2 cup dried herb to 4 cups of water. Boil gently for about 40 minutes, then strain. It will stay fresh in the refrigerator for several days. You can drink it warm, about 1/2 to 2 cups per day, just build up to that. This herb is a neuroprotectant. Sweeten only if needed (you don't need any more sugar because of the candida). This is meant to be a medicinal tea, and it's pretty mild in taste, but if you need a sweetener, use a high-quality honey, something local and organic, or the brand Manuka.

Think Outside the Doc Box

Electricity for Health has been around for decades. This was before the advent of prescriptions. In 1991, microcurrents as applied using the Beck Protocol, were re-introduced to 'zap' bugs in the blood stream. It's an option that is "beyond the doc box" but if you are unable to take any antibiotics, I think a little hand-held device may help eliminate some bugs in your blood stream over time. I feel confident recommending it. The unit I like is the Silver Pulser by SOTA. It is gentle. The unit can also be used to make ionic silver, and silver is a natural anti-microbial. More information can be found at sota.com and it is sold directly to consumers.

I'm a Pharmacist, Let's Talk Medicine

Lyme is one of those situations where I feel the use of a strong analgesic may be helpful. Talk to your doctor, and family about this. There is the potential for addiction, however, if you can stop the pain I recommend it, even with that potential because I have compassion for you. Lyme headaches can be disabling. I want you to hold on and take anything you can to relieve the pain, while at the same time, taking an antimicrobial (or several in combination) to address the underlying cause. Medications in this class include oxycodone, hydrocodone and codeine. Use the lowest effective dose and be sure to try an anti-inflammatory first, or in combination with your narcotic (ibuprofen, acetaminophen or high-dose curcumin). You and your physician can settle on what is right for you, the point of the anti-inflammatory is to reduce swelling, while the narcotic works to reduce pain.

When you combine different analgesics you have the potential to really suppress your central nervous system. You have to make sure these are combined properly. For example, it's an absolute no-no to combine Vicodin with Oxycontin, but it's okay to combine either one of those drugs with an anti-inflammatory like ibuprofen. Check with your pharmacist and physician before combining anything.

Killing Lyme

The balancing act here is to kill the organisms without killing yourself. You think I'm kidding but I'm not. Antibiotics can be terribly harsh on the system, causing dozens of side effects, some life-threatening. It's no easy task to get rid of Lyme. Since this is not a Lyme book, but a headache book, I'm only going to highlight some drug names for now, rather than launch into a full discussion. There are lyme books out there, and lyme doctors out there to help you sort through which medication is right for you. The medications listed here may address Lyme itself, a co-infection, or both. Here are some ideas:

Clarithromycin (Biaxin)
Doxycycline
* Ciproflaxin
* Levoflaxacin
Mepron
Malarone

Metronidazole (Flagyl)
Minocycline (better brain penetration compared to doxycycline)
Rifampin
Sulfamethoxazole with trimethoprim
Tinidazole (Tindamax)

*Levaquin is listed it here for completeness sake but I can't recommend this for you, since there is a dangerous drug-induced reaction associated with it that could change your life forever. See section "Been Floxed?"

Herbs

Andrographis
Banderol and Samento (both together)
Cryptolepis
Japanese Knotweed
Resveratrol

Been Floxed?

This is the term given to people who suffer problems, sometimes disastrous and disabling as a result of taking antibiotics from the fluoroquinolone category. In 2008, the FDA added a "black box" warning to Levaquin, Cipro, Avelox and all fluoroquinolone-class drugs.

"Fluoroquinolones are associated with an increased risk of tendinitis and tendon rupture. This risk is further increased in those over age 60, in kidney, heart, and lung transplant recipients, and with use of concomitant steroid therapy. Physicians should advise patients, at the first sign of tendon pain, swelling, or inflammation, to stop taking the fluoroquinolone, to avoid exercise and use of the affected area, and to promptly contact their doctor about changing to a non-fluoroquinolone antimicrobial drug."

Kill Fungus Naturally

Antifungal supplements may help because they reduce yeast, a common problem in Lyme patients. Yeast gives off acetylaldehyde, and this will contribute if not cause chronic headaches. Natural anti-fungal supplements are sold at every health food store:

Grapefruit seed extract
Monolaurin
Brazilian Green propolis
Oregano oil
Rosemary Oil
Caprylic Acid
Pau D'arco herb

Weirdest Pain Relief Yet!

Use the "OSIM uCrown 2 Soothing Head Massager with Music." It looks like a helmet, so don't strap it on and go to the community pool. This battery-operated device uses a combination of patented air pressure technology, soothing music, vibration massage, magnetic therapy and gentle heat. Let me circle back to that "soothing" music. The setting my husband put it on sounded like crickets, but he only did that for a giggle. It does have different music options. He likes to get a rise out of me. Between the squeezing, pulsing, rolling and "crickets" I made such a fuss, he videoed me and posted it on youtube.

Lyme headaches sometimes cause a "vice grip" sensation, and this causes counterpressure, it may feel good. It may also quell tension headaches. It's the closest thing I've found to two real human hands on your head! It's sold at Brookstone, and online. It has an auto-timer that allows for a 5, 10 or 15 minute massage. Portable and cordless. I think I paid $130 U.S. dollars.

Labs

First let me say there is much more about testing for Lyme in Appendix I. People with lyme have headaches and almost always have several MRIs run on them before they are diagnosed properly. Your MRIs and CT scans could be perfect, so don't expect brain imaging to show Lyme germs.

There used to be a vaccine for Lyme that injected proteins into you (think of them as dead bands because they were not really living germs). The goal was to desensitize you to Lyme germs, should you come into contact with it. The vaccine was being offered publicly and they didn't want everyone and their brother in the population to come up positive for Lyme (when they didn't have it). Long story short, the lyme vaccine was eventually discontinued, but the laboratories still do not test for the most popular bands. This is why testing for Lyme disease is a huge challenge. The germ's DNA sequence in Western blot tests (termed "bands") are not tested for thoroughly. Bands associated with Lyme germs that are commonly found in the blood of a Lyme patient will not necessarily show up using conventional labs which detect only a few bands (because they eliminated some when the vaccine came out). This medical horror has left millions of people with Lyme thinking they do not have it, when they do. Then there's the trouble of "false positives" where these bands light up due to cross-sensitivity with other bacteria. For more information regarding labs that test for lyme disease, refer to Appendix I "Labs."

Lyme Headaches - Let's Talk to the Einstein's of Our Time

First Up, Richard Horowitz, MD...

I interviewed Dr Richard Horowitz, a board certified internist in Hyde Park, New York, who has treated over 12,000 chronically ill patients with Lyme disease. This expert physician has noticed the trend of varying symptoms. He's dubbed it "Lyme-MSIDS" short for Multiple Systemic Infectious Disease Syndrome.

According to Dr. Horowitz, "Just about all of the co-infections can contribute to headaches, not just Borrelia, but also Babesia, Ehrlichia, Bartonella, Rocky Mountain spotted fever, Q-fever and Tularemia. Unfortunately, the complexity of treatment is due to overlapping factors on the MSIDS map which can include adrenal fatigue with reactive hypoglycemia, environmental toxins, detoxification problems, mitochondrial dysfunction, mineral deficiencies, food and chemical sensitivities and lack of restorative sleep. Of the mineral deficiencies, magnesium is critical because there is a direct association between magnesium deficiency and headaches. To give people narcotics and anti-inflammatories only treats the symptoms. You have to also treat the underlying cause of the headaches." If you recall, emerging studies suggest mitochondrial damage as a cause migraines (see Chapter 2).

Dr. Horowitz went on to explain that while not foolproof, one approach to reducing the incidence of Lyme headaches is to reduce the microbial load. He explained, "you can do this with targeted treatments for Lyme and associated tick-borne co-infections." While reducing germ load on the body, it is equally important to get adequate sleep, support the body with a high quality nutritional supplements, such as mineral supplements with magnesium and adaptogens like licorice, rhodiola, shisandra and ashwagandha for adrenal support."

He also emphasized to me the importance of eliminating food triggers like MSG and sulfites as well as common food allergens, such as wheat, gluten, dairy and eggs (or whatever you are sensitive to). Eating small frequent meals with adequate protein, complex carbs and healthy fats in a balanced diet to prevent blood sugar swings can also be beneficial since reactive hypoglycemia is a common overlapping cause of headaches. I highly recommend Dr. Horowitz's book, *Why Can't I Get Better? Solving the Mystery of Lyme and Chronic Disease* (St. Martin's Press, November 2013).

Next Up, Connie Strasheim...

According to Lyme disease survivor, Connie Strasheim, who is also the author of "Insights Into Lyme Disease Treatment: 13 Lyme-Literate Health Care Practitioners Share Their Healing Strategies," *"Headaches are a common symptom of chronic Lyme disease, but because headaches can be attributed to many causes, most people don't consider Lyme to be a potential reason why their head hurts. Of course, a person with chronic Lyme will usually have other symptoms, in addition to headaches, such as joint or muscle pain; brain fog, fatigue, cardiac problems, and/or mood disorders, but if these or other Lyme symptoms accompany the headaches, Lyme may be a potential cause."*

Lyme disease is a complex infectious syndrome involving at least three types of microbes, like Babesia, Bartonella and Borrelia. As you've learned, all of these bugs cause headaches. According to Connie, *"The different microbes/infections involved in Lyme can cause different types of headaches. For instance, Babesia, which is a parasitic microbe with characteristics similar to malarial organisms, causes severe pressure and migraine-like headaches all over the head. Bartonella, a bacterial organism involved in Lyme, causes frontal lobe headaches or headaches on the top of the head. Bartonella headaches are often confused for sinus headaches. Borrelia, the most commonly recognized organism in Lyme disease, and which lives in the body in three different forms (as a spirochete in the blood, cyst in the tissues, and cell-wall deficient form in the blood/tissues) most commonly causes headaches at the back of the head and neck. A fourth Lyme organism, ehrlichia, causes sharp, knife-like headaches behind the eyes."*

When all of these infections are present in the body, it can be difficult to sort out which infection is causing symptoms, but let it be known that all can cause headaches! I recommend a copy of Connie's book, *Insights Into Lyme Disease Treatment: 13 Lyme-Literate Health Care Practitioners Share Their Healing Strategies* available at: www.lymeinsights.com.

Next Up, The Healing Arts Partnership

Next, I interviewed Dr. Marty Ross and Tara Brooke ND. The dynamic duo are integrative medicine specialists based in Seattle Washington and together, they founded "The Healing Arts Partnership" where they see people with complex disease. They find the best treatments for infections are ones that integrate prescription and holistic medicines approaches. I asked them why a person can be infected with Lyme as a child, but not get sick until adulthood. I wonder why people carry the disease, but don't show it (because many of you do). "In many people the germ can live for years kept under control by the immune system. Then at some point in time due to stress causing immune suppression or other suppressors building up like environmental toxin build up or heavy metal toxicity, the germ can take off. Another cause of the germ becoming active is receiving general anesthesia, and we do not know why." Another burning question I have is what natural antimicrobials can help unravel the biofilm, because that is where the Lyme germs hide. "There are major voids in treatments when prescriptions alone are used. Cat's claw and Otoba bark extract eradicate the biofilm and the various forms of the lyme germ." Just so you know the brand names I recommend for those are Samento and Banderol, respectively.

Drs. Ross and Brooke provide many useful free resources, interesting articles and videos. There is a great explanation about antimicrobials that treat Lyme called "Kills Lyme Germs: A Brief Antibiotic Guide" found at Treat Lyme and Associated Diseases at www.treatlyme.net.

Drug Muggers that deplete Vitamin A and D

Some medications used in the treatment of Lyme disease rob your body of vitamins. One very popular medication called Rifampin has the ability to cause a deficiency of fat soluble vitamins such as vitamin A and D. For a more comprehensive list of medications that zap vitamins and minerals from your body thus increasing your risk for other health problems (which will most likely get diagnosed as a new disease unless you know this), please refer to my *Drug Muggers* book (Rodale, 2011).

How to Remove a Tick

Don't burn it, that is a myth, and the fastest way to make it 'spit' germs into you!

1. Use tweezers or forceps.
2. Grasp the tick mouthparts close to the skin.
3. Avoid squeezing the tick which may spread infected body fluids.
4. Pull the tick straight out. Do not twist.
5. Save the tick (you can have it tested for B. burgdorferi and co-infections)
6. Wash your hands with soap and water.
7. Apply antiseptic to bite site.

Your Plan of Action: A Dozen Ways to Minimize the Pain

If you have Lyme headaches, here are some options, you should discuss all of these with your doctor:

1) Find an LLMD. An absolute must, you need a good doctor, preferably a lyme literate medical doctor that has a high success rate. Termed an "LLMD" they will recognize the pathogen you that is acting up, and treat it correctly. I prefer LLMDs that know how to balance holistic treatment with conventional ones. You might try ilads.org

2) Hydrate. Sip hot water with lemon or lime every 15 minutes, this helps hydrate you, and move lymph.

3) Rescue herbs. Pinella and Burbur by Nutramedix. These are two different herbal detox formulas made by Nutramedix. My

friend and lyme-literate doctor Lee Cowden, MD suggests using them together, you can take 5 to 10 drops of each in 2 ounces pure water. Let it sit for a minute, then drink. Repeat if necessary at periodic intervals as a "rescue" aid, about every 15 minutes up to 2 hours. Stop if you get dizzy. Make sure this rescue aid is right for you by asking your own lyme-literate doctor.

4) Move Lymph. Get acupuncture, or "cupping" this helps restore balance in the body and get lymph flowing.

5) Bathe. Take a warm bath with Epsom salts, use about 3 to 4 pounds in the tub

6) Bind toxins. Try bentonite clay or activated charcoal to bind neurotoxins. These should not be taken within 2 hours of medication or supplements. As an alternative, the supplement "Calcium D glucarate" can bind toxins in the gut and it's not constipating.

7) Eliminate. Never get constipated, you'll hold toxins. Keep bowels moving with fish oil, probiotics and fiber.

8) Eat Greens. More alkaline foods, like raw kale salads or lightly steamed Swiss chard. The point of this is to quickly alkalize your body.

9) Massage. Hands-on massage or pressure on your temples or the base of your head might feel good. Stretching your temples in an upward motion (while squeezing) might feel nice too.

10) Buy a hat. Wear a tight baseball cap, the counter pressure feels good.

11) Reach for pain relief. Take analgesics or anti-inflammatories or both together to help get you through the day.

12) Calm the brain. Glutamate, an excitotoxin runs very high in Lyme patients. The drug clonazepam is prescribed because it blunts glutamate, and raises GABA. Anytime you raise GABA and calm glutamate you help a headache, while reducing anxiety. Clonazepam is addictive so I don't recommend it as a long-term solution, in fact, I hope you can do without that drug. It's mentioned here because many LLMDs prescribe it, based upon the fact that it quells glutamate, a toxin that fires up your brain. Low doses of GABA and L-theanine can help neutralize glutamate.

Chapter 7

Mystery Headaches Solved

Some of you reading my book may not fit into one particular category such as migraines, clusters or tension headaches. You are still searching for an answer to your head pain. That's why I wrote this chapter, I believe you. Just because no one can see it, I'm sure you can still feel it! And what about your child? This chapter includes hard-to-find information about a natural herb that can ease your child's headache and I'm thrilled to share that. You'll learn about some fascinating causes for headaches including gelato, toothaches, sex, perfume, lightning and minor injuries. My hope is to uncover the hidden cause for your mystery headaches.

Mystery Headache Solved: Is it Perfume?

While that *Euphoria* by Calvin Klein might smell sexy to you, it is far from "euphoric" to a headache sufferer. The scent can buy you one way ticket to bed for 24 hours with a triptan! A 2011 article published in *Cephalalgia* confirmed that many migraineurs are affected by strong odors and perfumes. This was confirmed again in 2013, in the same journal that looked at various odors including perfume, paint, gasoline and bleach.[11]

In this study, researchers studied 200 migraine patients and 200 tension headache sufferers. Headaches were triggered only in the migraineurs, in 70% of them, and it only took about 25 minutes, plus or minus 2 minutes. The tension headache sufferers did not have odor-triggered headaches. Migraineurs reacted mainly to perfume (76%), then to the odor of paint (42%), then gasoline (29%) followed by bleach (27%). It's clear from this that perfumes are the primary trigger to avoid, but all strong odors can affect you. If you step into an elevator where the odor is very strong, I'd recommend holding your breath, or stepping back out and waiting for another elevator. Sometimes it's more awkward, like when you get to your seat in the plane, and your seated next to someone that has sprayed a bucket of perfume on themselves (I've noticed this with older women, who may have a reduced sense of smell, so they spritz the Chanel #5 on heavy) and then you're faced with an awkward problem. You have to sit next to them and pray you don't get a migraine, or you have to ask the airline attendant for a different seat. I'd do it, gather up your strength and ask to be seated elsewhere, or settle in for a very long painful flight.

Snack Yourself!

Feeling hungry can trigger a migraine, complete with aura and flashing lights, according to a 2005 study in *Cephalalgia*. If this fits you, carry a snack bar and some almond butter in your purse.

Mystery Headaches Solved: Is It Your Child?

In the past 50 years, the prevalence of headaches has been increasing throughout the population. Headaches have become a big problem in school-aged children, especially girls. The statistics that I've perused show that headaches are reported in 10-20% of school-aged children and 27-32% of adolescents. The reports indicate these kids experience a headache at least once per month. Migraine headaches are prevalent in 4-19% of the adolescent population by the age of 15. That is nothing to sneeze at. Some kids get migraines once or twice a week!

You probably wish these headaches on yourself as you watch your beautiful child suffer with them, feeling helpless and confused about how to ease their pain. I understand, even my own son Michael (now an adult) used to get headaches from time to time. Luckily they responded to some powdered magnesium that I gave him, (I used a powdered form that tastes good like *Natural Calm®*, and a little liquid ibuprofen. I got rid of them entirely by removing eggs and dairy from his diet for 5 solid months. It was tough but worth it. He was 5 at the time. Despite the increasing reports of the number of children suffering from chronic migraines, I feel hopeful and excited to share good news with you, leave it to me to dig this one up, it wasn't even published in the United States! Drum roll, please.

Researchers from the *University of Heidelberg* (Heidelberg, Germany) designed a prospective, randomized, partly double-blind, placebo-controlled, parallel-group trial. This just means it's a really tight, intelligently done study, so that no one could ignore the results. This study was designed to evaluate whether butterbur root extract (also known as Petadolex) and music therapy was an effective treatment for children suffering from migraines. Pretty cool huh? We already know that butterbur root extract promotes relaxation of the smooth muscle lining in the cerebral blood vessel walls, and it helps adults with migraine. And as an added benefit, it reduces some of those pain-causing pro-inflammatory cytokines you might read about if you venture into the more complex chapter at the end of my book, Chapter 12 "Reduce Pain-Causing Cytokines." Butterbur reduces inflammation extremely well.

During the 12 week trial, published in 2008 in *European Journal of Pain*,[36] people were randomized into specific treatment groups; 19 received butterbur root extract, 20 received music therapy and 19 were placed in the control group. These participants were measured by the reduction of headache frequency at 8 weeks post treatment and again 6 months later.

After data analysis, researchers found both music therapy and butterbur root extract were superior to the placebo group. The music therapy and butterbur root extract groups documented a significant reduction in attack frequency. Less headaches experienced by these kids, just by listening to soothing music! That means less headaches for mom and dad too! Therefore, I conclude (and the researchers did too) that music therapy for relaxation and/or butterbur root extract are excellent options for pediatric migraines.

> **Wine, Chocolate & Cheese**
>
> That combination gives me a craving but it can trigger headaches. Most people blame the sulfites, but it could also be a fungus, as in Candida krusei. In chocolate, this fungus is used to ferment the cacao beans to remove the bitter taste.

And there's more good news for your sweet child . . .

In a recently open label trial published in *Neurological Sciences*, researchers found they could significantly reduce the number of migraine and tension headaches in school-aged children using nothing but natural supplements (no drugs, no music, no diet changes).[2]

During the trial which lasted 3 months, 119 children were given a combination of Ginkgolide B (an herbal extract from Ginkgo biloba tree leaves), Coenzyme Q10 (CoQ10), Riboflavin (Vitamin B2), and Magnesium. These nutrients were selected based upon their safety and efficacy histories. If you decide to try this yourself, you'll have to speak to your pediatrician to find the best dose for your child based upon age, weight and severity of headaches. The kids in the trial had *not* been using any regular pharmaceutical medications or interventions for the prior 6 months to enrollment in the trial. There was nothing in their bloodstream to confuse the results. Participants were evaluated by clinical interview, examination, as well as subjective wake and sleep EEGs. The participants also kept journals documenting the number and intensity of their head pain.

After evaluation of the data, the researchers saw that they had been able to do something rather amazing, at least "amazing" from where I sit! They decreased the 'mean frequency' of the children's headaches from 9.71 all the way to 4.33. Another way to say this is that they saw a reduction of 50% in migraine and tension headache frequency! They got these glorious results all the while using the specific nutrients described above.

Now, we all know there are a variety of pharmaceutical drug treatments available for both kids and adults, however, the side effects can be a problem, especially for kids! Based upon this study, which suggests a handful of nutrients, I think we have an effective and safe approach to chronic migraines in your child, with minimal if any side effects. Certainly, it's worth discussing with your child's pediatrician.

Mystery Headaches Solved: Is It Lightning?

If you develop a headache when a storm rolls through this is not your imagination playing tricks on you. This can happen, and the article appeared in the April 2013 edition of the journal *Cephalalgia*.[3] Researchers aimed to determine if lightning was associated with a higher frequency in migraineurs.

Lightning Strikes a Headache

A 2012 study found that you're almost 30% more likely to suffer migraines on days when lightning strikes near your home.

The research consisted of 90 people from Ohio and Missouri who fulfilled the diagnostic criteria for *International Headache Society* defined migraines. In other words, these were not just volunteers saying, 'Yeah I have headaches." These folks truly experienced headaches and specific symptoms that met strict criteria. The participants were about middle age, mostly female (91%). Researchers tracked the participants over three to six months, who recorded their headache activity in a diary. Weather factors, such as thunderstorms were noted. The probability of having a headache on days with lightning was increased. So lightning is a trigger for headaches in some people. If you live in Florida, the lightning capital of the world, and you have headaches when storms roll through, I give you my blessings to get out first chance you can! Living there 35 years myself, I can vouch that the lightning storms there are frequent, and at times, violent.

While this study shows that lightning represents a trigger for your headaches, we cannot completely explain why. It is not known whether it's the electromagnetic waves, or it's the production of ozone (a bioaerosol) that sparks the migraine. Some theorize that the lightning induces fungal spores too, so we know that lightning is a trigger, but we don't know the mechanism why.

Mystery Headaches Solved: Is It a Post-Concussion Headache?

This type of headache isn't random; it comes after a traumatic brain injury, or TBI. The onset of headaches can be immediate, or may come on as much as a year or more after the injury. You would be stunned to know that a TBI doesn't have to be so "T" as in "traumatic" and yet, the headache can be debilitating. Long-term pain can occur if you hurt your head, face, or neck.

It could be a minor traffic accident that jolts your head or a fall. Yeah, seriously a fall! In fact, this is the number 1 cause of TBI, according to the Centers for Disease Control (CDC) accounting for 35% of cases.[5] The CDC estimates that up to 3.8 million cases of TBI occur in the United States each year, compare that to breast cancer which is 176,300 cases, and you hear about this from skateboarders or mountain bikers who crash, football injuries and even 'Shaken Baby Syndrome." I wonder how many moms are reading my book right now, whose sons play high school football, and suddenly have frequent headaches and trouble concentrating or sleeping. (Yes, it could be!) We have to make nice with our head or trouble ensues, remember, it's housing our precious brain! Luckily not everyone with an injury or TBI gets long-term headaches.[4]

They can have any number of causes, including trauma to the brain and skull, injury to the neck and/or back, medication side effects, anxiety and tension. They may also be exacerbated by a history of migraines or other types of headaches.

Speaking very generally, your odds for this go up if you're a senior, or have some other disability or underlying infection, or if you engage in activities that could cause it (think 4 wheeling). All this talk just gives me one more excuse not to bungee jump. Anyway, the symptoms following a concussion can persist for weeks, months or longer after a TBI and one of the symptoms can be a headache. The headache may be accompanied with difficulty concentrating (what some might call brain fog), irritability, emotional instability or trouble thinking, reading or processing. A study in July 2012 points out that concussions age our brain faster, causing faster cognitive decline.[6] This same article also suggests that being smarter or having greater "cognitive reserve" reduces long-term consequences.

Misdiagnosis is common because the symptoms may occur days or weeks after the TBI so the connection isn't clear to you. People with post-concussion headaches are usually just medicated with analgesics. Yeah right. While the majority of post concussion headaches resolve over time, not all of them do. And by that time, you may get addicted to hydrocodone and sleeping pills.

A study published in the September 2013 issue of *Journal of Rehabilitation Medicine* examined long-term effects of TBI.[7] The researchers just wanted to see the difference between men and women, and see how their quality of life had been, how they were fairing out with symptoms and how stress had impacted them. To find out all of this, the participants, all patients with mild TBIs were given one sort of questionnaire or another. 163 patients answered the questionnaires, and of those 21 were given a medical examination. Years passed, 11 years to be exact. And then these patients were contacted again. Researchers determined that some of the patients had "disabling post-concussion symptoms" even after 11 years following their TBI. The 5 most common symptoms reported were as follows:

Fatigue	*53.4 %*
Poor memory	*52.5 %*
Headache	*50.9 %*
Frustration	*47.9 %*
Depression	*47.2 %*

The researchers concluded "Long-term consequences were present for approximately 50 % of the patients 3 years after mild traumatic brain injury and were also reported 11 years after mild traumatic brain injury." Wow! Doesn't say much for our ability to help this subset of folks, and my heart just goes out to you. If you have a headache that is unresponsive to typical headache medicine, and you can think back to a time you suffered a TBI, this may be the cause of your mystery headache.

I feel so fortunate to have connected with a real expert on this issue, Ginny Lazzara, RN, BSN, CRRN who is the Board Chair of the *Brain Injury Association of Illinois*. Part of her career has been facilitating a hospital brain injury support group for more than 26 years. She is compassionate and caring and I asked her what weighs heavy on her heart. She said, "So often, the patients fail to get good care post-TBI. I have been able to follow such great people over the years, listen to them, and learn from them. The biggest complaint I've heard from TBI patients is that once discharged from the hospital, and rehabilitation is completed, if they are lucky enough to get it, they feel no one cares that much. They feel the attitude of many, not all, practitioners is that 'it has been treated' and 'you're done now' which is frustrating to me because I know they feel ignored, and need long-term care. Many do not have the luxury of returning to their rehabilitation centers, or to neurologists due to insurance issues, geographic location or major disabilities that prevent them from getting back for adequate care."

So what happens next? You go to your primary care physician, and your actual brain injury is probably not addressed at all. This is not a judgement against doctors but even the kindest well-meaning, skilled physicians do not fully understand the complexity of traumatic brain injuries . . . they are not brain specialists and are ill-equipped to deal with the serious neurological and cognitive issues that linger. This creates more issues because TBI patients often stop paying attention to their health, and start to withdraw, losing friendship and relationships. They tend to eat easy-to-prepare (and affordable) meals that are not healthy; they often can't afford a proper wheelchair or other walking aid. Lazzara shared with me an interesting story. She had a TBI patient with headaches that were musculoskeletal in nature, and this was the result of an ill-fitted wheelchair.

The problem is there is no magic bullet in treating TBI. You should partner with the right healthcare professional who will give you adequate time and attention so that all your needs are met, and you are not ignored. It's the smallest of tweaks that make a big difference, like proper glasses, maybe the right shade on your glasses (some prefer grey, others prefer bronze or rose), sometimes it's a better fitting wheelchair, or routine massage therapy, a great support group where you feel validated and you can share your stories with other courageous, caring persons who are dealing in ways similar to you. I want to thank Ginny Lazzara for her assistance; the following are some of her suggestions for you, if you think you might have headaches from a brain injury:

* Get a correct diagnosis. Seek out a healthcare provider who understands brain injury and has treated headaches.
* Know how to describe your pain. Have someone assist you, if needed, to write down exactly the nature and character of the headache
* Keep a list of medications and supplements that you take. It helps if you can keep a history or calendar of prior headaches and what helped relieve them. If you're uncertain about whether something helped or not, write it down anyway. Your healthcare provider can never have too much information.
* Contact your state Brain Injury Association, if you have one, or contact us at the Brain Injury Association of Illinois 1-800-699-6443 You can visit their site here, www.biail.org

Treatment Modalities

Depending on your injury, energy levels and degree of endurance, some of the following treatments and supplements may help you reduce tension, anxiety and musculoskeletal pain.

Ask your healthcare provider what is right for you, as some of these are perfect, and some are contraindicated based upon your injury and current health status. You may also want to get in with a Neuro-Ophthalmologist and pain specialist for follow-up.

* Physical Therapy
* Biofeedback
* Exercise
* Meditation
* Yoga (no Crow, or other inversions, protect that head!)

* Ice packs
* Heating pad

Options, options!

Ginkgo or vinpocetine (two different herbs sold at health food stores) may be used to improve cognitive function and memory, however these are blood thinners so they may not be right for everyone. They also enhance the effect of anticoagulant drugs like warfarin, Plavix and aspirin.

Strattera- a prescription medication known generically as Atomoxetine, it's often used for people with attention deficit disorder (ADD), but it can also be used "off label" for symptoms related to concussions and TBI.

Mystery Headache Solved: Is It Ice Cream?

Some people call it an "ice cream headache" a "cold headache" or "brain freeze" but it's scientifically called Sphenopalatine gangleoneuralgia. It's a type of headache that occurs immediately after drinking or eating something cold like iced tea or ice cream. Gives 'Rocky Road' a whole new meaning. When you consume something cold, and it comes in contact with the roof your mouth, your blood vessels overreact, the nerves sense this and send pain signals back to the trigeminal nerve cluster which then causes pain in your forehead, temples, underneath or behind you eye. It's referred pain, meaning your mouth feels the sensation, but refers pain up to your head compliments of your well-functioning, or perhaps in this case, touchy trigeminal nerve. But it may also have something to do with blood flow, depending on what study you read.

Researchers induced brain freeze in 13 otherwise healthy adults by having them drink ice cold water. They monitored blood flow in the brain with a Doppler test and found that the headaches were triggered by an abrupt increase in blood flow on the brain's anterior cerebral artery. The pain dissipated quickly, right after the artery constricted (which occurred when they drank warm water). The temperature of the drink really impacted the headaches. Luckily, you only feel stunned by this for 20 or 30 seconds, perhaps for some it can last a few minutes but that's it. If you're prone to these headaches, avoid slurping smoothies, Fraps, sorbets, ice cream, anything cold. If you're experiencing one, you can abort it faster by warming up the roof of your mouth with your tongue, or sipping something lukewarm. You can also cup your hands together, and place over your nose and mouth and breathing in the warm air can quickly abort it. Probably the quickest way to abort it is to suck your thumb, I've seen it done!

Nothing's ever really simple when it comes to head pain, and I'm aware that some of you get different kinds of headaches. Is there a connection between ice cream headaches and migraines? What about ice cream headaches and tension headaches? That's a good question. Researchers looked at exactly that in 76 migraine headache participants and 38 tension headache participants.[8] The researchers documented the pain duration, location, and quality (throbbing) of the headache each patient felt during their ice cream induced headache. It's pretty interesting, 74% of migraineurs and 32% of the tension headache sufferers got a headache around the temple region. Seven of ten migraineurs (the majority) experienced throbbing, but that sensation only occurred in about 8% of the tension headache participants. Based upon this data, researchers concluded that ice cream headaches are more frequent in migraineurs. Like, you don't have enough to deal with already, now you have to microwave your Pralines n' Cream or take your chances on eating it cold.

Three years later, another article[9] appeared in Cephalalgia, entitled *"Ice Cream Headache, A Large Survey of 8,359 Adolescents."* This article was based on the results of data collected by asking questions to teenagers in Taiwan. These were 13 to 15 year old students who filled out questionnaires. A little over 40% of these kids confessed to ice cream headaches. Boys got them more frequently than girls. The researchers also found that students who suffered from migraine headaches had substantially more bouts of ice cream headaches than students who did not suffer from migraine headaches. The take home point? If you are prone to migraines, you are more likely to get brain freeze, so minimize or avoid cold drinks and ice cream. That mint chocolate chip swirl simply isn't worth it!

Mystery Headaches Solved: Is it Bright Light?

Light sensitivity or "photophobia" is common among migraineurs and research proves it worsens your situation. I can spot you quickly because you are the ones wearing sunglasses in normal daylight, or in a doctor's office, or inside the mall. You're the one that doesn't want to be in any photos, or you'll oblige to just one, and only if the flash isn't used. You are never the one to photobomb a picture. I'm actually a little light sensitive myself, but not in any big way, I just like my Maui Jim rose-colored sunglasses and wear them at all times. Luckily, I do not get repercussions like some of you. Bright sunshine glaring off a car, bright headlights, or sun reflecting off the snow (or beach) will sometimes spark a short-lived migraine for Sam, and if it doesn't, the possibility exists that he'll temporarily lose his vision in the periphery, much like optic neuritis.

Headache sufferers have so much more to deal with on a daily basis than just the hours during their headache. I'm sorry this is part of your life, and I'm doing my darndest to help you uncover causes, and give you real solutions.

For some of you, the slightest change in lighting can can trigger a migraine. A 2010 study published in *Nature Neuroscience* showed that even blind migraineurs have a painful aversion to flashes of bright light. The researchers think that migraines are tied to the part of your brain that identifies light as light, not the part of your brain which gives you eyesight. So the legally blind people who can still detect light suffered, but the totally blind folks (who don't detect light) were not at all affected by the flashes. Researchers think that's because legally blind people still have functional melanopsin receptors, whereas totally blind folks do not.

Do you have a relative whose eyes are always closed in pictures? This could be another expression of light sensitivity. According to a study published in the journal *Headache* (2008), migraine sufferers are more likely to blink when a camera flash goes off, and they're also more apt to wear sunglasses in normal daylight. Twenty six percent of participants surveyed answer "no" to the question, "Does light bother you?" but when asked if they prefer a dark room, 91% of them said "yes." That's basically the quick fix. Avoid bright lights.

Here are some other tips for you:
Don't look directly at the sun

Invest in sunglasses, the polarized lenses are a must; the bronze or rose tones are my favorite, however, you may prefer grey or green tinted lens.

* There are computer eyeglasses you can wear that are specially tinted
* Change your light bulbs in your home, from fluorescent to incandescent
* Avoid flickering lights, strobe lights and camera flashes
* Install "Flux" on your computer. Flux is downloadable (free) software that automatically makes your computer screen look like the room you're in, and it adjusts itself constantly. Because I work on my laptop about 18 hours a day, I have this installed. When the sun sets, it makes my computer screen go almost 'sepia' but it's very subtle. In the morning, it makes things look like sunlight again, but it's not bright. I highly recommend Flux, it has made a huge difference for me in terms of eye strain. It's downloadable from the website: justgetflux.com
* Take a dietary supplement BioAstin astaxanthin 6 to 12mg once daily (www.Nutrex-Hawaii.com). Many studies10-15 show it reduces eye fatigue, and I think it could only help. Use coupon code "suzy" for 25% off the price.
* Put a lavender eye pack over your eyes
* Eyebright (which is an herb) maybe a natural eye tonic that helps you and it is rich in vitamin C. This can be purchased at any health food store as a liquid extract or capsule. I've seen it sold as a tea by various makers, and of course, if you're a tea junkie like me, you can make your own if you buy some dried herb and steep it in water.
* Rich's "MSM Water Drops" for general eye health, it's an eye drop.
* Tulsi tea or supplements support eye health and capillaries in the body.
* If you don't mind looking a bit like a fly, buy yourself "Pinhole glasses." These don't prevent migraines but I think they'll reduce eye strain. It's a cool phenomenon that I wouldn't believe unless I tried it. They allow you to see clearly, without corrective lenses if you have blurry vision.

Astaxanthin & Macular Degeneration

We all know about lutein, zeaxanthin and beta carotene . . . well, astaxanthin is a relative newcomer in this category of "carotenoids" so it should support eye health just as well, maybe better. I asked my friend Stuart Richer, OD, PhD who is the Director of Ocular Preventive Medicine at the *James Lovell Federal Health Care Facility* in North Chicago to weigh in. I think Dr. Richer is perfect to ask because he is actively involved in primary care optometry and clinical antioxidant research. He literally studies this very topic! Dr. Richer has a passion for the aging eye, and how you can utilize nutrients to help age related macular degeneration (ARMD), low-tension glaucoma, diabetic macular edema, prevention of cataracts and dry eye. He is sweet enough to enlighten us with these comments:

"In the front of the eye, research has shown that astaxanthin improves ocular ciliary body function that controls accommodation or focusing. This would be particularly important to aging baby-boomers who often experience heavy visual (screen time) demands. For older patients, astaxanthin could be added to an age-related macular degeneration (AMD) regimen, as this carotenoid helps to mitigate damaging UV and blue light. It is a potent anti inflammatory and crosses the blood-retinal barrier unlike many larger molecular weight dietary molecules. A recently published study suggests that astaxanthin improves the primary ocular vascular circulation, known as the choroid - supplying 95% of the blood delivered to the back of the eye." What he's saying is that this study proves astaxanthin sends more blood to your delicate ocular tissue and this in turn, nourishes and protects your eyesight.

Mystery Headaches Solved: Is It a Fake Sweetener?

You know to avoid artificial sweeteners altogether, don't ever ever consume anything with those if you have headaches. But what about the sugar-alcohols like sorbitol? Sorbitol naturally occurs in fruits like plums, peaches, pears, prunes and apples. It's produced commercially from corn syrup, not these lovely fruits, and it's used as a sugar substitute in many foods. You'll find sorbitol in foods labeled "sugar free" or "lite" or "reduced calorie." For example, jams, cake mixes, snack bars, candy, whipped topping. It's in a lot of gums, toothpaste and mouthwash! It's a laxative for most people, and can cause diarrhea, bloating and stomachache. It's found in many drugs even those used for headache such as "Advil Migraine." But the joke here is that sorbitol, like many of the artificial sweeteners can trigger migraines, at least that's what my friends tell me. No one is sure of the link, it could be that sorbitol causes some minor irritable bowel issues, and that is a trigger. However it happens, my migraineur friends have reported episodes of either diarrhea or migraines soon after eating foods with sorbitol. If you suspect sorbitol is tied to your head pain, get it out of your diet, along with all the artificial sweeteners like sucralose, saccharin and aspartame.

Aspartame is a popular artificial sweetener sold under the brand name of Equal. It's found in hundreds of thousands of foods, you have to read the ingredient list because it's not always clear on the label. Aspartame has been linked to pediatric and adolescent migraines. After you eat or drink foods containing aspartame (usually found in blue-colored packets), it is broken down, converted and oxidized during a chemical reaction where it forms formaldehyde. They use formaldehyde to embalm bodies you know. This toxin goes into various tissues all over your body, including your brain. The quick fix? Eliminate every beverage and food that contains aspartame, as well as any other artificial sweetener.

Mystery Headaches Solved: Is It a Chiari Headache?

Sometimes the headache stems from the back of your head, especially on exertion. This is one of the hallmark symptoms of a condition called "Chiari Malformation" and the headache often has neck pain associated with it. The brainstem or cerebellum is involved and whenever that happens, all sorts of painful or unique symptoms occur, all over the body.

I've included this type of headache in my "Mystery" headache chapter because you may have Chiari, and not realize it. Chiari isn't given enough attention, and people who suffer with it have very little information and research. It's important for me to help raise awareness for this condition. Information is power. When I say Chiari, I want you it's more officially known as "Arnold-Chiari" and there are actually 4 main kinds, named I through IV using Roman numerals. Since this isn't a Chiari book, I'm not going to put time into describing those. I'm specifically interested in talking about the headaches associated with Chiari.They almost always cause pain in the back of your head, but it could radiate to the front of your head and/or behind your eye(s). If you exert yourself, the headache may show up, or worsen.

For example, you take a heavy bag of trash out for your wife and your head suddenly hurts, or you bounce some basketballs around with the guys and notice a headache soon after. It doesn't even have to be that pronounced, for example, you sneeze, cough or bend forward to pick up something and the pain begins.

I've been very forthcoming in this book, sharing with you many stories about my husband Sam who has had every headache in the book, literally! We thought he had Chiari for a time too, even though his imaging scans did not prove it. But some of the symptoms were there, so we sent his MRI images to a specialist in New York, who told us to come, they assured us they could help him. With great relief, we charged everything to get there, during the worst hurricane in history (Hurricane Sandy), flight cancellations, then countless delays, flooding, crazy cab drivers, subway delays, and so on. When we walked into the office, we waited 4 hours to see the doctor. He looked over Sam's MRI for about 1 minute, asked him 2 basic questions about his health and said, "Why are you here? You don't have Chiari and I'm sorry that we can't do anything for you." Whaaaat?!

Tears fell for the next hour, all of our hope gone, and the frustration of having been told to come and buy a hotel stay for a week (to do the surgery). I had even called the office (one of the nation's leading clinics in Long Island, what a joke) to make sure everything was set, and make sure they'd read the MRIs, because traveling was a challenge. But when a cure is in sight, you do anything, don't you? Sigh . . . Looking back, Sam only had a few symptoms involving his cranial nerves, he had insomnia and visual changes; fortunately, he was living headache free at this point and had been for a few years. Still after many years of dealing with nonsense, you hear what you want to hear, and when you live with changing symptoms that affect your cranial nerves, and someone tells you, "Come over, I will help you," you tend to believe.

I share that story because I truly understand your trials and tribulations, the heartache of not having a diagnosis, or having one for a few weeks and then suddenly *not* having it! Incompetent doctors, rude staff at times, the roller coaster of emotions, the constant outpouring of money to people who are supposed to heal you, and don't. Many don't even have a clue what's wrong with you, and just pretend. I want you to see how easily headaches and other brain pain syndromes can be misdiagnosed. Some so-called experts mistake Chiari for migraines, go figure, they are not even close. They give Chiari patients lots of triptans that don't work, and harm you by altering your brain neurotransmitters (something you don't need to touch).

Other "experts" tell you they can help, and layer one drug on top of another, until you are a zombie with the same symptoms you started with, plus more from the medication side effects. Never submit yourself to surgery for Chiari unless it is absolutely proven and visible on your scans. In retrospect, those crazy people in New York could have soaked us and done surgery on Sam, and it wouldn't have helped him one bit, so we do count our blessings in that regard. As you know if you've been reading my book, his countless headaches were tied to an infection (Lyme and co-infections).

Chiari can be diagnosed at any age, and in fact, it may become more evident after a head or neck injury, such as one you might get from a car accident, a fall or a sports injury. Every now and then I hear that a person develops Chiari (or symptoms that look just like Chiari) from their epidural, spinal tap or after surgery.

Some other symptoms of Chiari that may be part of the clinical picture include hoarseness, difficulty swallowing, times of the night where you stop breathing temporarily, termed "sleep apnea," problems balancing, clumsiness, weakness, numbness or weakness of an extremity. In an infant, the symptoms are pretty general and could look like many other symptoms. Nevertheless, I want all you new moms and dads to be aware of Chiari because your infant can't talk yet, so the signs and symptoms become more important. They include trouble feeding and swallowing, excessive drooling, very noisy breathing especially with crying, apnea (stop breathing spells), head banging, stiff neck, irritability, and nighttime awakenings (which could be a sign of headache). These infants have trouble crawling due to poor arm strength. As a result, the diagnosis of Chiari is often delayed until more severe symptoms occur or after current symptoms persist for some time.

Symptoms are caused by disruption of the CSF (cerebrospinal fluid) flow and compression of the brainstem tissue. For this reason there are literally hundreds of symptoms, and I will list a few of them now, but remember, having these doesn't necessarily mean you have Chiari, it's just possible. Imaging is key to proper diagnosis:

Neck pain, across your shoulder blades
Chest pain,
Joint hypermobility (Ehler-Danlos syndrome)

Dizziness
Tinnitus or hearing loss
Blurred or double vision
Light sensitivity
Floaters and jerking eye movements (nystagmus)
Fatigue
Snoring
Insomnia
Facial pain, numbness or tingling
Changes in voice
Chronic cough
Weakness, numbness or poor coordination of arms and legs
Difficulty finding words
Memory problems
Depression
Irregular heart beat
Passing out or "drop" attacks
Urinary problems
Cystitis

The take home point for you is to be aware that Chiari malformation can trigger headaches and that may be the cause of your pain. Proper diagnosis is important becuase bony and soft tissue abnormalities may compress the spinal cord, brain stem, blood vessels or cranial nerves resulting in a wide variety of symptoms, not necessarily Chiari. Infections that get up in there can do it too! Tethered cord syndrome is different than Chiari, so correct diagnosis is important. Accurate diagnosis is key to effective treatment, which is usually surgical. I won't lie, there are no herbs or vitamins that I know that will cure this. In fact, most sufferers spend boatloads of money on migraine medicine, antidepressants, muscle relaxers, TENS units, acupuncture, chiropractic, and other modalities to no avail. Your best bet if you don't do surgery, is a licensed Physical Therapist who is very familiar with Chiari patients, and perhaps gentle massage. No chiropractic! You can certainly try any of the palliative remedies and teas listed in the Migraine and Cluster chapter, but again, there is no quick fix or supplement that helps this structural issue (you need a neurosurgeon), and an experienced one at that! For more information, visit www.ConquerChiari.org or www.cfsingo.org. There are also Chiari thrivers on facebook if you care to search those individual pages out.

Mystery Headaches Solved: Is it a Sinus Headache?

I bet you think that when your headache is accompanied by a stuffy or runny nose or itchy, watery eyes that you have a sinus headache. Not necessarily, these symptoms can accompany a migraine too. The pain is in the forehead, and it's often associated with movement just like a migraine. The way to tell if your headache is migraine or sinus related is by the following:

Do you have nausea or vomiting?

Are you highly sensitive to light, noise, smells or touch?

Is your pain on one side?

Is your vision affected?

If you answered yes to any of those questions, you probably have a migraine not a sinus headache. If you have a genuine sinus headache, then the order is that you got sick, developed signs and symptoms of a cold, *and then the headache began.*

Sinus headaches happen because you have an infection, or chronic allergy. The ducts that connect the sinuses to the back of your nose get irritated and inflamed and then your sinuses can't drain properly so the pressure builds up in the blocked sinus cavities. The lining of the sinuses become swollen and inflamed with excess fluid and mucus. This is termed sinusitis, and it's what sparks the sinus headache. Keep in mind a sinus headache doesn't have any neurological feature like a migraine, nor is it connected to a damaged trigeminal nerve like a cluster headache is. There's no issue of referred pain like a tension headache.

It's a completely different type of headache, and as far as headaches go, it is not that bad. Frustrating yes, painful absolutely, but dangerous? No. Chronic, in some cases yes. To completely relieve a sinus headache, you need to start by removing the allergen (bedding, food, mold, pollen) or by treating your infection with an antibiotic, herbal or prescribed. Samento is the brand name of a good broad-spectrum herbal antibiotic made from Cat's Claw. It's my go-to remedy if I even so much as feel a sniffle coming on, or if I have to take a plane trip. Planes are full of recirculated germs. Samento is made by Nutramedix company, and it's sold at their website. You can use whatever you want. This is a good time to remind you of the importance of probiotics because those increase immunity, and reduce pathogen load.

For me, my go-to probiotic is always Dr. Ohhira's Probiotic, it restores my own microbiome, and the blend is guaranteed to be live and viable. I take this every day. I can't even remember the last time I got a cold or dealt with sinusitis. In my 20's, I had sinus headaches once or twice a month easily. For me, the cure was to eliminate dairy for 6 months. Now, I eat some kind of dairy (perhaps cheese or ice cream) only once or twice a month with no trouble at all. But there was a time I lived on doxycycline and Afrin, no more, not in 20 something years. If you want to read more about this particular probiotic, turn to page 198.

Intranasal steroids like Flonase are often prescribed for a short period of time to reduce swelling in the passages. Unlike migraines and tension headaches, sinus headaches are short-lived. If they are chronic for you, you've missed something. Perhaps you are allergic to dairy, this is a biggie for sinus headache sufferers. Every person that I've ever suggested to go dairy-free has reported to me that their sinus headaches completely cleared up. Sometimes it's your bedding, are you allergic to down? Are you allergic to dust mites? You can buy covers for your pillows and mattress to protect yourself from dust mites. I did this for all the beds in my own home. You have to determine what the driving factor is for your own sinus headaches. Triptans and ergotamine drugs are not at all helpful for a person with chronic sinus headaches. Anti-inflammatories like acetaminophen or ibuprofen can help short-term, but again you have to find the underlying cause.

As a pharmacist, I've seen people buying nasal sprays 3 or 4 bottles of Afrin at a time! That is not your solution! That only tells me you are addicted to these drugs, and you are having rebound headaches when the spray wears off.

The condition is called "Rhinitis Medicamentosa" or RM and it will cause a chronically stuffy nose. It happens from overuse of nasal decongestant sprays... the ones with active ingredients in them, not the ones with pure saline. You can develop RM by overusing Afrin or Neo-Synephrine (the ones which contain oxymetazoline or phenylephrine). I know it provides relief for you, but if you use these for more than 3 or 4 days (in full dosages) you run the risk of getting RM, and it's really hard to break the habit. It happens because the underlying cause of your condition wasn't addressed, so you keep using the spray, and after a few days, you need the spray for relief. When it wears off, you need to spray again, and before you know it, you are addicted, literally. Breaking this habit is almost as hard as going off caffeine, which some of you need to do also.

With nasal sprays, you'll need to wean off very slowly. I would alternate nostrils with each use, or use one spray instead of two. You can fill the gap with menthol nasal spray, or saline. You can also run a steam vaporizer or humidifier. Adding a little eucalyptus essential oil to the water may help. If you really need assistance because you've stuck on these nose sprays for months, then ask your doctor for a prescription of a nasal corticosteroid, like Nasonex, Flonase, Nasalide, and use it for a week or maybe two, not forever. The best thing you can do is find out what the underlying food allergy, or structural problem, or infection is. Only when you uncover and fix that will your sinus headache pain go away for good. Also, check out www.FluNada.com.

Mystery Headaches Solved: Is It Related to Testosterone?

A study led by "Check and Cohen" at the *Cooper Medical School of Rowan University* found that DHT or dihydrotestosterone plays a role in migraine headaches. So they the gave a drug called finasteride (Proscar) to a young woman with chronic migraines to see what happened since the drug lowers levels of DHT in the body. The drug finasteride is sold under two brand names, one is "Propecia" for male pattern baldness, and the other is "Proscar" for prostate enlargement. So it's kind of interesting to me, since she has no prostate, that they'd choose a woman for their analysis versus a man but I'm not in charge of these decisions. I suspect, they're working off the fact that finasteride is a powerful DHT inhibitor and DHT is present in females too. So it makes sense from this standpoint. Lo and behold, *"The chronic migraine headaches almost completely disappeared shortly following therapy."* That quote comes straight out of the study which was published in 2013 *Clinical and Experimental Obstetrics & Gynecology.*[10] I'd like to say this has a happy ending, but she gave up the finasteride due to dry eyes, a side effect. Then her headaches returned!

I conclude from this one-person study, that we need more studies, bigger ones! Especially because there are anecdotal reports of people using Propecia for baldness and getting headaches, just the opposite of what one would expect. Nevertheless, the researchers conclude that DHT plays a role in the development of migraines, or that perhaps the resulting increase in testosterone from finasteride does. They're not sure, and neither am I so I can't recommend this drug to you yet. Discuss it with your physician. I asked my go-to guy on all things confusing to lend his insight. He is very smart, and studies all the time to help his patients feel their best. I'm referring to my good friend and Functional Medicine doctor, Douglas Hall, MD who has been in the field of obstetrics and gynecology for more than 4 decades. He pointed out, "Another possibility that was not considered in this study is how DHT increases Thromboxane A-2, a strong vasoconstrictor. One theory in migraines is the alteration of blood flow in the brain, so DHT can indirectly cause vasoconstriction. This results in elevated intracranial pressure. The finasteride would make sense because it lowers DHT, and reducing Thromboxane A-2. It's a back door way to controlling the hormonally-induced vasoconstriction which affects the brain."

All of this made me wonder about natural DHT blockers. Why not? The argument against them is that we have one case study of one woman who responded to a drug that blocks DHT. I know this is enough for some of you to want to try it yourself too. But drugs are potent and they have side effects galore. Why couldn't we capitalize on natural herbs or foods that do a similar thing, that are weaker but still block DHT? It couldn't hurt you to try eating a few more pumpkin seeds right? And oysters, and green tea . . . these are all natural DHT blockers. I eat those foods all the time. Keep in mind green tea has some caffeine and that's a trigger for some of you.

DHT, Testosterone & Estrogen

Testosterone is converted into dihydrotestosterone (DHT) and Estradiol (E2). Imagine opposite ends of seesaw, that's how these two hormones are in your body. DHT blockers can increase estradiol, which exacerbates hormonally-driven cancers in the reproductive tract. Too much estrogen in men leads to man boobs, low libido and erectile dysfunction.

There are supplements that naturally block DHT, and you should ask your doctor if these are okay to experiment with: Saw palmetto, eleuthero roots, pygeum extract and beta sitosterol. Zinc is another one that is easy to find in tasty lozenges.

Herbs are plant-derived drugs so remember to use low dosages and start slowly. With your docs blessings, you can pick up one of these at any health food store, and try taking it for 1 week of each month and see if you note a difference, or maybe 3 times per week for an entire month; these don't have to be taken every single day to get an effect. I worry about you doing that because these could alter your hormones in a way that doesn't serve you. They are effecting testosterone levels, DHT, estrogen, and so forth, all of this impacts the rest of your hormonal system, and your entire body. I like to 'think outside the pill' but I always want you to be safe.

Mystery Headaches Solved: Is It a Toothache?

A common cause of headache is an abscessed tooth, which occurs from a crack in the tooth, and subsequent infection. You might not even realize your headaches are coming from your mouth so I recommend routine dental check ups. Dental headaches are quite common. Did you know that the trigeminal nerve has a branch called the lingual nerve which is in the mouth, and it's a major nerve pathway. It allows for your tongue to have sensation. The trigeminal nerve is the very same nerve that sends shockwaves of pain during attacks of trigeminal neuralgia, or cluster headaches. So if the lingual nerve is irritated, inflamed or infected from a cracked or infected tooth, this branch sends its throbbing, shooting and stabbing signal from the lingual nerve, up through the trigeminal nerve, all around your head, especially the top and sides of your head. It could totally cause your head pain! One person described his pain like this:

I had a wisdom tooth that was eventually removed. Before it was removed I had the worst migraine that it felt like my left side was pounding louder than a bass drum. It felt like I was numb on that side not to mention that I wasn't able to concentrate.

The only way to relieve this type of pain is to clear the infection. If that is not possible, I recommend an extraction. I don't really believe in root canals, I worry that they harbor germs which can enter your bloodstream. There's a lot of controversy surrounding root canals and I can't decide what's right for you so talk over the pros and cons with your dentist. You can always seek the advice of a biological dentist, they are more holistic in their approach and they have a different tool box from which they draw their cures from. A dental thermography can detect areas of inflammation in your mouth, in case you are opposed to X rays. Thermography is completely painless, it's a picture. It's hard to find a place that does this, but you're luck improves if you get in with a biological dentist. Biological dentists recognize the impact of toxic materials and relate it to dental and physiological health. They do not use mercury. To find a dentist like this, visit the website for *The International Academy of Oral Medicine and Toxicology* and put in your zip code. Here's the site: www.iaomt.org

I interviewed my favorite dentist Elliott Higgins, DMD, of *Pearl Street Dental* in Boulder, Colorado, who has over 30 years experience. He's my "favorite" because he is super nice and kind-hearted. His lovely staff has worked my loved ones and I in quickly during times of need, plus he uses breakthrough technology like digital microscopes, digital X-rays and laser technology which means fewer needles, numbing and drills. Who here isn't happy with that?! Dr. Higgins isn't just a dentist, he's one of those forward thinkers, and caters to cowards like me by making every procedure quick, comfortable and painless. I didn't need this, but I think it's cool he can do same day crowns using amazing same day "chairside restoration" technology which produces all ceramic crowns, inlays and veneers at the same time.

What about mystery headaches related to your teeth? Yes, he's seen it many times. According to Dr. Higgins, "Some of my patients have experienced headache relief after I've addressed their infected tooth so this is definitely an underlying cause of headaches for some patients. If a patient comes to me with a failed root canal, that should be considered for extraction rather than re-treatment. Further, implants may provide the most dependable result for some patients, although it's a case by case situation since everyone is unique. Since dental health plays a major role in your general health and well-being, I want to emphasize the importance of good nutrition and the avoidance of refined and processed foods, artificial sweeteners, GMO products and sugar. Remember, your teeth are a reflection of the health of your body." To learn more about Dr. Higgins and his minimally invasive techniques visit www.PearlStreetDental.com or find him on Facebook.

Teeccino: Coffee Drink Without Caffeine

Love the taste and smell of coffee, but can't drink it because of the caffeine?

For some of you, caffeine is a trigger for your headache, even the decaf sort which still has caffeine, and has similar effects on your nervous system because caffeine isn't the only compound in coffee causing sensitivity and migraines. No food is worth the pain, that's why I suggest Teeccino. That's a brand of herbal coffee that tastes like the real deal, but it is completely free of caffeine and other headache-inducing compounds including dairy and gluten. I love the chocolate flavor but it also comes in hazelnut. Leave it to me to find you something amazing that does not compromise flavor! Other benefits are that Teeccino does not cause the jitters, anxiety, sweaty palms, insomnia or reflux. Here's a testimonial from Jamie:

I have always liked the flavor of coffee, but after realizing that caffeine was one of my headache triggers I knew I needed to find an alternative to coffee (even an alternative to decaf). I also wanted an alternative that wasn't as acidic as coffee. I'm so happy I found Teeccino! My favorite flavors are chocolate and hazelnut. I will definitely be a lifelong Teeccino drinker!

Mystery Headache Solved: Is it Caffeine Withdrawal?

I know you love your coffee, so do I. I affectionately call it my 'brains in a cup.' I probably drank no less than 100 in the making of this book with all the long hours I put in. Sam makes me the best with organic Kona coffee and almond milk, along with natural maple sugar and grated cacao on top. I'm fully aware that it can be a double edged sword because if you're used to your morning cup of coffee, and you miss it one day you'll get a headache within hours. I don't get many headaches at all, but I confess I fall into this particular category. I will feel the effects of not having coffee within a day or two.

For me, the pain is dull, constant and one sided, and it won't go away until I drink some coffee. Rarely it is stubborn and I need 200mg of ibuprofen. This kind of headache isn't dangerous in my opinion, there's no vision loss, nausea or vomiting, it has no aura and it is not neurologically based.

I'm going to take a lot of flack for what I'm about to say, but I've seen ugly headaches before, the kind that are horrendous and so I'm not going to worry about you if you get caffeine withdrawal headaches. If you are otherwise healthy, and eating well, including lots of healthy greens and you juice, and you exercise. I do all of that myself, and I'm in good shape. I love the aroma of freshly brewed coffee, in fact I'm having a cup right now.

So we are guilty of loving a latte, so what?! You can stop anytime you want to. I know I can, I've stopped a dozen times just to try out different diets. Far be it from me to preach to you to give up your morning coffee in order to avoid the caffeine withdrawal. Do I wish you'd wean off and get off caffeine completely? Sure, because caffeine can be a trigger for some of you.

But I'll leave that decision up to you. If it's a habit you want to break, I commend you, and recommend that you wean yourself off coffee slowly, and onto an alternative such as Teeccino herbal coffee, which tastes as good but does not have caffeine or other stimulants in it. If you are allergic to the components in that, then just drink herbal tea.

And contrarily, if that piping hot drink is part of your happy day, and you offset the acidity of that treat with a healthy, organic diet full of leafy greens, then go ahead and enjoy yourself. I'm all about enjoying your life, and like I said, caffeine withdrawal headaches aren't that big of a deal in my book. Probably because I've seen the ugly ones up close, like migraines and clusters, and trigeminal neuralgia . . . now those are major headache syndromes!

If you have heart disease, diabetes, high blood pressure, anxiety or insomnia it's better for you to avoid caffeine, and I advise you wean yourself off. And if we're talking about a serious addiction of coffee, like 4 to 8 cups per day, that's a totally different story, and one that requires you to change your lifestyle because it's crashing your adrenals. I'm imagining one, perhaps two cups a day. Let me say it outright, I'm tired of reading articles that make you feel guilty for small pleasures and I'm not going to do that to you. Cheers!

Time to Clean Out Your Medicine Cabinet - Just Do It!

Some of you need to clean out your medicine cabinet because you may have expired or recalled pain medicine. After a flurry of studies proving increased heart attacks among patients using certain anti-inflammatories, several drugs went by the wayside. Among them, over-the-counter Orudis KT (ketoprofen) voluntarily discontinued their drug, and in 2004, Vioxx (rofecoxib) was withdrawn from the market. Then in 2005, Bextra (valdecoxib) was withdrawn. If you have any of the withdrawn medications, I would throw them out immediately so check your medicine cabinet today.

Mystery Headaches Solved: Is It Lovemaking?

You know the standing joke "not tonight dear, I have a headache" well in this case, sex gives you the headache. And it's not just sex, I could easily retitle this section for headaches induced by coughing, or exertion, because it's all related to the same thing. So if you have headaches that are triggered by coughing, or by exercising or overexertion, read on. I'm still going to talk about this situation openly because sex-induced headaches are not frequently discussed. I'm not sure if it's because you, the patient, is too embarrassed to bring it up with your doctor, or if your doctor just blows you off and focuses on something else during your visit like your thyroid or glucose levels. Regardless, sex headaches, also called "orgasmic headaches" are common. It is estimated that 1 in 100 people will suffer from a sex headache at some time during their life.[12] I think it's higher than that because reporting is slack. Typically, sex headaches occur in men between the ages of 20 and 25 years old and in men between 35 and 45 years old.[13] I'm willing to bet migraineurs and clusterheads are more prone to these.

It's an unfortunate phenomenon, the joy of sex colored by the gloom of a violent headache. Termed "coital cephalalgia" "benign coital headache" there's nothing really benign about a headache sneaking up at you at the point of no return! These are brought on by sexual activity (and like I mentioned, also exercise or coughing). Some of you notice the dull achy headache during sex, and it may build up with excitement. If you've had this headache, you've probably wondered if you were going to die from an aneurysm. I can imagine this is quite scary.

Sex headaches are the result of increased blood pressure and heart rate as the fun continues. It's a terrible catch 22 isn't it? The pain often begins at the base of the brain, but not always; the pain may radiate to the front of your head at any point. It may last a few minutes then dissipate, or linger for a few hours. Most don't get a headache at all, until you get to the Big O, as in orgasm. Yes! Yes! OH NO! At that point, the headache comes on suddenly, and is rather severe. That's why they're referred to as "thunderclap" headaches. They have nothing to do with thunder, or weather. Thunderclap headaches just mean the intensity builds quickly, and the headache comes on suddenly . . . no aura, no warning, and rather painful. The pain may subside within a few minutes, but if it's "postural" it will reoccur as soon as you get out of bed and stand up. Lots of you have sworn off sex.

In a Russian study, researchers found 19 participants who suffered from sex headaches.[14] Fifteen men and four women were evaluated. The researchers discovered that 58% of these participants reported the headaches developed during foreplay, before orgasm and 26% of the participants developed the headaches during orgasm. The remaining 16% of the participants developed their headaches after their orgasm. The duration of the sex headaches varied for all participants, however, most headaches lasted for several minutes. In one participant, their sex headache lasted 24 hours! The researchers suspect that sex headaches are caused from a *"disturbance of venous outflow and dysfunction of antinociceptive systems."* Essentially, something is amiss with your blood vessel around your brain and your pain perception. Experts also wonder if it happens from an increase in blood (arterial) pressure combined with tension from big event.

That makes sense to my good friend, Douglas Hall, MD, a Functional Medicine doctor who has four decades experience in obstetrics and gynecology in Ocala, Florida. He says, *"Endothelial dysfunction with low nitric oxide (NO) can cause vasoconstriction with resulting headaches. You can check NO levels with urine testing strips. NO is stimulated by estrogen and thyroid so you might have to increase these hormones to a physiologically normal level in order to prevent the headaches."*

So to make sure you understand, it is low estrogen in this case, or perhaps, low thyroid hormone that needs to get raised to physiologically healthy levels then the NO goes up. It's not a slam dunk though (why is everything so complicated in health?) because in the presence of endothelial dysfunction, the endothelial cell would be unable to respond and make nitric oxide. Over time, this will raise your risk or cause all sorts of problems including diabetes, hypertension, peripheral artery disease, thrombosis, high homocysteine and atherosclerosis. If you have any of these symptoms, do what Dr. Hall does, ask the question, "Why?"

One way to test for endothelial dysfunction is called "Flow Mediated Dilatation" of the brachial artery. Special equipment is required which Dr. Hall and other progressive docs have in their office. You monitor the blood flow through the brachial artery with special Doppler for baseline. The nurse or doctor puts a blood pressure cuff on you, and pumps it up above systolic pressure until you feel some numbness in the fingers indicating you are creating oxygen debt in those tissues. Then you let the cuff down. In normal cases, the endothelial cells will produce increasing amounts of nitric oxide to dilate the brachial artery which increases blood flow to replace the oxygen debt. Failure to see proper dilatation, indicates endothelial dysfunction. What do cardiologist usually do in this case? Say something like, " I think you should go on some Lisinopril." Supplements that increase nitric oxide may be helpful instead. Well, it's an idea for you.

I talked candidly with two people who had experienced sex headaches, and they were deeply frustrated because they were told to lose weight (neither one was more than 10 pounds above normal), and/or to refrain from sex. That "solution" doesn't sound like it would make either partner in the relationship very happy. I felt sorry for these guys, both sweet and just terrified to have a relationship again. It causes too much pain.

And to pay $150 or more for a doctor's visit and labs, and work ups . . . for what, to be told *"Don't have sex if it makes your head hurt."* That's what they were both told.

Duh. Thankfully, many doctors do take you seriously, and offer medications for pain or to reduce blood pressure like the prescription, propranolol.

I can offer you a few other suggestions, and you don't have to pay me a doctor's visit. Try the following and see if this helps:

* Be honest with your partner if you've been avoiding intimacy. I'm not sure, but I suspect your relationship will suffer more if you don't say why the two of you can't have sex.
* Take an anti-inflammatory about 1 hour before the big event, such as 500mg acetaminophen or 400mg ibuprofen. These will have no effect if you take them once the pain begins.
* Don't be so active during sex, try to take it easier if you know what I mean.
* Maybe race a little faster to the finish line as opposed to lingering for an hour to get there, stopping and starting, stopping and starting . . . while tantric sex has it's virtues, it's probably going to exacerbate the situation because it keeps your blood pressure up for a longer time.
* Drugs known as "beta blockers" like propranolol are sometimes used, but not with great success. You can certainly ask your physician to try medicine in this category. And you can eat foods that have natural beta blocking activity in the body. Those foods include bananas, potatoes, raisins, white beans, celery, orange juice, spinach, and chamomile.
* Progesterone. Guys, you can buy this as a cream over-the-counter at health food stores, or online, or take it as a prescription pill such a Prometrium. Progesterone is the pregnancy hormone, produced naturally when a woman is pregnant. You must think I'm crazy to suggest this to you but why not? There's a case study that proved its benefit to a man who suffered 27 years with severe sex headaches! His wife got pregnant. His condition was "spontaneously relieved in the first trimester of his partner's pregnancy. This relief continued through the remainder of the pregnancy term, returning only after the birth of their child." The timing of his relief, and subsequent return of headaches after delivery suggests that progesterone helped him. His doctor tested the theory and prescribed "norethisterone 5mg" a medication that contains a synthetic form of progesterone. The brand name of this drug is called Micronor. The drug derived from peanuts is Prometrium, it's more natural than norethisterone, there are no studies to support it, but it is a type of progesterone so I want you to have it as an option.

Probiotics, Probiotics, Probiotics!

Antibiotics are so over-prescribed so I want to preface this section by acknowledging that fact. I don't advocate pill-popping for every itch and scratch, in fact, I find the big commercial push for medications rather annoying. But I'm responsible, and do think it's important to stay on your medicine if you're treating a dangerous pathogen such as Borellia, Bartonella, Babesia, certain species of Clostridium, E. Coli, MRSA, West Nile, Legionella, Anthrax, Strep pyogenes and others. Just FYI, that last bug eats flesh!

People with Lyme disease notoriously take antibiotics, sometimes 3 or 4 at a time. These drugs harm your gastrointestinal tract. Everyone knows antibiotics can harm your GI tract and annihilate beneficial flora, but so can any other drug going through your GI tract. If it's prescription or over-the-counter, it has the ability to harm your probiotic stash, and that can affect brain pain.

You're intestines, especially the large intestine is a major warehouse for your immune cells, which help you fight infection. There are about 10,000 different kinds of microorganisms living inside you, and these 'germs' weigh about 2 to 3 pounds. There's about 100 trillion little organisms which outnumbers your own body's cells. Freaky, but in a good way! And here's the craziest part, your genetic material is made up primarily of these beneficial bacteria, located mainly in your intestines (and skin, vagina, nose and mouth). Think of your gut flora as a garden, one that you need to maintain with 'fertilizer' and 'weed killer,' by that I mean high-quality probiotics.

Everyone has their own microflora, what I call a 'flora fingerprint' and it's unique to you, kind of like a thumbprint is, and where 70 to 80% of your immune system lives. Your gut flora makes natural antibiotics. Beneficial flora is the first thing to be compromised when you take prescribed antibiotics, in fact, if you take any medication. New studies shows that probiotics can modulate your immune system and offer you strong anti-inflammatory effects. Remember, with headaches of any sort (and Lyme disease) there is an upregulation in certain pathways that causes you to make more pro-inflammatory cytokines. Probiotics are an inexpensive way to reduce inflammation, support immune function and put back what the drug mugger stole. Drugs mug probiotics, all of them. Other than keeping bad bacteria under control, what else can probiotics do?

Improve energy and metabolism- Adequate flora helps you convert T4 hormone to T3 hormone which is active thyroid hormone. You want that conversion to take place because thyroid hormone is what gives you energy, helps you lose weight and grow beautiful hair and nails. Probiotics improve levels of T3 hormone without giving you any kind of jolt, the little "bugs" do the work for you.

Help obesity- Your Microbiome helps you extract and absorb nutrients from your food, thus 'feeding' your cells. They also improve thyroid hormone, which in turn burns metabolism.

Improve allergies- Probiotics retrain your immune cells to tell the difference between harmful and non-harmful things that you get exposed to. This could also benefit asthmatics.

Improve auto-immune conditions- Probiotics help your immune system differentiate between "self" and "non-self" particles so that you don't over-react to your thyroid gland, for example.

Absorb vitamins and minerals- Probiotics improve gut flora and the healthy microorganisms are able to do their job which is to help your body absorb healthy vitamins and minerals.

Detoxification- A healthy Microbiome can support healthy elimination, many say it stops the constipation. If you can eliminate properly, and routinely, you are getting rid of waste material that contains toxins. This is great.

Improve mood- Your gut Microbiome is partially responsible for production and breakdown of neurotransmitters. If you are stressed, nervous, sad, overwhelmed or you cry easily, I suggest trying probiotics. It helps modulate serotonin and other brain neurotransmitters.

Gene expression- If you do not get adequate microflora during birth and infancy, your genes are permanently affected into adulthood. Researchers have found that poor probiotic status alters genes and signaling pathways that help with cognition, memory and movement. Probiotics influence hundreds of genes in your body including the genes that help you fight infection, and maintain healthy blood pressure. And you thought probiotics were only good for constipation!

You should supplement with probiotics even while taking antibiotics, just separate the administration times by 4 to 6 hours. It's harmful to your health to take antibiotics without also taking probiotics, and yet many of you have never been warned of the dangers. Once the antibiotic goes off like a shotgun in your gut, killing the pathogen as desired, but also the innocent bystanders (your beneficial bacteria), then any bad yeast, parasites, worms or dangerous organisms that the antibiotic missed become opportunistic and start proliferating. "C'mon everybody, let's get this party started!" Unfortunately, it's a party for them and sheer misery for you. Some women get uncomfortable yeast infections, others get tongue coating, or any one of a hundred symptoms associated with whatever germ is having the party. You can't see what's going on, so you just have to trust me on this. Probiotics help by running damage control. Probiotics push out pathogens, including yeast. This is huge for a headache sufferer because when yeast breaks down it forms acetylaldehyde which is a potent neurotoxin known to cause a drunk feeling, and a headache (and hangover for that matter). You can starve yeast by cutting off their food supply, carbs, processed or refined foods, vinegar, high fructose corn syrup, and refined sugar. Probiotics help detoxify you by getting rid of waste. This is important for any kind of headache or migraine you have, not just Lyme-related headaches.

Probiotics and liver-supporting herbs and nutrients will help minimize the Herx reaction during antibiotic therapy. A Herx reaction is short for Herxheimer, and refers to the misery one feels during antibiotic therapy, as bugs die in your body, forcing your liver to contend with and clear all those dead "bug parts" and toxins released upon their demise.

There are many good probiotic supplements that you can try and I've recommended many over the years. The one I personally take, and give to my family is Dr. Ohhira's. I love their product so much I agreed to become part of the Scientific Advisory board for the makers. They guarantee their product is live and viable, and fermented using 12 microorganisms that make my "flora fingerprint" grow. In other words, this brand fertilizes my own garden, helping me to make the organisms I got at birth, without adding foreign organisms to my body.

My fans get a substantial discount with this product, free first-class mail shipping and a trial size beauty bar of Kampuku, use coupon code "freegift" at www.drohhiraprobiotic.com.

Dr. Ohhira's Probiotic supplement is fermented using the following 12 strains of Lactic Acid Bacteria (LAB):

Bifidobacterium breve ss. breve- Aids in the prevention of diarrhea and in the production and promotion of natural antibodies.

Bifidobacterium infantis ss. infantis- Protects against inflammation of the bowels and stomach; fights E. Coli.

Bifidobacterium longum- Among other things, it helps to eliminate the negative effects of nitrates in food.

Lactobacillus acidophilus- Neutralizes yeast, campylobacter, and various flu's, while helping to lower cholesterol levels.

Lactobacillus brevis- Helps produce natural antibiotics and promotes cellular immunity.

Lactobacillus bulgaricus- Transient bacteria helps alleviate digestive problems and acid reflux.

Lactobacillus fermentum- Builds immune system and promotes nitrogen activation.

Lactobacillus caseii ss. casei- Protects against deadly Listeria bacteria; inhibits activity in tumor cells.

Lactobacillus helveticus ss. jagurti- Promotes anti-tumor activity.

Lactobacillus plantarum- Blocks receptor sites for gram-negative bacteria and produces natural antibodies.

Streptococcus thermophilus- Produces antitumor activity and the antioxidant superoxide dismutase.

Enterococcus faecalis or TH-10- Has proteolytic power which helps digest proteins and reduce allergic response, and pro-inflammatory chemicals.

Migraine headaches can be caused by many mysteries, so it's important to find out what your trigger is. I talked to my friend, Pierre J. Brunschwig, MD, the medical director of Helios Integrated Medicine in Boulder, Colorado about migraine headaches. He has been in practice for twenty years and tirelessly studies inside and outside the medical box. He said, "Many of my migraine patients have benefited from natural migraine prevention. They use magnesium (orally and intravenously), folic acid, vitamin B2 and feverfew, just to name a few important options. Other migraineurs have discovered how to adjust their hormones or eliminate food allergy triggers to control their migraines. They find that they can minimize and sometimes eliminate the use of migraine medications and their side effects."

Headaches & Hypertension

Sometime the first sign of high blood pressure is a headache. It is usually dull and sometimes it is worse in the mornings. It may also occur in the back of the head, but it could be anywhere. Monitor your blood pressure, because this may be the cause of your mystery headache.

Part II
Solving the Pain Puzzle

Chapter 8

Detoxification Matters

It was bizarre. After 32 years without headaches, Janice, one of my fans, wrote to me seeking help. In 2010 she had moved with her family from their home in Ohio to a townhouse in California. About 2 weeks after moving, she developed throbbing pain in her head. Like most people, she didn't think too much about the headache. No big deal. She simply popped some over-the-counter pain-reliever, and the headache went away. It revisited her the next day, and the day after that, and the day after that. After 10 days, the headaches had reached an intensity that frightened her, and prevented her from taking care of her children. They were coming on more frequently, and not responding to any pain medications.

After spending close to seven thousand dollars on medications, MRIs, intravenous vitamin drips, hyperbaric oxygen, and countless visits to specialists, Janice found out her headaches were caused by mold in her home. Mold is a fungus, and a known biotoxin that can cause hundreds of symptoms, including migraines. Just because you inhale mold, doesn't mean it stays in your lungs. Fungus is a tenacious organism, and it spreads quickly throughout the body.

Janice is not alone. Her symptoms improved, though unfortunately did not completely abate, after taking prescription anti-fungals and replacing her carpet with natural wood floors. It wasn't what I'd call a quick fix, but at least it was a fix that allowed her to get on with her life. There's more about mold in Chapter 10.

Clean Out the Toxins

If you experience headaches on a regular basis, you are likely focused on relieving your pain, and for good reason. But I need you to think big picture for a few minutes. Relieving your pain temporarily, only to have it come back again and again, is not the answer. Long term, the answer is clearing poisons from your body. Detoxifying it. That's why I've divided this chapter into several sub-sections, all identified for you with the words "Big Picture." Unless you have a structural problem in your brainstem, headache pain is usually caused by toxins.

Think of toxins as left-over compounds from chemical reactions, or as toxins you somehow take into your body. You have to filter them out. Drinking pure, clean water is the simplest way to help remove water-soluble toxins. They won't all be removed, but some will. If you fail to drink enough water during the day, you will become dehydrated, and the toxin ratio to your internal body fluids increases. More toxins could mean more pain.

My goal for this chapter is to teach you an important point: *If toxins back up in your blood, they back up in your head.* Keep that in mind as you read this particular chapter because I will be repeating it throughout. The more toxins we can get out of you, the better you should feel.

I'll also share little known information about a metabolic pathway in your body called "methylation." Think of methylation defects as your body's trash building up and not leaving your body properly. Imagine piling all your garbage bags outside your door, and you have a dumpster full, but the sanitation truck only takes half away for you. By the end of the month, you have made more trash than was picked up, so it piles up out there, and it starts to smell and rot. Get the picture? You want to open up the methylation roadblock so that the sanitation truck can take ALL of your garbage away, not just some of it. Later on, I will tell you how to find out if you methylate well, and what to do about it if you don't.

Pollutants You Can't See

Many people experience chemical-induced headaches from the air they breathe. You might think this problem is limited to air pollution and mold, but it isn't. Headaches can be triggered by dry cleaning chemicals, weather patterns, pesticides, food additives, and synthetic fragrances. You can't get away from all of these things, so your best hope is to do the quick fix I offer in each section. And try the detoxification ideas I list later in this chapter, things like dietary supplements to support liver health, castor oil packs, colon hydrotherapy, and saunas.

There are pollutants and chemicals that affect your head everywhere. I mean everywhere! Think about those perfume strips in magazines that you can open and smell. Taking a whiff of the latest new celebrity-endorsed scent can send you to the hospital if you are an asthmatic.

Researchers conducted a study and found that asthmatics had a significant reduction in the amount of air they could exhale compared to most people, who can breathe in and out just fine. Chest tightness and wheezing occurred in more than 20% of folks tested. For asthmatics, the sensitivity shows up as bronchospasm. For people like yourself, the problem manifests as a headache.

Remember what I said earlier? *If it backs up in your blood, it backs up to your head!* In Janice's case I believe, though I cannot confirm, that she has a methylation defect. I suspect this because many people breathe in mold spores. In fact, we all do. So did Janice's husband and teenage son, but only she experienced the headaches. I suspect she could not clear toxins out of her body created from the mold. There's much more on methylation coming soon. First, let's look at all the unseen pollutants that confront us every day.

Your Geography: Air Pollution

Persistent Organic Pollutants, otherwise called POPs, move around the world. They do not just disappear. These chemicals do what's called "leapfrogging." So for example, a pesticide sprayed in West Africa for a grasshopper epidemic ends up in Florida five days later, then it moves up the Gulf Stream and across the Atlantic Ocean over to Great Britain. No kidding. Sensitive folks (especially people with a PON1 gene mutation) can get very ill, and get headaches from pesticides.

You can see toxaphene sprayed on cotton fields in the southern United States, and within 3 days, it is detected in the northern United States and Canada. Please don't buy a one-way ticket to Skopelos Island in Greece (unless I can come along). POPs are everywhere; I'm betting even there too! In case you're wondering, Skopelos is that pristine village on the coast of Greece where *Mamma Mia* was filmed. POPs build up in everyone; however, people who have trouble methylating or detoxifying feel the effects of these poisons much worse than lucky folks who detox well.

You are not going crazy. If I had a solution to the problem of leapfrogging POPs, I'd be a millionaire. The best solution we have as residents of a world full of chemicals is to use air purifiers and HEPA filters wherever, whenever we can. You are not immune to air pollution no matter where you live. It's true there is less pollution if you live closer to the equator due to volatilization and wind patterns.

Smoking Cigarettes: Does Tobacco Cause More Headaches?

We all know that smoking dramatically increases your risk for lung cancer, but headaches? Yes, more than 5 cigarettes per day triggers a headache according to research published in the *Journal of Headache and Pain*. Migraineurs are more greatly affected by tobacco, even if it is second hand. A group of 361 medical students were given questionnaires. Sixteen percent of the participants were migraineurs, and 20 percent of them smoked. The rate of migraines was highest (almost 30 percent) in the group that smoked and had migraines. The migraineurs noted that smoking worsened their migraine and over half assumed that smoking precipitates a migraine. Clearly nicotine is a migrenade. Why would they continue smoking then? Heaven knows, it would take only one migraine for me to step away from a cigarette! I'm sure it's difficult to break dependency, and I'm aware tobacco withdrawal in and of itself triggers headaches.

It may feel like a no win situation but even reducing the number of cigarettes is a "win." Smoking kills more people than HIV infection, alcohol, car accidents, illegal drug use, suicide and murder put together. Smokers die 14 years sooner than non-smokers. Look at your precious kids and imagine them grieving your death. Conjures up quite a visual, doesn't it? I'm trying to motivate you because I care. I know you have the courage to do anything you choose to. It is a choice after all isn't it?! The first step you make is the decision to quit. That's it, first decide. Then make a plan, and prepare yourself mentally for it. One day, you will feel ready. For more information visit www.smokefree.gov.

Carpets Can Be a Trigger

Carpets are full of chemicals. Rubber-backed carpets can be high in formaldehyde[2] which takes up to 15 years to off-gas. So when you put in new carpets, for the next 15 years (about the time you're ready to replace the carpets), you inhale all those off-gassed toxins. Formaldehyde is also something you can get from chewing gum, coming up in the next section.

It's not just formaldehyde (used in preserving dead bodies) that your body needs to deal with from carpets. There's another chemical called styrene butadiene found in rubber backing on carpets. One or both of these inhaled toxins can easily trigger headaches in certain individuals. The quick fix? Replace carpets with tile or wood; these are less allergenic.

You might think replacing your carpets is too expensive, but I think it's easier and less painful to replace your flooring, than to attempt to detoxify your body over 15 years with expensive supplements, drugs, and treatments, not to mention enduring all that pain!

Stop Chewing Gum and Drinking Sugar Free Soda

You will hate me for saying this until your headaches go away, and then you will think, splendid, and fall in love with me for the tip. I don't know how many people (in the hundreds now) who I have told to avoid artificial sweeteners and cured them of their chronic migraines. Artificial sweeteners (all of them) have been tied (at least anecdotally) to migraine headaches. Aspartame itself may not be a problem, but upon ingestion, the molecule of aspartame is broken, converted, and oxidized into formaldehyde in various tissues. It's the formaldehyde that is a problem for living people (okay for dead ones, it's a preservative). I found a case report on PubMed (a database of medical articles, created and maintained by the *National Library of Medicine*) identifying sucralose (different than aspartame) as a cause for migraines.[6]

The problem is that artificial sweeteners create excessive glutamate in the brain, and that harms (kills) your delicate glutamate receptors and neurons connected to it. This has long-term implications for your memory. There are studies tying Parkinson's and Alzheimer's to excessive glutamate production. The same could be said for MSG (monosodium glutamate, key word "glutamate") again, it has the potential to damage your brain cells. You can offset glutamate with a little theanine or GABA supplements. Doctors like to prescribe benzodiazepine drugs to raise GABA, but these are highly addictive and very hard to get off.

Your Clothes: Dry Cleaning Chemicals

Can you just say no? There was a study[3] called TEAM (Total Exposure Assessment Methodology) conducted in 9 homes, using 2 "control" homes. Researchers collected clothing from each home and had them dry cleaned. The dry-cleaned clothes were later brought back into each home. Then, very carefully, using highly specialized equipment that measures levels of compounds, the homes' air was monitored for 3 to 5 days after the clothing was returned.

Researchers found elevated levels of the dry-cleaning chemical tetrachlorethylene in 7 of the 9 homes, with concentrations reaching 300mg/m3. That amount is just crazy. What's worse, the elevated levels persisted for about 2 solid days. And when the breath from the homes' occupants was analyzed, their levels of tetrachloroethylene were increased by 2 to 6 times!

The quick fix? Don't dry clean at all. Give those clothes away if you can't wear them anymore. Reducing headaches is more important than how you look in a particular pair of slacks! If you must dry clean certain dresses, coats, or other clothing, allow the garments to air out for 3 or 4 days, ideally out of the plastic wrapper outside in the fresh air. Only after that, bring them into your home and put them in the closet. This won't remove the chemicals completely, but it's a good start, and does keep your breathing space a bit less toxic. *Remember, if it backs up in your blood, it backs up in your head!*

Activities Create Toxins

Plenty of ordinary, every-day activities and substances release toxins into your environment. Here are just a few:

Smoking	Benzene, xylene, styrene, ethylbenzene
Driving	Benzene
Gas station	Benzene
Dry cleaning	Tetrachloroethylene, styrene
Hot showers	Chloroform
Painting	Ethylbenzene, styrene, xylene
Vegetable oil	Bromine (ingested)
White flour	Alloxan (ingested)

Swimming Pools	Chlorine
Moth balls	Dichlorobenzene
Deodorants	Dichlorobenzene
Gasoline	Chloroform, bromodichloroform
Insulation	Tetrachloroethylene
Plastic	Styrene
Foam Rubber	Styrene

Naturopath Walter Crinnion is one of the world's leading experts on pollutants, heavy metals, and toxins, such as the ones we've been talking about. He has devoted his life to keeping you "clean, green, and lean," which is the title of a book he wrote. *Clean, Green and Lean, Get Rid of Toxins that Make You Fat* (Wiley 2010).

I highly recommend you pick up a copy of Dr. Crinnion's book and also visit his website, www.drcrinnion.com, to access all of his free website information. Dr. Crinnion also offers a newsletter you can sign up for. Health care practitioners interested in environmental pollutants and ways to detoxify their patients can buy his course, "Environmental Medicine for Healthcare Professionals." I've taken this course myself, and it is very enlightening. The way I think about cosmetics, personal care items, cleansers, and everyday household items has not been the same since I viewed his training course, which is on DVDs.

I'm going to switch gears now, and talk about specific ways to detoxify your system.

Big Picture #1: Get Toxins Out of Your Lymph

Your lymph system is twice as big as your circulatory system. Your circulatory system delivers blood to every cell in your body. And your lymph system drains your body of toxins. We're always obsessed with what's in our blood. But we need to pay attention to what's in our lymphatic system as well. To be frank, we need to deal with the equivalent of clogged drains. It's number one in my opinion because the better your lymph system works, the cleaner your blood is.

The main job of your lymph system, which consists of lymph nodes and lymph vessels, is to soak up toxins, germs, excess fluid, fat, and debris from your body. If the lymph gets overloaded, it becomes congested, which can lead to frequent infections, joint pain, chronic fatigue, tender breasts, swelling in the belly, cellulite, uterine fibroids, and ovarian cysts. And . . . headaches! If your doctor suspects you have an infected lymph node, he or she may order a lymph node culture. This lab test identifies the culprit bacteria, fungi, or virus responsible for the infection. Your lymph nodes could swell up if your immune system is trashed from allergies or poor diet.

If you have a toxin build-up in your lymph system, you don't necessarily get headaches right away. One of the first signs that your lymph is stagnant shows up in swollen hands or feet. You hold onto more water, causing weight gain. Rings get tighter on your fingers. You might get rashes on your legs, hands, or feet and experience joint pain, especially in the hands or feet. What's causing all this? With stagnant lymph, toxins can't get out.

Lymph systems don't drain well in an acidic system, so avoid foods that acidify your body, such as soda, carbonated water, cream cheese, pastries, vinegar, refined foods, energy drinks. And avoid acidic emotions and stress, which produce excess amounts of the hormone cortisol in your body.

You simply cannot detox your body without doing some kind of lymphatic detoxing, or you miss a big piece of the puzzle. Your goal is to get that lymph flowing again.

Try this 1-Day Lymph Cleanse. Sip hot water with a squeeze of lemon every 15 to 30 minutes all day, for at least 10 hours. Just sip the warmth. This beverage will get your lymph moving. It hydrates, dilates, and detoxifies you. If you are dehydrated, this will be an amazing, cheap, and simple way to rehydrate. I notice more energy on the days that I do this. Here are other ways you can move lymph:

Get hydrated. You need to drink plenty of fresh, filtered water.

Relax. Try your best to live in harmony. Get as much sleep as you can.

Get moving. Bouncing is great, like on a mini trampoline. If you can't do that, you can buy a jump rope. Jumping just 5 minutes a day does the trick. No trampoline or jump rope? Just have fun doing your favorite exercise. Yoga is fabulous for lymph drainage; all the squeezing and twisting releases many stored toxins.

Eat seasonally. Eat more brightly colored fruits in the summer, such as berries and cherries, and then in the winter eat organic beets. Leafy greens are necessary to alkalize your body. All of these foods can help get your lymph moving and unclog those drains.

Heat 'em up. The fewer toxins that your lymph has to soak up from your body, the better. If you can tolerate some heat, relaxing in a sauna or steam bath will help flush them out.

Get a rub down. Massage gets your entire body relaxed, and prevent lymph congestion. There are specialized massage centers with therapists who do nothing but lymph massage.

Clean up your diet. Avoid preservatives, artificial food additives, and refined foods. Eat more organic leafy greens, such as kale, chard, and spinach. All these foods make your body more alkaline. I like Hawaiian Spirulina, too. It's a green algae that you can take by mouth as a tablet or use as a powder in smoothies. (Use coupon code "suzy" for 20% off at www.nutrex-hawaiil.com.)

Brush your skin. Do dry skin brushing. Always brush your skin so that you are moving the brush (and lymph) towards your heart. So brush from your fingertips to your shoulders, from your toes to your hips. Do this gently, you don't want to scratch yourself to death! It should feel nice and comfy.

Big Picture # 2: Get Toxins Out of Your Liver

Unless it misbehaves, you probably don't think about your liver much at all. It just quietly does its many jobs, and one of the most important is detoxification. Your liver is the primary organ for removing toxins from your body, and there's a lot you can do to help it carry out that important task:

Apply a castor oil pack. Castor oil packs can be made at home, and they are applied to your abdomen, usually over your liver because they are thought to detoxify the liver. I think these are a safe, natural alternative to relieve many aches and pains. I think it's great for monthly cramping or fibroid pain, and any kind of situation where toxins have been accumulating. The more toxins you can release, the lower your risk for head pain.

I frequently recommend castor oil packs because they're non-medicated, so they have no side effects, and the moist heat on your belly feels good instantly. Castor oil is rich in oleic and linoleic acid; it contains a strong anti-fungal, anti-microbial compound that's why it helps with certain skin problems (keratosis, ringworm). People with ligament strains, muscle aches, headaches and backaches may reap benefits. It's used most frequently by people who suffer with abdominal discomfort such as constipation, inflammatory bowel disease, gallbladder disease, pancreatitis, spleen or liver problems.

An ideal location to apply the pack is on the right side of the abdomen over the gallbladder and liver, because this promotes bile flow, which relieves pain from digestive disorders, Mittelschmerz (ovulation pain) and pancreatitis flare-ups.

You will need a bottle of castor oil and a piece of wool cloth, about 12 by 12 inches. These items are sold at health food stores and natural grocers. You'll need some clear plastic wrap, or a plastic bag. Squirt the castor oil onto the wool pad. Saturate the cloth, but don't make it dripping wet. Warm the castor oil-saturated cloth by microwaving it 30 seconds. Careful, it gets hot very quickly. Apply the pack wherever your pain is. Cover the wet cloth with the plastic wrap, and then put a little dish towel over it. Then, put a hot water bottle on top to keep the pack warm while you lay back and rest. Leave it on for 30 minutes to an hour, and repeat applications several times a week. Never apply to open (bleeding) wounds. To remove the oiliness from your skin, use a mixture of water and baking soda.

Smoking, drinking alcohol, exposure to environmental pollutants, food additives, artificial sweeteners, dry cleaning chemicals, pesticides, cosmetics, household cleansers, emotional stress, pharmaceuticals and home building materials can all kill liver cells. Here are some herbs known to support intestinal and liver health.

Milk thistle herb- contains silymarin that block absorption and neutralize toxins

Artichoke extract- stimulates bile flow, removing toxins before they do damage

Dandelion root- stimulates bile flow and removal of toxins

Astragalus- contains saponins that protect against chemically-induced liver damage

CoQ10- protective antioxidant found that nourishes liver and helps detoxify

Triphala- an overall digestive and liver cleanser

Big Picture # 3: Get Toxins Out of Your Skin

This section is a no brainer, so I'll keep it short. The best way to get toxins out of your skin is to sweat. You can do that with any kind of exercise, whatever you can handle. You can jog, you can do Zumba®, yoga, pilates, swim, anything you want. The goal here is to sweat so that you can remove poisons from your body, and reduce total toxic load. You can also use a steam room, sauna, far-infrared or FIR sauna, or full-spectrum sauna.

Keep in mind one thing: As you sweat, you lose electrolytes, so you want to replenish those important molecules with an electrolyte capsule or drink. Restore your electrolytes with E-lyte Balanced Electrolyte Concentrate by BodyBio or with Re-lyte Electrolyte Capsules by Redmond. I don't recommend Gatorade because of the additives and sugar and/or food coloring.

Big Picture # 4 Unglue Toxins From the Gut

I'm not recommending gastric lavage here, so don't worry. I was thinking of simple solutions like drinking more water, eating more fiber, taking probiotics, and cleansing your bowels with colonics or enemas. All of the following can be used with your physician's blessings to bind toxins directly from the gut. They are widely available without a prescription. These agents absorb and bind to bile acids in addition to toxins in your intestine to form an insoluble complex that gets excreted in the feces. Think of these as a rescue remedy, not for chronic daily use. All of them are potentially constipating except psyllium husk.

Bentonite clay

Activated charcoal

Psyllium husk

Your Colon is Connected to Your Head

If you think your gastrointestinal tract has nothing to do with your headaches, you are wrong. Just go with me on this okay, your gut is your second brain, in fact, it's sometimes called just that, "your second brain."

Your goal is to do three things:

Eliminate foods that are bad for you
Clean out your gut
Restore probiotics and enzymes

Coffee Enemas: Some Take It Black And In The Backend

For decades holistic physicians have recommended coffee enemas to treat all sorts of conditions, even migraines. I am aware that there are anecdotal reports that they help. Likewise, there are reports of them triggering migraines. If you're a migraineur, I see no benefits of taking a coffee break in the bathroom.

Colonics Help With Detoxification

I don't blame you if you're a little gun shy about colonics. Most colonic practitioners use a speculum that looks very intimidating. Thankfully, I've not seen one of those up close but if I did, I'd run too. Google to see what I mean. However, I promise you that the newer, thinner nozzles are much more comfortable. These look about no bigger than the width of a pencil. You can handle that, I'm sure!

Clinics that do colonics cannot make headache-cure claims because the FDA is always breathing down their throat, but I can say what I think because I'm a writer, and I do not sell these units, or administer therapy. So I'll tell you exactly what I think about colonics.

Remember what I said earlier? If toxins back up in your blood, they back up in your head? Well, I could say it this way too: *If it backs up in your colon, it backs up to your head.* Did you know that at times there is food rotting inside you? You need to get it out. Removing as many toxins as possible from your body can make a big difference in your general health. And it can make a big difference in when and whether you get headaches. In fact, colonics (and enemas) can improve your health in a number of ways:

✓ Helping remove toxins from your intestine
✓ Rebalancing your digestive system by removing rotten material, like meat, from your intestinal tract

✓ Relieving constipation

✓ Reducing bloating

✓ Restoring natural intestinal flora (After the slate is clean, good bacteria can recolonize.)

✓ Repairing damage done by antibiotics, poor hygiene, and unhealthy lifestyle habits

✓ Boosting immune function

✓ Hydrating the body

I interviewed Francis Gonzalez, ND, who is an I-ACT certified colon hydrotherapist instructor and founder of Fluid Water Therapy in New York, www.fluidwatertherapy.com. The therapists at her clinic use a state of the art system for their colonics called The Angel of Water Surround® Colon Hydrotherapy System. The name alone makes me feel more comfortable.

According to Dr. Gonzalez, many colonics are performed by untrained personnel using unregulated, home-made systems referred to as "Woods Gravity" method. To ensure a safe, effective and hygienic colonic, I recommend that patients insist that their colon therapist meet stringent criteria." Dr. Gonzalez provided the following list of criteria:

* Be certified and trained by the *International Association of Colon Therapists* (I-ACT) and/or the *National Board for Colon Hydrotherapy* (NBCHT)

* Only utilize FDA-registered Class II medical devices to conduct the therapy. A Class II medical device has been cleared by the FDA for use when medically indicated, such as before radiological or endoscopic examination. Just so you are aware, some colonic providers advertise the use of Class I medical devices like Colenz enema systems and Colema boards. While it is true that these devices are FDA-registered, they are intended for home use only (non-prescriptive) and should NEVER be used for clinical or commercial purposes.

* Only use disposable rectal nozzles that have been sterilized.

* Can ensure that the water that is used to cleanse the patient's intestinal tract is properly purified to eliminate any water-borne microorganisms.

* Use colon hydrotherapy equipment installed with back-flow prevention valves so that fecal matter from one patient can't contaminate another (heaven forbid!)

I think colonics can help improve the environment in the lower intestines if you happen to eat certain foods. Some of the major culprits are dairy items, animal protein (meats), white flour, processed, refined foods, milk chocolate, coffee, and alcohol. For some reason, after a while, these foods encrust the intestines with a sludge made up of thick mucus and fecal material, as well as other trapped debris. You would think this is bad enough, however, the sludge promotes the growth of pathogens adding to the intestinal mess. So if you're prone to headaches, you have to consider internal pollution, not just environmental pollution! Digestive enzymes, probiotics to the rescue! Before those, you should consider colonics or cleansing enemas. According to vegetable juicing pioneer, Dr. Norman Walker, "One colon irrigation is equivalent to 30 enemas."

The Angel of Water Surround® Colon Hydrotherapy System

This is a very simple, safe, comfortable, and hygienic way to irrigate the colon.

The tank is filled with pure water that is comfortably kept around 99 -103 degrees Fahrenheit and is monitored by a temperature gauge. You position yourself on the basin (with the pillow and cushioned backrest in place) and insert the nozzle into the rectum, and then water flow is activated. A typical colon hydrotherapy session lasts approximately 30-40 minutes and uses approximately 10 gallons of water. After the treatment, you can back off the nozzle so that it naturally drops away from your body. You can now drain comfortably on an ergonomic basin, sitting up erect or leaning back in a lounge position to fully drain your colon. Then you rinse, use a personal shower sprayer and towel dry. You can then leave the privacy of the colon irrigation room and get on with your day.

I'd like to thank Dr. Francis Gonzalez for assisting me in writing this section, for I do not claim to know all about colonics when my profession is a pharmacist. But I do know what questions to ask when teasing out what treatments can help you. One of the first questions I always ask, is what are the cautions and contraindications for colonics. I always want you to be safe, so ask your health care practitioner if you have any concern about the appropriateness and safety of colonics, especially if you find yourself in the following list.

Contraindications and Cautions for Colonics

Recent colon, rectal or abdominal surgery
Congestive heart failure
Intestinal perforations
Carcinoma of the rectum
Fissures or fistula
Severe hemorrhoids
Abdominal hernia
Renal insufficiency
Ulcerative colitis
Crohn's disease
Colon cancer
Diverticulitis
Blood in the stool
Pregnancy
Cirrhosis of the liver

The main point of this section is to help you realize that detoxing your gut can affect the frequency of your headaches. I could summarize it this way: Clean yourself out, and restore healthy intestinal bacteria with probiotics. The absence of probiotics in the small and large intestine will contribute to the sludge buildup in your colon. Then, the digestion is hampered because of poor probiotic status, and slower transit time in your lower bowel. The longer that gooey food bolus takes to get through your colon, the more likely gunk sticks to your colon wall. Nasty bacteria and fungus just love this, and when you have more of those, you could have more headaches. Bam! So the quick fix here is to clean yourself out, and restore healthy probiotics.

Clean Yourself Out

Colonics
Enemas
Fiber
Steel-cut oatmeal

Probiotics Optimize Gut Microbes

High-quality probiotics are incredibly important to people with a
methylation problem and once you've cleaned out your intestines (with
colonics for example), the next most sensible thing to do is reinoculate
with healthy intestinal flora. We all have untold millions of bacteria
living in our gut. A probiotic supplement supports the right kind and
helps eliminate the wrong kind.[4] If Candida yeast overrun your gut, for
example, you get excessive amounts of the Candida toxin called
acetylaldehyde, which is also a break down product of drinking
alcohol. Obviously, another way to repair the digestive tract is to stop
drinking alcohol.

The less Candida you have, the less acetylaldehyde. You may have
yeast overgrowth and not even know it. It makes you feel drunk. And
it can give you headaches too. It should come as no surprise that the
symptoms of hangover are exactly the same as the symptoms of yeast
overgrowth. For example, headaches, brain fog, anxiety, weakness,
soreness and melancholy. Interestingly enough, these symptoms also
happen in people who have reduced methylation!

If you've taken an antibiotic for more than a week, you are
automatically low in probiotics. If you have had your appendix removed,
you are deficient in probiotics, and thus at higher risk for Candida
overgrowth. If you drink a lot of coffee, if you have recurrent vaginal
yeast infections, if you have a lot of flatulence, if you crave sweets or
have a white coating on your tongue, you have signs of probiotic
insufficiency. You can take whatever probiotic supplement you like. The
one I recommend is Dr. Ohhira's Probiotic. If you buy it online,
www.drohhiraprobiotics.com, you can get free first-class mail shipping
and a trial-size beauty bar of Kampuku by using coupon code "freegift."

Restore Healthy Intestinal Flora

Take high-quality (living) probiotic supplements
Eat fermented foods like sauerkraut
Avoid junk food
Pass on the yogurt, cultures may or may not be live and viable

Eat a great salad, like **"Dr. Mercola's Daily Raw Salad"**
By Dr. Joseph Mercola www.mercola.com

You'll need:
5-6 ounces fresh sunflower seed sprouts
1-4 tablespoons organic pastured raw butter
1/2 to 1 avocado, sliced
* Kinetic Kulture vegetables
1/2 to 1 red pepper
1/4 chopped red onion
** Optional: Protein of your choice, suggest 3 ounces sashimi grade salmon.

* You make your own vegetables and the the starter culture to make them is available at www.mercola.com

** If you don't want "raw" sashimi, you could substitute 4 ounces pastured sautéed grass fed organic ground beef, or wild-caught smoked Alaskan salmon

Directions: Place freshly cut sunflower sprouts on plate, layer avocado, red onions and red peppers. Top with Kinetic Kulture vegetables and butter. I've had the pleasure of lunching with Dr. Mercola, and he made this for me and my husband. It is delicious and healthy, and will leave you craving more. Learn to grow your own sprouts at home, it's easy and fun. It's okay to spritz Dr. Mercola's salad with some organic lemon or lime juice if you want a fresh zing!

My friend and colleague Leonard Smith, MD of Gainesville, Florida has openly stated his support of colonic therapy. He has practiced as a gastrointestinal surgeon for decades and seen it all including operations for colon cancer, colon diverticulitis, appendicitis, hemorrhoids, and many other internal organ problems.

The Connection Between Corn Flakes and Colonics

J. H. Kellogg was a medical doctor in Michigan, and he passed away in 1943. He's most famous for his invention of corn flakes. But he popularized colon hydrotherapy when he published an article in the *Journal of the American Medical Association* praising the procedure for saving someone's dysfunctional large bowel.

"I also believe that normally healthy people will find it valuable to take colon hydrotherapy every couple of months in order to experience how well one feels when the colon is truly empty. It's a fact that most people fail to fully evacuate the colon, something they don't realize. People undergoing colon hydrotherapy on a prevention basis, are quite

surprised at how much waste is removed by the procedure," Dr. Smith says.

Just the fact that colonics alleviate constipation is a good thing. Toxins that build up in your body have the ability to cause headaches of all sorts. Getting them out is critical to you getting well. It doesn't matter to me how you choose to get these toxins out, just as long as you start doing so, and on a regular basis.

Big Picture # 5: Get Toxins Out of Your Bloodstream

"Methylation" is a big word that you probably don't think applies to you. However, read on, because knowing about methylation could improve or save your life. My editor didn't think it was that important that I include methylation in the detox chapter. After all, it sounds so terribly complicated doesn't it? But I fought for this section because so many of you have the genetic problem that causes poor methylation and don't know it. If you have the problem, you are holding onto poisons. Equate it to the sanitation truck not being able to get to your house and take your garbage!

My concern is that you may be heavily medicating yourself to relieve symptoms, when what you really have is just a problem of methylation. And methylation can be addressed by a physician in-the-know, using dietary supplements, not drugs. Are you surprised by that? Only key nutrients and minerals, cofactors, and enzymes can fix this pathway, not drugs! In fact, some drugs make it worse.

Methylation is a complex metabolic pathway in your body that converts folate from your food into glutathione. Folic acid is a B vitamin supplement that you can buy, which is meant to act like natural folate found in foods. If you can't convert folate (or folic acid) into glutathione you have a big problem, because you have less glutathione to neutralize toxins. *Remember, if it backs up in your blood, it backs up in your head.*

Poor methylators have trouble with hormone imbalances. Let's take the female hormone estrogen as an example. You make it in your body; men produce a little bit, too. And you also get it from xenobiotics—shampoos, pesticides, chemicals of all sorts. If you can't break down estrogen (because you don't methylate well) then you can't get it out of your body and you suffer hormonal imbalances; that translates to dozens of problems including menstrual headaches, fibroids, endometriosis and prostate trouble for men. Oh, and if you are extremely sensitive to medicine or to nitrous gas (given by the dentist), you might have a methylation problem too.

Methylation also plays a role in making and breaking down various neurotransmitters, such as energy producing epinephrine and melatonin (the sleep hormone). If there's a problem breaking neurotransmitters down, then they will hang around in excess, possibly causing insomnia, anxiety (the kind that is evident to all), seizures, bipolar and schizophrenic-like behavior. See how important it is to have a well-functioning methylation cycle? I would never bother you with crazy scientific jargon if I didn't think it applied to you or someone you loved.

When you have excessive or imbalanced neurotransmitters, you can have terrible migraines. For example, high levels of your passion hormone dopamine may cause migraines. Low levels of serotonin are tied to migraines in some people. Triptan drugs for migraines are useful because they increase the relative amounts of serotonin; that's how they work. Imbalances in your brain chemistry give you brain pain!

Glutathione, the downstream end product of the methylation pathway is supposed to be made in all of your cells, especially your liver. It detoxifies chemicals. Glutathione is huge, huge, huge! It is a downstream product, made at the very end of the complex methylation pathway. Let me walk you through the key points in this process. At the very top of the pathway is the folate that you get from your food. An enzyme called MTHFR (methyltetrahydrofolate reductase) helps turn folic acid into methylfolate, sometimes abbreviated like this: 5-MTHF.

You might think taking a methylfolate or "5-MTHF" supplement would be a simple fix for this problem, and for some lucky people it's perfect but not all. Methylated folic acid supplements, such as "5-MTHF" are sold online, you don't find them at pharmacies (which usually sell only folic acid and I don't recommend that). You see, 5-MTHF is an activated form of folic acid. The problem with taking 5-MTHF is that you can get too much and begin overmethylating. Then you've tilted the see-saw the other way. Symptoms that you are getting too much 5-MTHF (or folic acid) are feeling wired, anxious, frantic, having nervous legs, insomnia and irritability.

In addition to taking a supplement of 5-MTHF, many poor methylators also take glutathione. Liver disease, Crohn's disease, irritable bowel syndrome, Candida infections and celiac disease deplete glutathione. You need to protect your precious glutathione supply, then you will be less likely to need a glutathione supplement.

If you do supplement with glutathione, you can get too much. The body is about balance. There's a feedback inhibition loop. This means you can take too much glutathione and it will block your ability to methylate (then you have to undermethylation). You may or may not need glutathione, I cannot make this decision for you, there is no way for me to know. Here's a clue if it's good for you or not. Do you ever get IV pushes of glutathione and then crash 4 to 8 hours afterwards? That's a sign you may not need glutathione shots or supplements. Feedback inhibition can also be caused by taking too much folic acid, 5-MTHF, dimethylglycine or SAMe.

Glutathione Gets Mugged

What can you do to make sure that your body doesn't run out of glutathione? Here's a look at what uses up this precious antioxidant:

Drinking alcohol, the more buzz, the more depleted
Medications like statins, acetaminophen and antibiotics
Diet high in sugar
Yeast overgrowth
Cigarette smoking
Poor probiotic status

Methylation: Unclogging the Drains

The most famous practitioner working on methylation is Dr. Ben Lynch, a naturopathic physician from Bastyr University who also has a Cell and Molecular Biology degree from the University of Washington. Dr. Lynch has devoted years to researching this intricate pathway. You should visit his website (www.MTHFR.net) to learn more about his work.

If your physician is unfamiliar with methylation but expresses curiosity, I would definitely point him/her to the work done by Dr. Lynch, who offers presentations and webinars. (You can watch them too). There's a ton of information on his site. He is my methylation guru, and after you visit his site, he'll be yours too! Another pioneer in this field is Dr. Amy Yasko. She works with autistic children, who often have methylation difficulties, as well as other genetic issues that affect their ability to detoxify. Interestingly, kids with autism are often low in homocysteine.

I know a lot of great doctors that think you can over-ride a methylation defect by simply giving high dose folic acid. Dr. Lynch says not to do that. In fact, he does not ever recommend folic acid. Ever.

So, because I subscribe to his teachings, I feel the same way: You should not just take a lot of folic acid! Again, I know many physicians who suggest this supplement to their patients, but I disagree. It doesn't usually work, at least in the long haul. And besides, it can cause more problems. You need to address problems with methylation. After all, it took you years (decades) to get to this point!

Opening up the roadblock after you've been storing toxins for years can quickly overburden your body. You want to open the roadblock slooooowly.

Support and repair. The supplements phosphatidylcholine and CoQ10 support your mitochondria and repair cell membranes. Mitochondria are the little power houses in each cell that produce energy.

> **Methylation Problems**
>
> *Many people with the following disorders test themselves and find out they have a methylation defect.*
>
> Autoimmune disorders
> Diabetes
> Fibromyalgia
> Chronic Fatigue
>   Syndrome
> Alcoholism
> Insomnia
> Neuropathy
> Autism or Down's
>   syndrome
> Frequent miscarriages
> Allergies
> Atherosclerosis
> Hashimoto's
> Attention deficit or
>   ADHD
> Dementia/Alzheimer's
> Schizophrenia/Bipolar
> Anxiety, Depression

Pay attention to sulfur. Taking the supplement molybdenum glycinate and following a low sulfur diet will help eliminate sulfur sensitivities. One thing though, and this will sound crazy. Sulfur-containing foods, such as cabbage, cauliflower, Brussels sprouts and broccoli, are fantastic if you can tolerate them, but many people cannot. If you cannot, molybdenum will help you. I've read where people with brain fog and a feeling of being drunk take molybdenum, and over time it helps relieve this problem.

Watch what you eat. Avoid foods that contain excitotoxins, such as

MSG. And minimize or avoid foods high in tryptophan or tyrosine (chicken, lamb, salmon, sardines, soybeans, nuts, seeds, milk, yogurt, chocolate, wine).

Take a methyl donating supplement. These include methylfolate, methylcobalamin, and MSM, S-adenosylmethionine, cysteine, taurine. You don't take them all. In fact I don't want you to take any of them until your physician weighs in and makes a suggestion. They are not right for everyone. If you get to a point of overmethylation (wired, anxious, insomnia, buzzing), you need to stop, and consider taking low dose niacin (to balance you). Folate and niacin work in opposition to eachother, like a see-saw, you have to keep tilting things back and forth until your level.

At this point, I've given you a number of steps that you can take to promote detoxification and encourage methylation. At the top of this list is taking a supplement of methylfolate, which works for most people. What else can you do?

You can also pay careful attention to improving your diet, taking supplements that replenish important nutrients depleted by pharmaceuticals, and to relieving stress. Here are some specifics: You need a physician skilled in this detox pathway, I can't help you through my little book so please go to functionalmedicine.org or acam.org and see if you can find a doctor in your area who understands this. Here are some things you can do:

Option 1

Take one of these formulas designed to support methylation:
>   HomocysteX Plus by Seeking Health (This is Dr. Lynch's formula.)
>   Methyl Guard by Thorne Research
>   Methyl Protect by Xymogen

You can buy HomocysteX Plus online at www.SeekingHealth.com and get 10% off your entire purchase by using this coupon code: Suzy10

Whichever product you choose, you should slowly ramp up the dose. Don't take the full dose all at once. For example (and this isn't right for everyone), you could take 1 capsule daily for a week or two, then 1 capsule twice daily for another week or two, then 1 capsule three times daily thereafter. The point is that you are slowly increasing the dose.

Option 2

Don't assume it, take a lab tests to see if you really have a methylation problem. The 23andMe genetic test is a saliva test which you can do in about a minute. It only takes a little bit of saliva. You do not have to have your doctor order it, you buy it yourself from their website. It can find out if you have any of 40 inherited conditions and it tests for almost a million genetic snps! I recommend gene testing through www.23andMe.com and when you get your raw data, generate a report from www.MTHFRSupport. com (for $20) or GeneticGenie.org (for free, but the report is not as good as the $20 one from MTHFRSupport.com).

I needed help to do this but I'm not the most technical girl; most people are able to upload the data pretty easily within a few minutes, especially teenagers who get around on the computer like whiz kids.

Anyway, after you get your report, don't panic if you have gene snps (mutations) that suggest you have a higher risk for risk for Alzheimer's or breast cancer. I have to warn you, we all have gene snps, thousands of them!

A snp (pronounced "snip") doesn't mean you're going to get anything. It just means the potential is there. In my opinion it's better to know your weaknesses and protect yourself than to not know and get a disease you could have avoided. If you're freaked out by the idea of knowing this type of information, skip genetic testing. Opt for a simple test to uncover just the methylation defect, which you can buy yourself at www.directlabs.com/suzycohen.

I'm a Pharmacist, Let's Talk Medicine

Along with genetic testing, you and your doctor need to take a close look at all your medications. Why? As a pharmacist, I need to tell you that many medications contribute to methylation problems and can make the problem much worse. Medications that can cause or contribute to methylation problems include:

Acid blockers and antacids. Even the over-the-counter sort deplete your probiotics and suppress your ability to make methylcobalamin. They reduce your ability to absorb nutrients needed to drive the methylation pathway.

Cholesterol-binding drugs. Cholestyramine or Colestipol are not only are drug muggers for vitamin D and A, but they also reduce absorption of folate and cobalamin from your food. This enhances the methylation problem, allowing for more toxins to build up.

Nitrous oxide. This one you get from the dentist. It inactivates an enzyme, causing more problems. Ask for an alternative sedative.

Niacin. It's a good thing to remember if you are over-methylating and cleaning out toxins from your body too quickly! You can put the brakes on with niacin. High doses deplete SAMe and reduce B6. But for people with methylation defects, steer clear of niacin.

Anti-seizure drugs. Do not stop any of these! You need to ask your doctor what to. Carbamazepine, oxcarbazepine, phenytoin, and valproic acid are "folate antagonists" that is, they are drug muggers of folate. That's how they work! They deplete folate. You cannot supplement because that inactivates your medicine, and you can't stop your medicine. I just want you to be aware.

Estrogen drugs. Birth control and menopause medications are drug muggers of folate. It should be fine to supplement with methylfolate (5-MTHF).

Sulfa-containing drugs. Septra, Bactrim, sulfasalazine, or triamterene inhibit the enzyme DHFR, which makes methylation problems worse. DHFR (dihydrofolate reductase) is an enzyme that changes dihydrofolic acid to tetrahydrofolic acid and ultimately allows for the creation of 5-MTHF.

Methotrexate. It is a drug mugger of folate. Do not supplement at the same time, it inactivates your medicine.

Metformin. As you may have learned in my *Diabetes Without Drugs* book, this is a drug mugger of methyl B12 (methylcobalamin). This makes neuropathy worse and it suppresses your ability to methylate.

Up to 45% of people have the genetic issue of poor methylation MTHFR defect,[5] so feel free to blame mom and dad for that. Genetic issues are not the only cause of methylation problems, in fact, more often the methylation pathway gets blocked from these problems:

Zinc deficiency
Vitamin B2 (riboflavin) deficiency
Magnesium deficiency
Vitamin B6 deficiency
Vitamin B12 deficiency
Poor diet
Probiotic deficiency
Xenobiotics (synthetic estrogen-like toxins)
Alcohol
Catechols found in green coffee bean supplements
Catechols found in coffee and tea
High dose niacin (like prescription medications for cholesterol)
Heavy metals
Smoking (because of the cadmium)
Catechols found in white and sweet potatoes

Chapter 9

The Adrenal Hormone Connection

Do you ever stop to treat yourself to something peaceful, quiet and soothing, or do you work and care for everyone putting yourself last on the list? We're going to explore how adrenal hormone affects your well-being, in particular the hormone connection to headaches.

Even though I'm discussing adrenal hormones now, your hormones are all dependent on each other and it's rare to see someone whose deficient in adrenal hormones but perfect in other hormones. Imbalances with one tilt everything. It's miraculous though, how when you correct one hormone, the others do a pretty good job at shifting themselves too.

No matter what type of headache you have, the place to start is with your adrenal hormones. My opinion, and this concurs with other practitioners, is that it doesn't usually matter much how aggressively you treat the other hormonal systems if your adrenals are still taxed and weak. You have to start there first.

Let's see if you have adrenal stress, sometimes termed "hypoadrenia." I call it adrenal fatigue, but you'll also see it referred to as adrenal burnout or adrenal insufficiency. Whatever you want to call it, the energy pattern is pretty much the same. Take a moment and answer these questions:

Do you have difficulty rising, and lounge around in bed until 10am?

Feel slightly more energetic after lunch?

Do you experience an afternoon low between 3 and 5pm?

Around 6 or 7 pm, you probably feel pretty good, right?

Are you tired by 9 or 10 pm, yet resist hitting the sack?

You stay up, catch your second wind at 11pm and stay up happily until 1am.

If you answered "yes" to most or all of those, it's a slam dunk for adrenal fatigue. Adrenal glands pump out cortisol hormone to help you deal with stress. If you have one big stressor (such as grief) or a million micro-stressors, then over time, your adrenal glands weaken and eventually become less able to produce adequate amounts of hormones.

Signs and Symptoms of Adrenal Fatigue

Depending on the phase of adrenal fatigue that you are in, you may experience any of the following:
Chronic fatigue
Crave salt and fatty foods
Increased menopausal or
    PMS symptoms
Allergies/Food sensitivity
Lightheadedness
Frequent sighing
Apathy
Low libido
Insomnia
Dizziness upon standing
Poor concentration
Depression or Irritability

Cortisol secretion occurs in a cyclic fashion. Normally, it's at the high point in the morning, and slowly falls by evening, reaching its lowest point at bedtime. Salivary tests for cortisol levels are ideal because this hormone concentrates in your saliva glands.

You will drag yourself through each day never knowing what is wrong with you. Physicians who fail to recognize this disorder assume you have depression and prescribe antidepressants or stimulants. Many people with undiagnosed adrenal fatigue, soothe their hormonal imbalance by binge eating or drinking, alcoholism or drug addiction. Only when a proper diagnosis of adrenal insufficiency is made, can you begin to support your body better.

Our bodies are not designed to remain in a high state of alertness or stress. We have a hard time coping with long-term, never-ending stressors. It helps if we can take periodic breaks for ourselves.

Some signs of adrenal fatigue include the need to lie down after emotionally stressful times, muscle weakness and mild depression. See "Signs and Symptoms of Adrenal Fatigue."

The symptoms of adrenal fatigue speak to the bigger problem of hormone imbalance throughout the body. You see, the adrenals have an impact on other hormones, especially thyroid. Hypothyroidism almost always goes with adrenal fatigue. Hypothyroidism causes a cascade of other uncomfortable symptoms and no amount of thyroid medication will correct hypothyroidism, unless you simultaneously nourish your adrenal glands with adaptogenic herbs. Saying you have adrenal problems is a bit of a blur, because you could be in 3 different phases, and saliva and blood tests help determine the phase.

The Stress Response, Where are You?

There are 3 primary phases you could be in if you have adrenal fatigue. The "alarm" phase may last a few minutes to hours while you're upset or worried about something, but your body really requires about 2 days to fully recover. I tell you this because if you are always in the "alarm" phase, imagine how this state of chronic stress affects you, it pushes you into the "Resistance" phase. Eventually, your adrenal 'pilot light' burns out. Then you have entered "burnout." Where are you now? Has your headache frequency increased or decreased since you entered this phase?

Phase	Duration	Cortisol Levels	Comments
Alarm	Minutes to hours	Very High	Fight or flight
Resistance	Months to years	High	Long term stress
Burnout	Years	Low	Depressed, Exhausted

Cortisol is your 'stress' hormone. All by itself, chronically elevated cortisol may be a risk factor for headaches. Stress out long enough and you will absolutely have adrenal exhaustion (low cortisol) and this will increase frequency of your headaches. It happens because adrenaline is released and there is activation of your HPA axis (hypothalamus pituitary axis) and you make cortisol. It happens with good stress, like when your sports team wins the game, and with bad stress like when you get fired.

You can develop headaches at any point during the adrenal imbalances. Your headaches are more likely to retreat if your adrenal hormone (and thyroid hormone) is balanced. Most people don't realize that these two glands (actually three glands if you are counting a pair of adrenal glands with 1 thyroid gland) directly influence how well you feel, how much energy you have, and how frequently you get headaches.

Anatomy of Adrenal Fatigue

Your adrenal glands are two small triangular shaped endocrine organs that sit just on top of your kidneys, like two small top hats. Each gland weighs approximately 3-6 grams but almost double in size during stress or pregnancy. The outer portion called the "cortex" secretes aldosterone which regulates blood pressure, cortisol and DHEA. This promotes more energy and supports immunity. Excess amounts stress can be harmful, and lead to belly fat, diabetes and heart disease. Sex hormones, like progesterone, estrogen precursors and testosterone are made downstream from the DHEA which is made there.

Yoga & meditation reduce anxiety and blood pressure by increasing "happy" brain chemicals, and reducing cortisol.[1]

The inner core of your adrenal glands called the "medulla" secrete epinephrine (aka adrenaline) and norepinephrine, which collectively are called 'catecholamines' better known as your 'fight or flight' hormones.

Your adrenal glands secrete hormones that regulate blood pressure and blood sugar, so anytime these glands are fatigued, you're more susceptible to drops in blood pressure or blood sugar, usually around mid-afternoon when they are most weak. This is also the most common time for a headache to kick in. With adrenal exhaustion, the picture looks like this: Mid-afternoon, your blood sugar drops, you feel fatigued or drowsy, you start to yawn, put your head on your desk and/or get a headache.

I interviewed my dear friend Jill Carnahan, MD, Founder of *Flatiron Functional Medicine* in Boulder, Colorado. She's an expert in complex diseases and a sleuth when it comes to detecting underlying cause. She's cared for thousands of patients and helped many recover from long-standing illnesses such as mold toxicity, autoimmune conditions, chronic infections, leaky gut, hormone imbalances and much more. She is a national speaker at medical forums too. This is one doctor that never stops studying! We talked about how two tiny adrenal glands (the size of grapes) could play such a huge role in the development of pain.

Dr. Carnahan explained, "The main role of the adrenal gland is to help the body cope with all stressful situations. In order to do that, they secrete adrenaline and cortisol, in response to internal and external conditions. Pollution, stress or illness activate the glands which just so happen to modulate and oversee every other tissue, organ and endocrine gland. Your adrenals interact with the hypothalamus and pituitary gland. In fact, they play the lead role in the symphony of your endocrine 'orchestra.' Our bodies are fully capable of coping with acute stress, but not the kind of stress that goes on and on. The more stress, the more imbalance in the whole orchestra, and then the more pain and inflammation in the body. For some, this is represented as headaches."

Right on! It's all the little micro-stressors that get to me. But it could be more of a jolt too.

This type of experience happened to me in a hotel once at 4am, and we had to evacuate immediately. I grabbed my laptop, iPhone, purse and boots! (Hey I really love those boots). All of us zombie hotel 'residents' tromped down the stairs and waited in the courtyard of the hotel in the dark. Talk about a wake-up call. Luckily, my morning taping at the local morning show included a professional make up artist who did magic removing the dark circles from under my eyes. Unfortunately, she could not "remove" the cortisol that remained high until about noon.

Another example is if someone cuts you off while driving. You feel the jolt of electricity (it's really adrenaline hormone being pumped out of your adrenals) whenever you experience sudden shock, fear or alarm. You know it well, if you wake up to the scent of smoke (and don't realize it's your husband having a midnight snack of hot toast and almond butter) your heart starts pounding, brain becomes alert and kicks into high gear and you proceed to quickly grab your most important belongings, your precious poodle, and run out of your home into the street for safety. Or out of your hotel room in jammies (lucky I had any on!)

Once you realize it was a false alarm and you are totally safe, your heart slows down, your body is awash with relief and you sheepishly creep back into the house as the neighbors peep out their drawn shades to see what in the world got into you! Ahhh, sigh, that is the deep breath you needed. But the pro-inflammatory chemicals and 'alert' hormones will linger in your body for a bit longer, it isn't over internally.

Dr. Carnahan explains, "Our reaction to this type of acute stress is normal, it primes us to react quickly and efficiently in order to protect us from harm. However, when our body is alarmed, from financial disaster, impending divorce, death of a loved one, overworking, looming deadlines, lack of sleep, training for a marathon or anything else, our adrenals have difficulty going back to a calm relaxed state of balance. Rather, we remain in hyper-alert mode, pouring out the stress response hormones of cortisol and adrenaline. Under stress for an extended period of time, the adrenal glands will start to malfunction and just like a tired worker on an assembly line, they just can't keep up anymore with the demands made on them." And then you have it, more inflammatory chemicals amok from head to toe, and definitely in the head. Elevated cortisol may be a trigger for migraines. Managing your stress levels can help reduce the frequency of your headaches and other symptoms. If you'd like to learn more about Dr. Jill Carnahan, visit www.drcarnahan.com. I highly recommend her free health blog, which you can subscribe to at www.DrJillHealth.com.

Healing Adrenal Exhaustion Headaches

There isn't a quick fix, this takes months to completely resolve. I wish I could give you a simple solution, like a pill, but adrenals don't respond easily to drugs. They respond a little better to nutritional supplements so read my Script section coming up next. Even though my Script section contains helpful vitamins and herbs, in order to become headache free, you'll have to make a commitment to reduce stress levels, add fun, sleep more, control your emotions, avoid caffeine and eat nutritionally dense food as opposed to sweets, soda and candy. You may also need short-term medication. Let's talk about all of this, starting with the most essential piece, the reduction of stress in your life.

Reduce stress.

This is one of the hardest elements because it means you have to really examine your life and everyone in it. You have to limit time with people that force you into a victim state and make you feel bad. That might mean making a hard decision like cutting back on hours at work or getting a different job entirely. It might mean limiting time with folks that push your buttons and cause you fear, anger, or stress. It might mean ending relationships with people who say they love you, but don't prove it with their actions. It might mean moving. I don't know what it means for you, but I know that if you can reduce your stress, you reduce your cortisol, and this puts the fire out in your body. It's huge in terms of having a direct impact on reducing stress chemicals that cause pain in your body.

Add Fun.

Healing adrenals entails adding joy to your life. The list is endless, and for some of you, this is very difficult. Maybe start with something simple such as time for yourself, perhaps a nightly ritual of Epsom salt bubble bath with a cup of warm chamomile tea. Go to a cooking class, or Pilates, yoga or Zumba. Anything that you consider "fun" counts. Take a few printed photos to Michael's on the weekend, they will teach you how to ScrapBook. (Now that could end up costing you money because it is so addictive). Fun could even be a girls night out, or take yourself out on a date by going to the movies (by yourself) and sneak in a chocolate chip cookie. Make sure it's a comedy, no blood and guts kinds of movies. Do whatever you want to do in order to break the pattern of the 'same thing different day' that keeps you locked in the same sad emotions. If it makes you smile it counts.

Control Emotions.

Scientific research supports the fact that anger and fear are the most toxic emotions to our physical health. Adrenals respond to emotion and if you are constantly thinking thoughts of anger or fear, you will be triggering release of hormones like adrenaline and cortisol, which are critical to healthy function but toxic if continuously released.

According to Dr. Carnahan, "The healthiest emotions to the adrenal glands are the feelings of love and gratitude. Perhaps you need to add a morning ritual of meditation or prayer of thanks to God. I urge my patients to keep a bedside journal and write down a few things they are thankful for on that particular day. This puts you in a place where you are reaching for the positive in life and the thoughts you ponder right before sleeping set the tone for the entire night. Why not give you brain good fuel right before dozing off?" And speaking of sleep, getting solid, refreshing sleep, about six to eight each night is one of the best ways to restore healthy adrenal function.

One of the simplest things you can do, right now, is to "Forget about it!" By that I mean forget whatever is eating at you, just let it go. If someone was mean, or treated you unfairly, stop yourself from playing into the victim mode and calling all your friends to dump that story on them. This drains your energy, as well as your friend who is probably only half listening. It's totally okay if some big deal occurs, and you have to share it with your closest, but it's not okay to go down the list of friends you have and call them, and start telling the same story over and over. It just keeps your cortisol high for hours because your body can't tell the difference from the actual event, and the story you're telling days later, and for some of you, years later! *Forget about it already!* Give your soul a rest, think of something sweet and keep redirecting your mind every time it wanders to that bad event. You can retrain yourself with time to forget about it.

Avoid Caffeine & Eat Well.

As I mentioned earlier, the things you most crave when the adrenal glands are weak are sugar and caffeine. I know how bad you want a Caramel Mocha Frapp, but this just keeps your doctor in business and your adrenals under stress.

However, this is a trap and will keep the vicious cycle going of over-stimulation and then a crashing blood sugar and fatigue. I'm not entirely against a little coffee, but if you're suffering from adrenal exhaustion, I suggest avoiding caffeine altogether. I realize I can't control you, so if you won't give it up entirely, would you please choose options that have lower caffeine, such as decaf or green/white teas. Caffeine is a stimulant that can't help your adrenal glands because it stimulates production of norepinephrine, which is a precursor of adrenaline.

Avoid Sugar?

Sweets and sugary foods raise insulin levels and this raises cortisol so your body goes into alert mode and signals for energy. This is why many experts including myself feel that breakfast is your most important meal, especially if you have adrenal insufficiency. Because your adrenal glands help to regular blood sugar, you should support them by avoiding simple sugar or fruit in the morning so no French toast with syrup, and a big glass of apple juice. You would be better off with organic eggs and smoked salmon or a rice protein smoothie with spinach and frozen organic blueberries. These high protein low sugar options will give your body a stable blood sugar to start the day and help you avoid the sugar cravings and crashes that occur two hours after the French toast. You can expect sustained energy, better focus and concentration, and fewer temptations for sweets.

Throughout the day, you should choose meals and snacks that contain lean healthy protein and no sugar. Great choices are turkey wraps with fresh guacamole, organic veggies dipped in hummus, a 'trail mix' of nuts and seeds mixed with shredded coconut, and lean organic protein such as wild-caught fish and free-range chicken. Big salads and steamed or sautéed veggies are yours to eat all day. Don't be afraid of fats! Healthy fats like avocado, coconut oil, nut butters and cold-pressed olive oil are a great way to boost metabolism and sustain energy between meals leaving you more satisfied and less apt to dive into the cookie jar.

I asked my good friend Andrea Donsky about the impact of food on headaches. Andrea has been on many morning shows and she is perfect to ask since she's a Registered Holistic Nutritionist. She said, "I've made it my mission to educate people on how to properly read food labels, and one of the biggest issues I see today when it comes to our food supply is the large number of chemical additives used to make our food look good, taste better and last longer."

I can hear you right now, and I know how much you want to eat that comfort food, especially when your head hurts. Andrea wants to assure you, "Chemicals additives are ubiquitous and are responsible for a host of side effects including headaches, anxiety, heart palpitations, allergies, and hyperactivity to name a few. Headaches specifically can be triggered by ingesting additives like artificial sweeteners and MSG as they can overstimulate the neurons in our brain so it's important to always read labels to ensure what you are buying is chemical free."

I know how hard it is to sit here and read how everything in your kitchen and fridge is bad for you, and that's not at all what me or Andrea is saying. We just want you to choose healthier options more often. Make better choices more frequently than you have in the past. Occasional indulgences are okay, and if you fall off the wagon, get back on. Be proud of yourself for tilting in the right direction. If you have an occasional indulgence, you're less likely to have a backlash (headache). For those times when you're craving that indulgence, *Unjunk Your Junk Food* (Gallery Books 2011) is a book I absolutely love; it's so much better than other books in that same genre and sold on Amazon and it's written by Andrea Donsky and Randy Boyer (with Lisa Tsakos). You can use it as a guide to help you choose better options.

Because Andrea did the research on *Unjunk Your Junk Food*, she explains, "Through our research, we found a group of seven chemical additives that can cause the most harm to our bodies. We called them "The Scary Seven." They are: High-fructose corn syrup, trans fats, MSG, artificial colors, artificial sweeteners, artificial flavors, and certain preservatives. So if you pick up a product at the grocery store with any of these 7 ingredients listed on the label, I would encourage you to put it back on the shelf."

Sensible advice! Andrea Donsky is the Founder of www.NaturallySavvy.com, which is a great site with awesome videos, candid opinions and very interesting articles like "Conventional Feminine Hygiene Products: A Women's Issue with Toxic Implications. This article is accompanied by a video where she sets feminine hygiene pads on fire! She has thousands of other archived articles there, plus a free newsletter you can sign up to recieve.

Suzy's "Energy Script" for Adrenal Fatigue

Before you take any of the following supplements, you must ask your doctor(s) if they are right for you. My intention here is to educate you about possibilities and options. Do not misconstrue my ideas for medical advice. I have no idea what is right for every individual reading this so take my list to your practitioner(s) to ask if they're right for you with your medical history. Dosages are also just basic guidelines, some people tolerate different dosages than what is stated here:

Pantethine
Vitamin C
Phosphatidylserine
Panax ginseng
Cordyceps
Licorice root
Rhodiola
Electrolyte replenishment

How This Helps A Person Become Headache Free

Pantethine.
Vitamin B5, also known as pantethine and pantothenic acid, turns into Coenzyme A in the body. The nutrient is absolutely essential for proper adrenal function, and it's supposedly helpful if you grind your teeth too. Sometimes people with TMJ and trigeminal neuralgia find some relief with pantethine too. If you are chewing through those rubber mouth guards like a termite on wood, there's hope with this nutrient. I

recommend pantethine for people who feel frazzled and tired because it helps you make cortisol. Your "coping glands" can handle the stress better if you are at the point of adrenal exhaustion and low in cortisol. For those of you who are at the "Alarm" phase, you already have too much cortisol so I wouldn't suggest this. *A deficiency of B5 has been linked to high blood pressure, rapid heartbeat, exhaustion, infection and a slow healing of wounds.* We also know that B5 is a powerful lipid nutrient to lower triglycerides. It supports heart function, energy and carbohydrate metabolism.

Vitamin C.

This may be the most important nutrient for people with adrenal fatigue because vitamin C is needed for both the adrenal cortex and medulla.[2] Besides that, when you are under stress, you urinate more vitamin C (but remember, you need it for adrenal gland health). You can't make this water-soluble antioxidant and your adrenal glands have an extremely high concentration of C. Run out of it, and your adrenals suffer and you may get symptoms like fatigue, depression, difficulty coping and emotional instability. You can certainly eat foods rich in vitamin C like citrus fruits, sprouts, tomatoes and greens but most people with adrenal burnout need to supplement. You can take supplements like "Vitamin C with bioflavonoids" or "Liposonal C." Taking C through the day is better than one big dose.

Phosphatidylserine.

Phosphatidylserine is an antioxidant that can lower cortisol levels by optimizing your brain's relationship with the overworked adrenal glands. After about ten days of high doses (600mg total daily dose) of phosphatidylserine, excessive cortisol levels can be reduced in healthy men.[3] Not only that, the ratio of testosterone to cortisol increased, which may be helpful too. It may enhance brain function and memory, help with anxiety and depression, improve your mood, and possibly speed metabolism. It is very difficult for the body to make phosphatidylserine as it requires many cofactors for its production. Supplementation is vital for optimizing adrenal function.

Panax Ginseng.

This herb can ease mental and physical exhaustion. It strengthens immunity so it may be particularly helpful for someone with Lyme related headaches. It revs up your body so if you take it too late in the day it may cause insomnia. Panax ginseng is liable to be used by people aged 40 and older, as a general health enhancer. I like this adaptogenic herb more for men than women because every now and then I hear how it increased facial hair growth and acne in women. I never hear that happening to men, however sometimes, with overuse, there is more irritability or aggressiveness or insomnia. Some people find Panax ginseng a little too stimulating so for these folks, the Eleuthero (Eleutherococcus senticosus) or Siberian ginseng may work more gently.

Cordyceps sinensis.

Cordyceps is an adaptogen and it's a Chinese mushroom known as Dong chong xia cao. This is one of best medicinal mushrooms because it helps with a wide range of adrenal issues such as fatigue, dizziness, stress, immune function, libido, lung function, heart rhythm disturbances and liver problems; it even helps with poor oxygen utilization. It may help you get over stress quicker. When combined with magnesium, the results may be even more immediate. Other than occasional allergies, there's no real danger but you should build your dose up slowly. Just like ginseng, cordyceps can also increase sex drive, endurance and stamina. Most supplements suggest 2 to 4 grams per day in divided doses.

Licorice.

Licorice known as Glycyrrhiza glabra is a remedy used for ulcers, sore throat, asthma, depression, menopause, arthritis, heartburn, gastrointestinal concerns of all sorts and various viral infections (like hepatitis and the flu). Unfortunately, licorice candy (mmm, Twizzlers) doesn't have quite the same effect. Licorice contains healing flavonoids, phytoestrogens, and glycyrrhizin. Some of these compounds block the breakdown of cortisol in your body which means there's more of it handy if you need to cope with stress. Licorice increases the half-life of cortisol making your cortisol act longer than normal, and there are some of you who are still at the phase where you have high cortisol (like in the alarm phase), and you also have low DHEA which is another stress hormone. In other words, some of you haven't totally petered out yet with cortisol, and in that case licorice wouldn't be right for you, it could make things worse. Since I'm not a doctor, and I can't advise you from here, I would have your cortisol, DHEA and other hormones evaluated to see exactly where you are. If you do have high cortisol, I'd skip the licorice.

Licorice boosts levels of natural interferon which helps with infection, plus it can soothe irritated mucus membranes from cough and cold.

Caution: Excessive intake of licorice root can exacerbate hypertension and other heart problems, by disrupting the salt and water balance that your body strictly maintains so ask your doctor if it's right for you. It happens compliments of the glycyrrhizin. Licorice is mildly estrogenic so it may help with menopausal symptoms, but be careful because anything estrogenic has the potential to drive certain cancers, especially those of the reproductive tract.

Most herbs are straightforward, but with licorice I need to tell you that some companies make a deglycyrrhizinated form of licorice root, called "DGL." This form won't help adrenals, it's better for gastritis, reflux and heartburn.

Rhodiola.

The herb rhodiola (Rodiolia rosea) has been safely used for centuries in Russia, Eastern Europe, and Scandinavia to help people deal with stress and bounce back from debilitating illness. It's well known to relieve stress, lift depression and improve attitude. It reduces cortisol levels and may support healthy levels of blood sugar. Because it gently increases energy, I recommend taking this in the morning or around your lunchtime low. It improves serotonin levels (by preventing breakdown of the compound).

Rhodiola is a plant that thrives in Siberia and withstands the harshest growing conditions on the planet. Siberian natives and other people living along the Arctic Circle have traditionally reached for rhodiola whenever faced with dauntingly stressful challenges, both physical or mental.

In a 2007 study published in the *Nordic Journal of Psychiatry*, researchers gave rhodiola extract to a group people with clinical depression, the kind that requires medical care and constant follow-up.[4] Of the 89 study participants, only the groups which received rhodiola supplements (two different dosages) experienced "a significant anti-depressive effect" over a period of six weeks as compared to the group who were given dud pills. Physical symptoms related to depression improved, such as insomnia, emotional stability and feelings of self-esteem.

It's just amazing that not one single study participant reported any negative side effects from taking the herb. Did you hear that? Zero side effects! Mind you, all prescribed anti-depressants currently available come with a whole gamut of potentially devastating side effects, everything from sexual dysfunction to brain fog. Rhodiola enhances levels of key brain chemicals such as norepinephrine, serotonin and dopamine. This otherwise beneficial effect may be detrimental to people who teeter on the edge of making or having too much serotonin (remember triptrans increase it, plus some of us make too much, or have trouble clearing it because of our genes). There is research to support its benefit on the heart, specifically certain cardiac arrhythmias. And in a Moscow study,[5] scientists gave rhodiola to military cadets who face mentally and physically demanding work, 24/7. The cadets receiving rhodiola performed better and experienced much less mental and physical fatigue than those who took the dud pill.

In the brain, rhodiola appears to be highly serotonergic (it increases serotonin) and reduces corticosteroids. It blocks MAO-A, an enzyme in your body creating higher levels of serotonin.[6] You would not want to combine this with drugs that do the same thing. If you have manic or bipolar disorder you should not use Rhodiola.

In a recent trial, using rhodiola and measuring stress response, all participants had a significantly lower stress response after taking 200mg twice daily of rhodiola for up to four weeks.[7]

Electrolyte Replenishment.

If you are experiencing low blood pressure or dizziness upon standing, it may indicate that your adrenals are "wasting" salt and not keeping your blood volume in balance. If you experience frequent dizziness with accompanying headache, then my suggestion for you is simple. Try starting your day with an sugar-free electrolyte solution like Elyte Sport (www.bodybio.com) or Thorne Catalyte (www.thorne.com). Another option is simple add ½ to 1 teaspoon of real sea salt to a glass of water and drink first thing in the morning. Be sure you are using mineral rich sea salt and not the chemical sodium chloride, which doesn't exert the same beneficial effects since it lacks all the essential minerals contained in sea salt. By making an effort to decrease daily stressors and choose love, and gratitude and incorporating healthy food choices, you will be well on your way to a headache-free life!

Testing for Adrenals

Testing for adrenals is simple. I recommend a "4 point" cortisol test, along with evaluations of other hormones such as DHEA for example. All of the following labs offer a 4 point test, which means you provide 4 saliva samples, one in the morning, noon, evening and midnight. Some of these companies also offer more comprehensive tests that include DHEA or other hormones.

Diagnos-Techs	www.diagnostechs.com
ZRT Labs	www.zrtlab.com
Neuroscience	www.neurorelief.com

> Astragalus may be helpful to relieve fatigue and improve blood glucose, blood pressure and blood flow.

The Quick Fix: Top 10 Adrenal Soothers

I can't possibly tease out exactly what you need to balance your hormones because this is done on an individual basis, by a trained physician, based upon your lab tests, blood, urine or saliva.

DHEA, short for Dehydroepiandrosterone is a hormone you make, that is sold as a dietary supplement too. DHEA levels peak at about age 25, then steadily decline as you get older. DHEA is inversely proportionate to cortisol, so when one goes up the other goes down, kind of like a see-saw. DHEA is anabolic, it helps you grow and make muscles, whereas cortisol is catabolic, and tears down muscle. Cortisol lowers testosterone, DHEA raises it. DHEA may cause headaches as a side effect. You have to be careful not to take too much DHEA because it may ultimately create more estrogen in the body. If you have a hormone-driven cancer, it could make it worse. I only mention it here because if you need DHEA to balance high cortisol, it can breathe life into you very quickly, but if you don't need DHEA and take it, it can be very bad. So I only want to hear that you're taking this if your doctor has proven that you are deficient in DHEA. I tell you this because DHEA is sold over-the-counter, but it's a hormone and has widespread effects in your body, head to toe.

What else can you do?

1. Separate from the mental stress. When you find yourself facing a stressful person or situation, you have to consciously pull yourself out of the drama, out of the moment. Even if you can't physically leave, you can do this mentally. It's worth a try. I would just take bigger, longer deeper breaths. Visualize yourself elsewhere as you politely listen, careful not to further engage or inflame whoever you are dealing with. Leave as quickly as possible.

2. Try relaxation exercises. You can lie down and hike your knees in as tightly as you can to your chin then extend them long. Hike them in again, try to curl yourself into a ball by bringing your head to your knees. Breathe in and out with the motions.

3. Wet a little washcloth in some ice water and wring it out, then apply to your forehead or your neck.

4. Biofeedback devices can help over time, if you just keep using them. Among the best are those made by Heartmath. www.heartmath.com

5. Rescue Remedy by Bach. This is a little dropperful of flower essences diluted 5X that is used for relief of occasional stress. I still carry this in my purse in case I feel overwhelmed at an airport from delays, missing flights, cranky TSA agents (the last one hiked her hands up so high I literally asked her, "Are you trying to give me a pap smear or was that an accident?") Rescue Remedy now comes in an alcohol-free version for kids. I wish I had the alcohol-free version when my son was little, he used to have terrible headaches when transitioning between households (divorce conflict) but I used the regular version. I found this to be a very safe remedy for my child, as he was (we all were) under constant stress.

6. Zyflamend. This is sold at health food stores and it naturally reduces cytokines that run amok. I don't think you need it every day, but once is fine with me if it makes you feel better, and it may also help with joint pain.

7. A cup of green tea. It's cheap, simple and free of side effects. The relaxing benefits of L-theanine found in green tea (and Matcha) can soothe stress literally within minutes.
8. Acupuncture is known to support the body's energy systems. You'll need more than 1 treatment though, this is for long-term support.
9. Adaptogenic herbs such as rhodiola or licorice.
10. Exercise. Nothing's better for some of you than decompressing at the gym, or jogging around the block. It gets it out of your system! Hit the punching bag, dance like nobody's watching or fold yourself up into a knot doing yoga, I don't care, just do something to release the stored ball of fire inside of you.

Yoga Reduces Headache Pain

Yoga helps with headache pain. I hear you wondering, "Why if my head hurts, should I twist myself into a knot?" Because research proves yoga can help certain types of neck and back pain, headaches, migraines, anxiety, high blood pressure and osteoporosis. Since you've probably tried addictive narcotics, anti-inflammatories, steroids, and possibly surgery spending thousands of dollars and suffering endlessly, I think yoga's worth a shot. It has no side effects other than making you feel refreshed, sort of like a human breath mint!

In a 2012 German study, researchers saw how a 9-week yoga program helped participants with chronic neck pain.[8]

This could be helpful for people with chronic tension headaches because trigger points in your neck may be referring pain into your head. Yoga has been around for centuries, and there's no harm so long as you don't push your body past its limits, but in your case, I would still get your physician and

Melatonin Hormone

Maybe you don't make enough? Supplements of melatonin help because they normalize the circadian sleep-wake cycle. This can help you if your migraines are triggered by abnormal sleep rhythms or insomnia. Melatonin is naturally made in your brain in response to darkness. It's possible to make it naturally increase by turning off the TV in your bedroom by 9 pm, and of course all the lights. Some of you may need a supplement. Drug muggers of melatonin include certain anti-depressants, sedatives, and pain medications.

chiropractor's blessings. And speaking of "blessings" I've never associated a religious connotation with yoga, the classes I've attended are 100% about stretching and breathing. As an added perk, you'll be the life of the party if you can turn yourself into a human pretzel!

Flexibility is also important in maintaining good posture, and the strength that yoga builds in your bones and muscles can help to protect you from developing chronic pain disorders and arthritis. A systematic review was performed earlier this year in New Zealand, and sufficient evidence suggests that regular yoga practice alleviates pain caused by musculoskeletal conditions and disorders.[9]

Dr. Loren Fishman runs a physical medicine and rehabilitation practice in New York, and he relies heavily on yoga therapy to treat his patients. For those of you who suffer from migraines or headaches, Dr. Fishman advises inversion poses. An inverted pose is any pose in which your heart is above your head, like a forward bend, or a headstand. Although we have not found a consistent and exact cause for headaches yet, many of them seem to be correlated to muscle tension that is held in the posterior part of the neck. By realigning these muscles, which is often emphasized in yoga, you can alleviate your head pain without all the pain medicine! If inverted poses aren't for you, you can try to pull your spine into a straight line, open your chest by bringing your shoulders downward and slightly backward, and allowing the crown of your head to pull ever-so-slightly to the ceiling. By doing this, you are stretching the muscles that work all day to support your head, and giving them a moment to breathe.

Choose classes carefully, when I walked into my first yoga class, it was 105 degrees! It's called "Bikram" yoga, or sometimes "hot yoga." What a nightmare for me, I despise heat. I could not get out of there fast enough. So call in advance and ask about the class you want to take. Classes labeled "restorative" or "yin" are gentle, and cool, also those labeled "Vinyasa" or "Hatha" are also fairly easy, at least for me. Start out slowly and with your doctor's permission if you've had surgeries.

Your Plan of Action: A Dozen Ways to Minimize the Pain

We've talked about adrenal hormone imbalances. My plan of action is less about rescue remedies and more about options that can identify them.

1) Find a doctor. You need one that can identify your specific hormone imbalance, rather than one who will give you a prescription for a symptom. Do you have a cortisol or DHEA imbalance? Are you flat-lined with cortisol, or is your cycle upside down? How are you sleeping, what are your melatonin levels? You can find these things out with proper tests. I would seek out a Functional Medicine doctor, such as those from www.functionalmedicine.org or www.acam.org. See Appendix 1 for suggested Labs.

2) Switch drugs. If you already know you have an imbalance in your cortisol, and you're taking a synthetic drug like prednisone, you should consider hydrocortisone, because it more closely matches your own cortisol. It's still medicine, but it's a better match to your own God-given hormone.

3) Reduce stress. This improves cortisol and adrenaline levels, offering a 'cooling' effect in your body due to reduced pro-inflammatory cytokines.

4) Clean up your diet. Greatly reduce or preferably remove foods that contain caffeine and refined sugar.

5) Switch salt shakers. Eliminate white salt, and substitute "real" salt, the kind with color such as Real Salt™ by Redmond or Himalayan salt which is pink. The white salt is more of a chemical, it is nutritionally stripped of all minerals, whereas colored, "real" salt has naturally-occurring minerals that cells are are starving for. The topic of salt is fully discussed in my *Diabetes Without Drugs* book. The reason it's important is because your body runs on minerals (real salt), not just sodium chloride (white salt).

6) Keep some cholesterol. Do not lower your cholesterol too much. I can't tell you to stop your statin cholesterol drug, I would never do that. I can only tell you to keep your cholesterol at a normal, healthy amount because you need it to make

cortisol. If you are in the burnout phase, you need to make more cortisol, not less.

7) Lose weight. In a study, men of healthy weight showed a 5% increase in salivary cortisol levels after consuming a meal, the cortisol levels of the overweight and obese men increased by 51 percent.[10] When your body has excessive fat, you secrete more cortisol and you're at a higher risk for stress-related disease.[11,12]

8) Get Zzzs. Do you realize sleep deprivation affects your circadian clock and ability to make brain neurotransmitters, cortisol and melatonin. Sleep helps reduce adrenaline and cortisol. Try to get to bed around 10pm, and wake up around 8am.

9) Relax. Routine massage or meditation reduces your need for medication. Both massage and meditation reduce cortisol and other stress chemicals in your body. This naturally reduces pain.

10) Exercise. It's great to hit a punching bag or go to kick-boxing if you need to let off steam. But if you are in the late phase of adrenal burnout, and you don't have enough energy on hand, then high intensity aerobics are not good for you. Exercise triggers adrenals to make cortisol and adrenaline under healthy circumstances, but again, if you are burnt out, then you should choose restorative, gentle exercises such as those that improve flexibility like yoga (as opposed to high-impact Zumba or a 3 mile jog).

11) Prioritize. Make a list of your most important activities, the things that you really need to do, not feel obligated to do. Let everything else fall away, and focus. Say no to new tasks until you complete the ones you've prioritized. This will recharge your batteries and help build self-esteem for having done what you set out to do.

12) Just say "Thank You!" Allow yourself a helping hand, and learn to accept nurturing loving, compliments or affection. If you didn't learn how to do this while growing up, start practicing now. Every morning before you get up, think of someone who you love, and loves you. Resist thinking of work and problems while you are still in that fuzzy sleep state, only sweet loving thoughts.

Chapter 10

Estrogen, Progesterone and More

Estrogen and progesterone, the principal female sex hormones, play a significant role in menstrual migraines, and facial pain. Testosterone is the primary male hormone, but women do make some and these three hormones must remain in proper ratios for optimal wellness.

A healthy woman will be able to maintain appropriate ratios of estrogens, progesterone and testosterone throughout life. There are biochemical feedback loops which help determine how much of each hormone to secrete at any time and the system is highly complex. Your brain can 'talk' to the ovaries and adrenal glands and produce hormones which support all your other organs.

We know that a risk factor for developing migraines is being female. Women are 2 to 3 times more likely to get migraines, compared to men. This striking variation begins to occur in girls, during adolescence, after menstruation begins. Before monthly cycles, boys and girls experience migraines at about the same frequency. Many studies have indicated an association between estrogen and progesterone fluctuations in females and migraines.

If women are more prone to migraines, there has to be some connection to estrogen and in fact there is. A sudden drop in estrogen hormone concentration is an important trigger for migraines in women.[1,2] And that drop in estrogen happens at the beginning of every new cycle in women who are pre-menopausal. There's no getting around this natural hormonal cycle. This is a trigger for menstrual migraines.

In a normal female hormone cycle, estrogen and progesterone levels are the lowest during the days of menstruation. Estrogen peaks during the ovulation phase which is mid-cycle, around days 10 to 14 of the female hormone cycle; you'd be counting Day 1 as the first day of bleeding, and count out 10 to 14 days from there to find out when you've ovulating (and that's assuming you're pretty regular). Estrogen and progesterone plummet towards the end of the luteal phase, beginning and during the menstruation phase and this is often the trigger for women who are prone to menstrual migraine.[3]

While steady estrogen levels may improve headaches, estrogen levels that fluctuate have been shown to increase migraine headaches.[4] So it's not about how much estrogen you have on a given day, it's more about keeping the levels from getting too erratic, or chronically elevated. You can modulate estrogen levels with one terrific natural compound from broccoli called Indole 3 carbonol.

Menstrual Migraines Feel Different

I found a population-based survey of 2,600 women very interesting. This article was published in the October 2012 edition of *Journal of Headache Pain*. The 2,600 women surveyed were between 18 and 65 years old, and the researchers were interested in evaluating the effect of hormonal changes on migraine headache symptoms. The women were asked questions regarding their hormonal changes and migraine frequency during menstruation. A total of 989 women were diagnosed with menstrual migraines and 73% of these women reported that they were still menstruating. After analyzing the data further, the researchers determined the likelihood of developing a headache during menstruation was considerably higher in patients with migraines.

High Estrogen Low Progesterone

Termed "estrogen dominance" or "progesterone deficiency," the symptoms include:

Irritability & brain fog
Breast tenderness
Water retention or bloating
Unwanted hair growth
Migraines and headaches
Irregular or heavy periods
Fibroids & Severe PMS
Cancer

Also migraineurs reported a notably 'different' feeling type of headache during menstruation in comparison to their customary migraine headache. The researchers found that normal changes during menstruation affect women with migraines more commonly than those who do not suffer from migraines. The researchers also discovered post-menopausal women experienced fewer migraines, probably the result of lower estrogen, or a balance between estrogen and progesterone levels, instead of the constant hormonal fluctuations seen in women who were still cycling.[5]

Are You On The Pill?

Some women experience a sudden drop in estrogen (and thus potential for migraine) by using monthly pill packs of oral contraceptives. When you withdraw the pill for that last week to allow your period to begin, you pull the plug on your estrogen intake. This may spark a migraine for some. Didn't anyone ever tell you that? No, it's not "all in your head" if you know what I mean.

One option for relief is to switch medications. You could try Seasonale, an oral contraceptive that you take long term before taking a break from it. In fact, its claim to fame is that it gives you only 4 periods a year. Another option is to find a different method of birth control that works for you so you are not subjecting yourself to the sudden drop in hormone. I'm not advocating long-term synthetic drugs for you, I'm just offering options so that you can make a personal choice that is well-informed.

Getting your doctor to prescribe natural progesterone could be helpful too. Natural progesterone is not the same thing as progestin drugs like Provera (medroxyprogesterone). The drugs are not what I'm suggesting due to side effects, I was thinking bio-identical natural progesterone, and only if you need it. Now, careful, if you reduce your estrogen too low, you know what happens, you can get that nerve sensitization I mentioned a minute ago. It's perfect if you can just test your levels instead of shooting darts in the dark! I recommend urine testing for hormones, unless you are already applying a hormone cream in which case, saliva testing is better. See Appendix I on Labs for more on them.

Estrogen and progesterone are two sex hormones that have widespread effects all over your body. The brain is highly responsive to progesterone. In fact, progesterone concentrations are sometimes up to 20 times higher in the brain than in the blood. This hormone is so calming that when you become deficient your brain responds with severe insomnia, anxiety, and migraine headaches, and that's the tip of the iceberg. In the brain and elsewhere in the body, progesterone counterbalances the effects of estrogen, think of a see-saw. Whereas estrogen has an excitatory effect on the brain, progesterone's effect is soothing. Clinical and anecdotal experience indicates that women with estrogen dominance sleep restlessly, and when progesterone replenishment occurs (like from bio-identical hormones), you might sleep like a baby.

Studies suggest that progesterone works as a natural anti-anxiety drug by improving GABA (gamma aminobutyric acid); GABA is an inhibitory neurotransmitter and you want more of that if you're trying to rest, or live headache free. You want GABA to be balanced with glutamate, think of that see-saw again. Progesterone improves GABA, that's how it helps with menstrual migraines.

I interviewed Kristi Wrightson, ND, RD, *Founder of Nest Integrative Medicine Spa* in Santa Barbara, California. She is a caring doctor with some fascinating success stories when it comes to her patients. She said, "All too often, people accept their diagnosis of chronic headaches and take medication indefinitely, never getting to a comfortable place. I see a lot of patients with methylation challenges and I feel this is an important piece of the puzzle. Methylation is a complex metabolic pathway that, once corrected, helps enormously. After this detox pathway is opened, hormonal imbalances, specifically progesterone deficiency need to be addressed."

Progesterone deficiency is also termed "estrogen dominance." Progesterone is so important, don't dismiss it just because it is the pregnancy hormone. And guys, news flash, you make it too! You can be as young as in your 20's and start to experience a progesterone deficiency. One of your clues is belly fat! You can also have poor sex drive, irregular or heavy periods, insomnia, irritability, bloating, moodiness, cravings, pain (yes, headaches!) breast tenderness, or benign breast lumps (termed "fibrocystic breast disease"). Women who have challenges maintaining pregnancy may be deficient in progesterone. Also, women who have a baby experience a sudden drop in progesterone right after giving birth. This is natural, as the body attempts to get back into equilibrium, termed "homeostasis." But as the body does this, you as a new mom notice the sudden drop in progesterone which can be marked by melancholy, or a more severe version of that like "Postpartum Depression." This reminds me of my dear friend and college buddy, Lorraine Mobley, RPh, who is a wonderful pharmacist in Florida. Lorraine and I share a long history and we've been friends since we were 20 years old (that's almost 30 years of history for us). She shared her heart with us, in the hopes it might help some of you recognize that your migraines are tied to reduced hormones and neurotransmitters after childbirth:

> "After the birth of my daughter, my first child, I experienced postpartum depression with migraines and I tried some supplements and a few different medications. Only after I started a medication in the antidepressant category (Zoloft), my migraines virtually disappeared! I stayed on it for 11 years because it worked so well for me. As a pharmacist, I am accustomed to weighing risk to benefits with drugs, and the Zoloft made sense to me because it increases serotonin, something you naturally make. Serotonin is reduced in both migraine disorders and depression. Today, I feel very lucky because I only get one migraine about every 6 months or so. I wish we had a pill that contained pure serotonin, if we did, I know we would be forever sold out!"

The picture of progesterone deficiency could include fatigue, pain and depression. The fatigue part is really hard to untangle because your adrenals and thyroid get in on the action, and then you've got all sorts of hormonal imbalances, all at once! Conventional medicine's answer to the progesterone deficiency-induced "fatigue, pain and depression" is Synthroid, Vicodin and Zoloft! You know I'm only half kidding right?! I wonder how my dear friend would have done if her doctor prescribed bio-identical progesterone after the birth of her baby, but we'll never know. What we do know is that we have medications to help fill in the gaps, and it's a blessing that they work for some of you. When Lorraine and I first graduated in the 80's, we only had ergot-related drugs and those had very bad side effects. Triptans, even with their side effects are blessedly safer than the original migraine meds.

Hormone Imbalances Cause Migraines

I'm completely 100% dead serious when I tell you that hormonal imbalances are a common cause for migraines and headaches in general. It's the most frequent finding Dr. Wrightson sees in her office in her headache patients. It makes sense from a scientific standpoint, since progesterone deficiency is linked with over-activity of pain receptors, as well as abnormally low production of the body's natural painkillers, called the endorphins. Low progesterone causes reduced production of serotonin, your feel-good neurotransmitter, the one that triggers melancholy, anxiety and postpartum depression. So what are you going to do if you think you have progesterone deficiency?

You can certainly test yourself to see what your levels are. And if you need to replenish it, you can ask your doctor the best way to do that because there is a lot of debate about it. According to Dr. Wrightson, "Transdermal progesterone is indicated for some patients with deficiency, and this can be made by your local compounding pharmacy. The concentration varies, for my patients, 50mg/ml is a good starting point, applied twice per day on days 14-28 of the menstrual cycle to your skin. The dosage varies based upon your body's deficiency, there isn't a one-size-fits-all dosage like most drugs."

Progestin Drugs are Not Natural Progesterone

If you've tried using natural progesterone cream or medications, and experienced a negative reaction, keep a few things in mind. First of all, the drugs (like medroxyprogesterone) are not the same as natural progesterone, you might need to switch to a bio-identical form. Also, progesterone makes your thyroid gland work harder, and this means that there's a shift in your immune system (doctors, it causes more of a TH1 dominance), and this attacks pathogens in your body. You could be experiencing a little bit of a herx reaction which is where your body is faced with, how can I put this nicely . . . dead bug parts! Also, if progesterone makes you lightheaded and dizzy, your dose may be too high. The solution may be to reduce the dose, stop it altogether for a few days, or switch from one type to another (for example, switch from Prometrium or Provera to bio-identical creams and all of those are prescription only). You need to work with a health care practitioner that's why I don't want you to buy progesterone cream over-the-counter, I want it prescribed for you, in the correct dosage that fits your body's chemistry.

Women with Hysterectomies Need Progesterone Too

Millions of post-menopausal women are taking unopposed estrogen medications (meaning, estrogen therapy without any natural progesterone to go with it).

Excess estrogen has been linked to breast cancer and other hormonally-driven disorders including migraines. Natural progesterone balances estrogen and I feel strongly that no woman should EVER be taking unopposed estrogen meds, even if she has had her uterus removed. Of course, everyone reading this should get physician approval to use progesterone, because my writings are intended for educational purposes, not to be construed as medical advice.

Sadly, some physicians insist that women who do not have a uterus (ie hysterectomy) no longer need progesterone, so they only prescribe estrogen drugs. This is short-sighted because there are progesterone receptors all over your body, not just in the reproductive organs. Progesterone protects the breasts, and may relieve fibrocystic breast pain and reduce risk of breast cancer, plus it supports healthy bones, heart, liver and brain tissue in both men and women. Progesterone is calming so when taken orally, it can help with sleep and anxiety. Remarkably, progesterone feeds the brain, and a new study points to its benefit during the first few hours after a stroke.

So even if your uterus is surgically removed, your other organs need progesterone. Does it make sense to deprive the body of the benefits of progesterone, just because one particular organ that used it was surgically removed? Let me hammer the point home, progesterone stimulates production of thyroid hormone, important to every aspect of life, whether or not a uterus is present!

Natural progesterone is not the same thing as progestin drugs like methoxyprogesterone (Provera) which is sold by prescription. The medications are not bio-identical to what your body makes, and there are no receptor sites on your cells that exactly match the drugs. Because synthetic drugs are not bio-identical, there is a higher risk of side effects. What you read about progestin drugs does not at all apply to bio-identical, natural progesterone hormone.

When you take unopposed estrogen, you could tilt yourself, hormonally-speaking and cause progesterone insufficiency or "estrogen dominance" which appears with symptoms such as chronic fatigue, depression, anxiety, brain fog, insomnia, hot flashes, inability to lose weight, dry skin, thinning hair, bone loss, PMS, fibroids or migraines. Progesterone is known to relieve these problems, whether or not a uterus is present. It can benefit men sometimes too.

In pre-menopausal women, you might expect PMS, breast tenderness, migraines, fibroids, mood swings, bloating, or heavy periods. Symptoms of low progesterone in post-menopausal women include anxiety, depression, irritability, hot flashes, night sweats, weight gain, insomnia, bone loss or low sex drive.

Natural progesterone is needed for brain health so much so that progressive physicians administer the hormone intravenously post-stroke in patients admitted to the hospital. In men (who don't have a uterus) progesterone inhibits 5-alpha reductase, which can help with BPH (benign prostatic hyperplasia).

Even though the current medical "standard of practice" still says to give unopposed estrogen, and most physicians still adhere to this, me and other health experts completely disagree. According to two large European studies, women with or without a hysterectomy who use bio-identical hormones have no increased risk of any disease. For the record, if people didn't disagree with "standards of practice" we'd still blame ulcers on stress, and use leeches for blood lettings. We are born with many hormones and they are best kept in balance. It's dangerous to mess with Mother Nature.

Applying Progesterone Cream

Creams are sold at health food stores. I don't usually recommend them, because I want your dosage tailored to your personal biochemistry, and prescribed to you by a doctor. That said, sometimes the doctors just tell you to go and buy the cream at the health food store! For this reason, I've put together a general outline of how to use the cream. Always follow your doctor's directions for dosage and application. It is generally expressed as "1 pump" usually equivalent to 25mg but this is not always the case, you have to read the label for the product you buy. Here is a general guideline that may be right for some of you, not all. Please note that if you get breakthrough bleeding or any kind of side effect you need to ask your doctor to revisit your particular dosage and application schedule. What I'm sharing here is not right for everyone:

Premenopausal women: Apply your dosage on days 14 - 21 of your cycle. You may increase dosage to twice daily on days 22 - 28. Stop when you begin bleeding and this is Day 1 for your next cycle.

Peri-menopausal women: Apply your dosage on days 8 - 21. Count first day of bleeding as Day 1. On days 22 - 28, you may increase dosage to twice daily if needed/directed.

Post-menopausal women, or uterus or ovaries removed: The first day of each month is Day 1. Begin application of your dose on days 14 - 30 of each month. Apply your dosage once daily to start with. If no relief from symptoms, 1 pump twice daily may be required. Progesterone will NOT work if a woman is estrogen deficient. Many post-menopausal women require BOTH progesterone and estrogen, in which case a physician can prescribe a bio-identical hormone prescription tailored to your needs and these are made by a compounding pharmacist.

Are We Born With a Higher Risk for Headaches?

Yes, according to my good friend, Shawn Bean, CN, a certified nutritionist. He insists there are more problems trickled from estrogen imbalances than just high estrogen. Shawn lives for metabolic pathways! I pulled him out of his research to discuss the relationship between hormones and neurotransmitters because it's crucial to getting you headache free. *You probably didn't realize that, most people don't . . . but your levels of estrogen, testosterone, and progesterone (and others) have a direct impact on your brain neurotransmitters, the same ones involved in the pathogenesis of migraines!*

It's gets complicated so Shawn will help us take a closer look. He says, "Men and women with elevated serum estrogen are reducing their magnesium levels and this contributes to headaches. Excessive estrogen can also deplete magnesium levels by influencing adrenal function. This extra estrogen puts the adrenals into sympathetic mode, which has the same effect of slamming down your adrenal gas pedal and going off to the races. Adrenal glands in overdrive can cause severe magnesium wasting. The typical American is already low in magnesium, and wasting their depleted inventory. Even children born in a developed country enter the world with some degree of adrenal imbalance."

He's saying we may be born with adrenal compromise and low magnesium so from day one of our life we have a risk factor for the development of headaches. And as you know I'm big on detox pathways. I asked him what he thought of our ability to clear poisons from the body because as you know, if it backs up in the blood, it backs up in the brain.

As a reminder, glutathione is our primary liver antioxidant and it's responsible for 'taking out the garbage.' No glutathione, lots of garbage in the body. And there's a direct connection between this powerful housekeeping glutathione and magnesium. Shawn explains, "Glutathione is a major antioxidant which maintains proper levels of magnesium in our blood or RBC (red blood cells). It's well known that magnesium deficiency is a risk factor for migraines. Back in 1970, the lower end of acceptable RBC magnesium levels in the blood was 5.6mg/dL. Today the lower end of this range is 4.0mg/dL. What does this tell you? The ranges today are based upon a magnesium deficient and adrenal depleted society!"

Interesting! The actual normal range isn't really a healthy one, it's based upon declining health of the population surveyed and used for compiling statistics. An estimated 70% or more Americans are truly magnesium deficient. The point here is in order to maintain genuinely healthy magnesium levels, one needs to also maintain good glutathione levels. Shawn Bean can read your genetic snps like he's looking in a crystal ball! Reminds me of Dr. House actually, he specializes in what he calls "Bio-Individualized Medicine," you can learn more about him by visiting www.matrixhealthwell.com.

Before leaving the topic of glutathione, it's a good time to tell you the popular analgesic acetaminophen is a drug mugger of glutathione. You may want to supplement with glutathione or it's precursor N acetylcysteine (NAC) but don't go overboard. It's about balance. If you take too much NAC (or glutathione supplements) it could backfire. Some people can't even tolerate NAC or glutathione because they have a sulfur intolerance and those supplements are sulfur-based (which is different than a sulfa drug allergy, by the way).

Let's Switch Gears . . .
What You Eat Affects Your Head

I mentioned Candida earlier in this chapter, as a possible cause for neurotoxin-induced headaches. The neurotoxin given off by that is acetylaldehyde, which I discussed in great detail in my ebook, *"Understanding Pancreatitis & Pancreatic Cancer."* Acetylaldehyde is your hangover substance, it gives people a drunk feeling and a bad headache. Candida overgrowth causes your body to make more of this, even if you don't drink at all. The offending headache inducer is acetylaldehyde, but the underlying cause of this is candida overgrowth (or drinking). That's why I always advise that you take probiotics. My favorite is Dr. Ohhira's Probiotic.

I have a story to share with you from one of my friends and colleagues, Martie Whittiken CCN, author of "Natural Alternatives to Nexium, Maalox, Tagamet, Prilosec & Other Acid Blockers: What to Use to Relieve Acid Reflux, Heartburn and Gastric Ailments." (Square One Publishers 2012). Martie's experience with migraines is interesting. Basically conventional medicine failed her for a long time. She eventually found relief, and this inspired her journey into the field of nutrition and natural health. She's not only an author, she also hosts a radio show "Healthy by Nature" which you can listen to, visit www.radiomartie.com

> *"Shortly after college started, so did the migraines. The pain was crushing but that wasn't all. I would retreat to a dark room and hope there was no noise or odor because every stimulus bothered me so much more than normal. Sleep was a blessing because I temporarily escaped the searing head pain and nausea. This scenario happened a few times a month and lingered for days at a time.*
>
> *At all my doctor visits, I asked about the headaches. I was then asked, "Have you tried _____ (fill in the name of the drug du jour)?"*
>
> *My answer was also always the same, "Yes. It didn't help much and made me sick to my stomach. What do you think causes the migraines?" The response was typically a blank stare. One doc did try to help and asked me if I had had my eyes checked. "Yes."*

Was I under stress? "Yes, always (by this time I was working, a full time student and a mom). But I only have headaches sometimes."

This went on for years until I noticed a magazine in a health food store with a cover story on migraine triggers. Shocking! It had never crossed my mind that my headaches might be related to something that I was eating (or not eating). Avoiding the triggers didn't help a great deal, but now at least I was on a path of discovery. A physician with some nutrition sense helped me realize I had a probiotic imbalance in my gut, some key mineral deficiencies and a few food sensitivities. Addressing these concerns was fairly miraculous, considering how many years I had suffered, and everything I had tried prior to making these changes.

I was thrilled to have a migraine only once a month . . . and it became predictable based upon my cycle, so I figured it must be hormonal. It was a progesterone deficiency, so I used progesterone cream to lock in the final puzzle piece."

Martie mentions the nutritional changes as key to getting well, and her "final puzzle piece" was progesterone cream. As you've learned, progesterone deficiency (estrogen dominance) is often a driving factor in headaches. Progesterone cream is sold at health food stores by a company called Emerita. This is a good brand, but I usually don't advise self-treatment with progesterone cream. It is a hormone, and the dosage must (repeat must) be based upon your specific needs. Some women need more than others. I almost always recommend your doctor call in your dosage to a compounding pharmacy where they can make it up for you in a dosage that fits your needs.

   Martie suffered many years, needlessly, she wasn't told about the food connection by her physicians, she learned about it from a health food store article. There are many migrenades as you know, the most famous are tyramine containing foods like wine, chocolate and cheese. But yeast is another due to the indirect link; Candida produces acetylaldehyde, and that can make your head hurt. The best way to kill candida is to starve them from their food source which is sugar, and starches. Then you have to replenish healthy gut microflora. Your gut can 'leak' if the permeability is altered, and it is with chronic yeast infection and a poor diet. You probably think this is no big deal but it is. In fact, an undiagnosed fungal infection can cause 100s of symptoms head to toe. I went straight to the expert on fungus-based illness, Doug Kaufmann, author of 8 best-selling books on fungal disease, and host of Know the Cause television.

Allow me to give you some history on this remarkable man, who is also my good friend. By his own words, *"I began studying fungus when I came home from Vietnam in 1971. I felt miserable, yet I had no outward signs that I was anything but a healthy 21 year old man. I felt as though a parasite had gained access to my body and was in control of both my body and my brain. I began studying parasitology, hoping to discover the '3-foot Vietnam worm that commonly enters human bodies.' Of course, no such worm exists. Rather, I learned that parasites run the gamut from large worms to tiny flukes, and even tinier fungi. To me, fungi were mushrooms, so I had never thought of them as having the potential to cause illness, but the books I read told of fungus parasitizing humans and causing many health problems. My own complete recovery has been the basis for decades of personal research, which I hope is useful to you."*

Of the millions of species of fungi that probably exist, scientists have identified and labeled about 70,000 species. Of these, perhaps a few hundred are now known to be "pathogenic," or disease causing in man. Doug and I, and a rare handful of other health experts are convinced that some fungal species cause headaches in people. There's absolute connection for some of you and yet, according to Kaufmann, *"No headache specialist in his right mind would recommend a 'fungal free lifestyle' to overcome migraines. Although the fungi themselves can be disease causing, it is secondary poisons that they produce called "mycotoxins" that are intimately linked with symptoms and diseases. Fungi make very powerful byproducts that are well linked to inflammation and pain. I hope that in a few minutes of reading this, you will feel inspired enough to give an anti-fungal program a 30-day trial."*

We already have literature to show that fungi and their mycotoxins can cause inflammation and elevations of a pro-inflammatory cytokine called C Reactive Protein or "CRP." You can have this evaluated with a simple blood test and the higher it is, the higher your risk of heart disease according to some experts. Elevated CRP goes hand in hand with systemic (full body) inflammation.

Doug Kaufmann's years of work has allowed him to witness fungus and their poisonous mycotoxins causing all sorts of diseases, everything from itchy skin, nail fungus, liver cancer and definitely headaches and migraines. He's been able to help people with migraine headaches by introducing them to either anti-fungal supplements or his Phase One diet plan which starves parasitic fungus. Kaufmann continues to explain, *"Fungi can cause a number of painful symptoms which can cause or contribute to migraine headaches. It gets worse for some, there's a mycotoxin called "aflatoxin b1" which has been associated with liver cancer in humans. These mycotoxins are nasty. There is no one book or website that I've found that gives all of this information on mycotoxins. It took a few years to assemble this list that shows how toxic these fungi are:*

Fungal mycotoxins can be:

1. Mutagenic-changes human genetic material
2. Tremorgenic-capable of causing tremors and seizures in humans.
3. Carcinogenic-causes cancer in humans
4. Teratogenic-causes (birth) defects to the developing embryo
5. Genotoxic-are poisonous to our DNA
6. Neurotoxic-are poisonous to our nerves
7. Nephrotoxic-are poisonous to our kidneys
8. Hepatotoxic-are poisonous to our liver
9. Hematoxic-like venomous bites, poisonous to our blood stream
10. Cardiotoxic-are poisonous to our heart and blood vessels
11. Lymphotoxic-are poisonous to our lymphatic system
12. Dermatotoxic-are poisonous to our skin
13. Immunosuppressive-impedes the human immune system

Still craving that candy bar and soda? I hope not. One more important aspect of yeast and fungi that is commonly known to those who brew their own beer, is a process known as "yeast autolysis." In essence, this means that yeast and fungi cannibalize themselves. You're making beer in your gut! While shocking to hear, I've long wondered if fungal cannibalism doesn't finally explain why chemists cannot create a class of drugs that successfully treats and stops migraine headaches. How can any drug work when you are continuously making mycotoxins in your gut?

Now here's something else to make you go hmmm. A very common medication for migraine headaches is the "Ergotamine" class of drugs which I discussed in Chapter 2 "Migraine Headaches."

Basically, ergot is the *mycotoxin* of the fungus Claviceps which is classified as a poison in the US! This mold (fungus) grows on grains particularly rye, wheat and barley, three grains that contain wheat gluten. That makes me wonder if you're gluten sensitive, or mold sensitive . . . it could be either!

Few people know that some of these same mycotoxins, according to a study published in the prestigious *Journal of the American Medical Society* (JAMA) in 2002, "commonly contaminate" the American grain supply. Interestingly, the mycotoxin drug ergot, offers thousands of people relief.

I asked Doug Kaufmann about this because I find it so strange that a mycotoxin could heal a headache, rather than induce it. He has a hypothesis, *"If fungi or their poisonous mycotoxins are causing your migraine headaches, based on their ability to cannibalize themselves, one justifiable treatment . . . is more fungus! Being able to parasitize man, fungi must then survive by eating mans food. Fungi hate steak and eggs and nuts, but love sugar of any kind. In human/fungal cell relationships, fungi always become the dominant partner, even to the detriment of human cells. Soon, the migraine headache sufferer finds himself craving pasta, potato chips, bread, alcohol and sugar. He is no longer feeding himself; rather he is satisfying the dietary demands of fungus without even knowing it. As wheat, rye, and beer (barley) become standard dietary cravings, the migraines occur more and more regularly. No one puts the pieces of the puzzle together."*

For more information about the fungus link to various diseases, I highly recommend Doug Kaufmann's books or the audio version if you prefer to listen, "The Fungus Link" and these are available at www.KnowTheCause.com. His website has free articles that help you discover anti-fungal drugs that are safe and effective, as well as anti-fungal foods and supplements. The cookbook, "Eating Your Way to Good Health" by Doug Kaufmann and Denni Dunham contains many recipes to help you starve fungus. It's all at the site. If you click on "Watch the Show" tab at the top of his home page, you might even catch me on his program since I am a regular and have a syndicated medical minute. I subscribe to Doug's free monthly newsletter because it's full of incredible health tips. You can do that too, the sign up is on his home page.

One such tip is to eat spices. All herbs and spices are anti-fungal.

Eat more of the foods that fungi cringe from. You see, fungi dislikes spinach, broccoli, cabbage and grapefruit, they have strong anti-fungal properties. And remember this, carbohydrates like grains and alcohol fuel fungal infections, these foods keep the mycotoxins growing. I'm in your head, and I can hear you saying that you're willing to starve your yeast of sugar, and you'll just start eating foods with artificial sweeteners. No! No no no no no nooooooo!

Artificial sweeteners affect hormones and I want you to eliminate them. Just try to change your palette to more "bitter" than sweet. Eliminating artificial sweeteners is important, they are not a substitute for real sugar in my book. I fully discussed this in my *Diabetes Without Drugs* book. Artificial sweeteners are known as endocrine disrupters, because they can affect your hormone system, meaning your ability to make and use estrogen and so forth. There are also case reports for the popular "Splenda" as a trigger for migraines.[14, 15]

One such case report was of a woman who had migraine attacks consistently triggered by sucralose, although she did suffer with menstrual migraines too. The interesting thing is that she had those well-controlled for several months after switching contraceptives from fixed estrogen to triphasic pills.[16] The sucralose was identified as the trigger. According to the article printed in *Headache* 2006, "Some attacks triggered by sucralose were preceded by aura, and she had never experienced migraine with aura before. Withdrawal of the compound was associated with complete resolution of the attacks."

Erin's Temptation Dairy-Free Chocolate Ice Cream By Erin Elizabeth, www.HealthNutNews.com

My sweet friend Erin gave me the recipe that she and her boyfriend Dr. Mercola came up with one lazy Saturday afternoon when they were craving something sweet but healthy. Coconut is a natural anti-fungal and if you have a break down, this hits the spot using clean, natural ingredients.

2 cups coconut milk (I used Vanilla flavor)
1 cup organic coconut sugar
1/2 cup cocoa powder (organic)
1/8 tea salt
4 ounces dairy-free chocolate bar (chopped up)

1/2 tea vanilla extract
1/2 tea Ceylon cinnamon
1/8 tea xanthan gum

Directions: Heat the milk, sugar, cocoa powder, salt and cinnamon over medium heat and whisk until smooth and dissolved. Cocoa powder tends to clump. Bring mixture to a low boil, and then remove from heat. Add the chocolate to the mixture and it will slowly dissolve, keep stirring until completely dissolved. Add the vanilla extract and xanthan gum until combined. Freeze.

Note: Erin's recipe is good as an addition to your afternoon smoothie, in case you don't want to eat it as "ice cream" because it triggers a headache (see Chapter 7 "Mystery Headaches Solved" for more on ice cream headaches).

Suzy's "Script" for Hormone Balance

This is very simple, the way to balance hormones is with the help of a doctor who can prescribe bio-identical hormones for you. This is based upon your levels. If you are expecting me to recommend you take a drug like Premarin, Provera or FemHRT, Estradiol patches or cream, or anything else like that you'll be disappointed. I do not ever recommend one-size-fits-all medications as a method of replenishing natural hormones. You may be wondering why not Estradiol-based drugs (such as Vivelle or Estradiol tablets) . . . but again, these are medications with very big doses of hormone that are probably all wrong for you.

Please understand that my ultimate best "script" for you would include hormone balancing. And this is nothing I can write in a book because the type of hormone and the dosage you get is 100% contingent on your body's chemistry. It's individual. There isn't a pill that corrects it. There isn't an herb that will work for every woman because you may be high in estrogen, low in estrogen, high in testosterone, progesterone, low . . . how could I possibly know?!

This is why seeing a doctor is ideal, preferably one who understands bio-identical hormones. Bio-identical hormones are creams and made-to-order and they contain various different hormones which depending on your needs, may include a type of bio-identical estrogen like estriol for example, some testosterone, progesterone or

DHEA. These creams are made on a daily basis for women, at a compounding pharmacy, and again, the exact ingredients and dosage is specific for you based upon your doctor's evaluation of your labs. See Appendix I for Lab information. The formula may need tweaking if you stay on it for months or years.

So my "Script" section can only include possibilities for you. Below I've briefly listed some of your options. The topic of estrogen and hormone balancing as well as breast cancer is more fully discussed in my ebook, Breast Cancer Protection which is available at my website. Please discuss the use of these with your doctor even though they are sold without prescription. Remember, they affect your hormones, and I always want you to be safe:

I3C or DIM
Chasteberry
Black Cohosh
Sage
Iodine
Calcium D Glucarate
Chrysin

How This Helps You Become Headache Free

I3C or DIM.

There are ways to help 'modulate' or regulate healthy estrogen levels. Many women (and men) could benefit from eating broccoli, or taking the supplemental form of broccoli extract called "I3C" which is short for Indole 3 carbonol. DIM or Diindolylmethane is a component of I3C, also sold at health food stores. You can ask your doctor about I3C or DIM, two dietary supplements sold at health food stores.

In order for you to change IC3 to DIM there has to be adequate stomach acid. People over 40 years produce significantly less stomach acid. DIM may be a better choice if you are over 40 years old. Low stomach acid is very common in our society and is also (surprisingly) responsible for the *increase* of acid reflux. If you are over 40 and eating lots of broccoli and Brussels sprouts to prevent cancer (because crucifers are known for cancer prevention) you may just be teasing yourself. You might be (and you need to ask your doctor) be better off on a DIM supplement. DIM and I3C affect estrogen ratios and this can be measured with hormone panels (done with an overnight urine catch).

DIM was discovered over 10 years ago and is a naturally occurring phytonutrient found in the cruciferous vegetables broccoli, Brussels sprouts, cabbage, and kale. DIM is completely natural, and it encourages formation of good estrogen metabolites, while decreasing the so-called bad estrogens that have been shown to be associated with migraines. These compounds are thought to have a normalizing action on estrogen.[6-11] In high doses, it may lower thyroid. Not only can I3C and DIM help to calm painful menstrual cycles where appropriate, these compounds support prostate health.[12,13]

Vitex Agnus Castus or Chasteberry.

This dietary supplement may help women with certain hormone imbalances, particularly low progesterone. This herb supports progesterone production. It may help with headaches, acne, breast tenderness, depression and pre-menstrual problems. It may help normalize irregular cycles by improving ovulation. In menopausal women, it may ease hot flashes.

Black Cohosh.

Cimicifuga racemosa, this herbal remedy is also known as bugwort. Insects hate it. It's used by women in menopause to control hot flashes. Some have told me it reduced their headache frequency too. It's a dietary supplement sold at health food stores by various brands, and at the pharmacy as Remifemin. Years ago, there was a randomized, double-blind, placebo-controlled trial[18] which found that black cohosh was more effective than prescribed conjugated estrogen (ie Premarin). Eighty menopausal women compared black cohosh extract (Remifemin taken twice daily) with sugar pills (placebo) and conjugated estrogen medication (0.625mg/day). Both anxiety and daily hot flashes decreased in the black cohosh group but not so much in the placebo group, or the group taking medicine (conjugated estrogen). It went from 4.9 per day to 0.7 in the black cohosh group, and reduced only from 5.2 per day to 3.2 in the estrogen group, and 5.1 to 3.1 in the placebo group. About the same change in the conjugated estrogen group and the placebo! Only black cohosh has a positive impact.

Sage.

Salvia Officinalis or sage contains saponins which may ease headaches, especially a headache due to nerves. Considered a plus, this herb is estrogenic, so it's not right for everyone, perhaps only good for post-menopausal women or peri-menopausal women whose estrogen is erratic (that's what sets off the hot flash you know). Your doctor can decide if this is right for you. Sage is used as a spice on poultry, so it's probably hard to conceive this as a headache remedy or a hormone balancer but there's research to back me. Sage is a known as a phytoestrogen like black cohosh. It also keeps blood vessels flexible to some extent.

Iodine. This mineral is a dietary supplement that is well known for thyroid support. Running out of iodine results in increased sensitivity of estrogen receptors in the breast, which affects breast health. Iodine has an anti-estrogenic effect, so it could be useful for "estrogen dominance" or progesterone deficiency, a common trigger for migraines. Iodine helps balance your estrogen hormones; you have three of them, estrone, estradiol and estriol. Iodine shifts them into a healthy balance by increasing estriol (considered a good thing) and reducing estrone and estradiol. Kelp has natural iodine, or you can supplement with it.

Calcium D glucarate. This dietary supplement is not the same as plain "calcium." The supplement I am talking about here is the calcium salt of D-glucaric acid, a compound that we actually make. It's also found in fruits and veggies with the highest concentrations found in oranges, apples, grapefruit, and cruciferous vegetables. Supplementation of this inhibits beta-glucuronidase, which is good because elevated beta-glucuronidase activity in your liver (Phase II detoxification) is actually tied to higher risk of hormone-dependent cancers such as breast, prostate, and colon cancer.[17] Supplementing with Calcium D glucarate may reduce risk for these problems helping your body bind up toxins and take out the trash.

Anyone with gut dysbiosis or digestive trouble could benefit from this supplement which helps reduce estrogen. Beta glucuronidase (an enzyme found in certain bacteria) activity is very pronounced within the gastrointestinal tract due to gram negative bacteria hanging around. If you have digestive problems (medically termed "dysbiosis") you may benefit greatly by using Calcium d glucarate because it inhibits beta glucuronidase activity, which allows toxins to get bound up and removed from your body. Anyone on the Paleo diet could benefit from this too because that diet sometimes increases LDL cholesterol, and this supplement seems to help lower it.

Chrysin. An herbal dietary supplement that acts as a natural "aromatase inhibitor" just like the more potent breast cancer drugs tamoxifen and raloxifene. The rationale here is that estrogen is produced by fat cells through the process of 'aromatization' and estrogen dominant women, overweight women, and aging men tend to all (collectively speaking) show excess aromatase enzyme activity, resulting in their testosterone being 'aromatized' into estrogen. You can block this with an aromatase inhibitor such as chrysin (or tamoxifen and other breast cancer drugs).

Chrysin calms excessive production of estrogen. It is often compounded right into the bio-identical formula that you get from the pharmacy that contains estradiol in it. You can buy oral supplements too. In summary, chrysin is a dietary supplement supplement as well as an additive to compounded hormone creams sold by prescription.

Chrysin has a controlling effect on estrogen. Ask your doctor if it's right for you though because it has an interesting side effect which I should caution you about. As it happens, chrysin is a potent inhibitor of an enzyme MAO-A (monoamine oxidase A) and this raises your serotonin levels and other neurotransmitters.

I study genetics on the side for fun, like a hobby when I'm not too busy studying drugs and herbs. Some of you don't even know this but you have a genetic snp (mutation) in your DNA sequence that is homozygous for MAO-A and that means you already make too much serotonin, and other brain chemicals that may leave you feeling anxious, panicked, wired, irritable or angry. I would never recommend chrysin for you if I knew you had this genetic predisposition. You can test for it through 23andMe.com, they offer a saliva test and also ask your doctor, it's a good thing to know.

ThyroScript™

This dietary supplement supports a healthy thyroid gland, energy production and metabolism. I'm proud to say it is my own personal blend of natural herbs and vitamins. I developed ThyroScript™ based upon my studies and every ingredient has scientific research to support a beneficial effect. Read Chapter 11 for more on the thyroid connection to migraines.
www.ScriptEssentials.com

My point really is: You don't want to raise serotonin with chrysin herb if you take a drug that does the same thing. Drugs that raise serotonin include triptan headache relievers (like Imitrex), and antidepressants such as Zoloft, Prozac, Celexa, Lexapro, Cymbalta etc. The supplement called "5-HTP" is another. St. John's wort is another. So in summary if you take chrysin, you should know it can raise serotonin and thus interact with all of these drugs. I'd avoid it if you take these drugs or others that raise serotonin. Ask your local pharmacist about this before taking chrysin.

Your Plan of Action: A Dozen Ways to Minimize the Pain

We've talked about estrogen and progesterone hormone imbalances. My plan of action is less about rescue remedies and more about options that can identify imbalances.

1) Find a bright doctor. You need someone who specializes in bio-identical hormones, that can determine your specific hormone imbalance, rather than one who will give you a prescription for a symptom. In other words, find a doctor that can figure out if you have a progesterone deficiency (which is much different than a serotonin deficiency). The reason is a prescription for Zoloft (that addresses serotonin) does

> Estrogen lives in fat cells. You naturally reduce estrogen, and can remove the migraine trigger by losing weight.

nothing for the progesterone deficiency. There are labs that can help determine this too, refer to Appendix I on Labs.

2) Go bio-identical. If you already know you have an imbalance in your female hormones, find someone that can switch you from synthetic drugs to bio-identical ones. Bio-identical hormones are a closer match to your own God-given hormones.

3) Install a nutrient security system. If you are on birth control of any sort, whether it's patches, pills or shots you should restore the key nutrients that are "mugged" by these drugs. For example, probiotics, vitamin B6, folic acid, zinc, selenium and magnesium are several nutrients that may be reduced by taking these drugs. If you run low on those, you could be diagnosed with illnesses you don't have.

4) Enjoy. Reducing stress suppresses pro-inflammatory cytokines. How do you reduce stress in your life? By adding activities that take you out of the 'think' mode, and into the 'feel' mode like art, dance, funny movies, enjoyable exercises, gardening, or a new hobby that you've always wanted to do.

5) Say no to fake estrogens. Greatly reduce or remove foods in plastic wrappers or containers. These provide fake estrogens, termed "xenoestrogens" which contribute to your estrogen load. Your body cannot easily get rid of these. Excessive estrogen disrupts endocrine function.

6) Keep some cholesterol around. I can only tell you to keep your cholesterol at a normal, healthy amount because you need it to make hormones such as estrogen, progesterone, testosterone, and memory molecules. When you reduce cholesterol to unhealthy levels, you will feel sick, lose your mind, your memory and comfort in your muscles.

> Spearmint Tea may raise your estrogen and reduce testosterone. It may not be right for women who have excessive estrogen because it can raise estradiol levels, something you don't want if you have estrogen-related headaches.

7) Lose weight. When your body has excessive fat, it automatically means excessive estrogen and other hormones that increase headache risk. There is a direct relationship to obesity and migraines. Clinical features of migraine increase with body mass index (BMI).[19, 20]

8) No fake sweeteners. Eliminate artificial sweeteners because they disrupt hormone production.

9) Avoid GMO. These foods may damage the gut and cause inflammation.

10) Eat organic. Pesticides disrupt estrogen and other endocrine hormones.

11) No fungus. Avoid yeast-containing foods such as some commercial baked goodies. They contain fungus.

12) Consider anti-fungal herbs. These kill yeast and mycotoxins, reducing toxic load.

Chapter 11

The Thyroid Connection

Approximately 12 million Americans have hypothyroidism[1] which is tied to hundreds of symptoms including migraines, infertility and diabetes. You're little thyroid is a small butterfly-shaped gland with a big function. Located at the base of your throat, your thyroid produces hormones that control your metabolism (as in fat-burning ability) and regulate the rhythm of your heart and your body temperature. That explains why you eat like a bird and gain weight, while your husband eats a horse and stays thin. People like that either have a healthy thyroid and good metabolism or they have intestinal parasites!

Most people think hypothyroidism is strictly about fatigue, cold sensitivity and weight gain but news flash, it causes misery head to toe. One glitch in your thyroid and dangerous consequences can ensue, ranging from encephalopathy[2] to heartbeat irregularities, schizophrenia which is sometimes termed "myxedema madness," reversible dementia and certainly headaches.

Low thyroid, termed hypothyroidism can be a contributing factor to headaches and migraines in some cases.[3] Low thyroid that is driven by an autoimmune process is termed Hashimoto's disease. With low thyroid your metabolism (and thinking) slows down from the sluggish thyroid production and then your circulation becomes stagnant, you may bloat or notice a little swelling in your hands and feet right before a headache. Brain fog sets in. Hypothyroidism means sluggish detoxification pathways so you accumulate more waste. Blood vessels may dilate all around your body. The blood vessels surrounding your brain may swell. Then you develop a headache, migraine or cluster.

I asked a friend and thyroid advocate, Mary Shomon, coauthor of "Beautiful Inside and Out: Conquering Thyroid Disease with a Healthy,

Happy Thyroid Sexy Life" about this, and she explained, "Because of the inflammation, swelling, and fluid retention that occurs in hypothyroidism in some patients, headaches can be a symptom of an underactive thyroid. I have also heard some thyroid patients state that chronic migraine disease had fewer flareups once their thyroid treatment was truly optimized."

No triptan drug is going to balance your thyroid hormone, so I want you to keep that in mind if you rely on those drugs; it's a clue that you've not addressed the underlying cause of your headaches, and I'm telling you (and Mary's telling you) that it could be undiagnosed hypothyroidism.

The treatment of low thyroid hormone is thyroid hormone! Your doctor could also prescribe any kind of medication, some are more natural than others. Among the most popular are Armour Thyroid®, Nature-Throid®, Synthroid®, Levothyroxine, Cytomel and Compounded T3. The Armour and the Nature-Throid are "natural dessicated thyroid" or NDT because they contain both T4 and T3 in one pill; they are both porcine derived. Additionally, with thyroid-related headaches, it helps if you lie down and rest. Excess fluid can be eliminated from the body and this helps minimize the pain and edema.

As a pharmacist, I've seen doctors prescribe Synthroid (levothyroxine) a million times. This drug provides your body with T4, a precursor to T3 or thyroxin your active thyroid hormone. Synthroid is not an active drug, your body has to convert the Synthroid (T4) into T3 which is what you want because T3 does all the good stuff for you, it provides energy and better metabolism. It warms you up if you're cold.

You can get terrible pressure headaches from too much thyroid hormone, and that situation can arise because your taking too much thyroid medicine (your dose is too high), or you're pumping out excessive thyroid hormone because you have hyperthyroidism which is too much thyroid hormone.

Let's talk about hyperthyroidism (and Graves' disease) for just a moment because headaches aren't the only signs you'll get with that. It's important for me to spend a moment here because so many of you take thyroid medicine, and you switch brands sometimes . . . or you switch the type of medicine you take, or the dosage . . . I'm worried that you may not realize your dose is too high for you so I want to talk about hyperthyroidism even though it's less common than hypothyroidism (low thyroid).

With hyperthyroidism (high thyroid), the headaches are hallmark, probably due to the chronically elevated blood pressure that goes with it. The medications used for this condition are either Propylthiouracil or "PTU" or methimazole or "MMI." Side effects of those medications may include bone marrow changes, liver damage or aplastic anemia.[4]

These headaches associated with hyperthyroidism are dull compared to clusters and migraines, and may be bilateral or unilateral. There is no aura, and they are not sharp. They can occur any time of day. You may notice going to the bathroom more than normal with looser, more frequent bowel movements. Your heart will race, and you'll sleep poorly. Your mind may race. You may develop tremors or feel like your body is shaking or vibrating or buzzing; you are hot or sweaty when others feel comfortable or cool. You may be flushed, or feel like you're on fire but it's not a hot flash. You may feel prickly sensations on the skin, or itchiness. These are some of the signs of hyperthyroidism, whether it's drug-induced from excess thyroid medicine, or the autoimmune condition. I want you to be familiar with it, because it's a common cause of mystery headaches.

Autoimmune thyroid illness means that your own immune system attacks the thyroid gland. The opposite of (low) hypothyroidism is hyperthyroidism, where excessive thyroid hormone is produced causing weight loss, rapid heartbeat, increased sweating and heat intolerance, nervousness, moodiness, weakness and hand tremors.

The size of your brain changes with thyroid levels too. There is a highly significant correlation between a reduction in brain size and a reduction in T4 hormone. Reduced levels of TSH (which mean better levels of thyroid hormone) are correlated to an increase in brain size. Basically the research suggests that your brain shrinks a little if you have poor thyroid hormone levels.[5]

Testing Matters

Never with Coffee

All thyroid medications should be taken on an empty stomach, first thing in the morning unless otherwise directed.

There's an epidemic of tired, overweight folks who don't know they're hypothyroid because of improper testing. Some old school physicians are still drawing blood levels of TSH (thyroid stimulating hormone) as the sole method to evaluate thyroid function. TSH is incapable of telling you or your doctor what's happening inside your cells. It's fine to check as part of a comprehensive profile, but not by itself. People are often told they have "normal" thyroid levels, based upon their "normal" TSH. TSH is a brain hormone and has nothing to do with intracellular (mitochondrial) levels of active thyroid hormone called "T3."

This is an important point: TSH may very well be normal, while T3, (the hormone you want) is desperately low. You will hold on to weight, experience migraines or other types of headaches, have dry skin, suffer with hair loss, fatigue, muscle aches, arrhythmias, depression, forgetfulness, anxiety and low libido. Regardless of your misery, you may still be told your okay, because your TSH is okay. Big mistake! Huge! The solution is thyroid support.

Reverse T3 Makes You Hibernate

Evaluating blood levels of Reverse T3 also called "Reverse thyronine" and abbreviated as "rT3" is equally important. Reverse T3 is a mirror image of active T3. Elevated rT3 causes all the symptoms of clinical hypothyroidism I just mentioned. It's often high in people with heavy metals. I lecture around the world, and still meet physicians who dismiss rT3. Did you know that hypothyroidism is a major cause for diabetes? When rT3 is high (greater than 24), that means it's poised like a pit bull on your cells' receptor sites preventing the real deal (T3) from entering the cell. The net result of elevated rT3 is you feel like zombie. But again, if your TSH is normal, or your rT3 is never measured, you will be dismissed as normal. If you have elevated rT3, you should not be taking levothyroxine because it will likely convert to more rT3 instead of active T3. Ask your physician if compounded T3 is okay for you in this case (until the rT3 comes down to normal).

Please refer to Appendix I for Labs, you will find information about testing a "Thyroid Profile." I also discuss this in my new Ebook entitled, "Wake Up Your Thyroid by Eating Right." You will not only learn which foods heal and which harm you, but you'll also discover the most important thing: *How you can reduce inflammation in your thyroid!* This is key to getting well. In addition, you will learn:

*   How toothpaste attacks your thyroid
*   Why Synthroid can worsen hypothyroidism for some of you
*   Which foods (that you probably eat every day) raise risk for thyroid cancer

* How avoiding just one food additive can reduce TPO antibodies and full-body inflammation
* Which supplements are the very best, and scientifically shown to improve thyroid production, absorption and utilization
* Which medications have the ability to suppress thyroid production
* Why it doesn't matter how much thyroid hormone you make, or take! Shocker, it really doesn't matter if it doesn't get inside your cell!
* How gut bacteria (probiotics) help you make up to 30% more thyroid hormone
* Why high dose iodine isn't always right
* How to lower Reverse T3

This book is available at my websites: www.DearPharmacist.com and www.ScriptEssentials.com

One Special Mineral: Selenium

Selenium is important to thyroid functioning. I love selenium because it supports your basic thyroid health, and it helps even with autoimmune types of thyroid illness like Hashimoto's or Graves'. Celiac disease sometimes occurs with autoimmune thyroid illness, so you should always test for Celiac if you have an autoimmune thyroid disorder.[6, 7]

The triggers are often food sensitivities, especially grains, which is why Doug Kaufmann's "Phase One" diet or Loren Cordain's "Paleo" diet

Eating for Hashi's

If you have Hashimoto's disease, eat gluten free. I've seen the diet reduce TPO antibodies in my friend by 75% in just 2 months of a strict gluten free diet. To that end, a study published in the *Journal of Clinical Endocrinology and Metabolism*, states, "Malabsorption of T4 may provide the opportunity to detect Celiac Disease that was overlooked until the patients were put under T4 therapy."

work so well for Hashimoto's and Graves' disease patients. Other causes for autoimmune assault of the thyroid include parasites, bacterial, fungal and viral infection. Women are more susceptible to thyroid illness compared to men. A goiter (swollen thyroid) in the neck can occur. Whether you have hypo or hyperthyroidism, selenium, is one trace mineral that may help this too. Once you correct your thyriod imbalance, your more apt to live headache free. You might be getting too much selenium if you get heart palpiations. Dozens of drugs steal it from your body. See "Drug Muggers that deplete Selenium."

The Iodine Controversy

The thyroid gland is the only part of the body that has cells capable of absorbing iodine, which it gets from food, iodized salt and seaweed but it doesn't get nearly enough. I was shocked when I learned that the *American Thyroid Association* reported that approximately 40% of the world's population remains at risk for iodine deficiency. I think part of the problem is that foods grown in mineral-deficient soils are less nutritious. Bring in chemicals called halides such as fluorine, chlorine and bromine. These halides are annoying bullies and race for the same spot on the cell that iodine does, the bullies win. You need iodine to produce thyroid hormone.

Who are the bullies? For example, a very popular sports electrolyte drink contains bromine, your pool and jacuzzi contain chlorine and most toothpastes contain fluoride. It's not any one punch, it's the cumulative effect. You know how you love that new car smell? Some of it is off-gassing of bromine, and you're breathing it in. Your thyroid gets upset.

> ### Drug Muggers of Selenium
> Hundreds of medications have the potential to rob your body of selenium, this is covered in greater detail in my *Drug Muggers* book.
>
> Acid reducing medication
> Antidepressants
> Corticosteroids
> Hormone-replacement therapy
> Birth control pills
> Breast cancer drugs
> Sulfonamides

These bully halides are drug muggers of your iodine, they could cause deficiency. This increases your risk for becoming hypothyroid: Hair loss, depression, always feeling cold, weight gain, brittle fingernails, constipation, pale, dry skin. Did I mention fatigue? Oh yeah, it's constant and you wake up only after that triple shot latte.

I interviewed one of the world's leading experts on thyroid health, Dr. David Brownstein, a medical doctor who has treated thousands of patients so he has many years of hands-on clinical experience. I asked him about the connection to headaches because no one really thinks of headaches as a classic sign of thyroid illness. When we think of a person being hypothyroid, we often think of other symptoms, not migraines or headaches. Dr. Brownstein said, *"My experience with headaches is that over 80% of people that suffer from chronic headaches, any type, cluster, tension, migraines . . . they all have a hormonal imbalance, and when you correct that hormonal imbalance the headaches often disappear."*

That begs the question, WHAT hormonal imbalance are you talking about, estrogen, progesterone, testosterone . . . what? Dr. Brownstein explained, *"The number one hormonal imbalance I see is thyroid hormone because that hormone is the one that regulates your metabolism and many other hormones. Many people suspect they have a thyroid problem, and this can be confirmed by doing proper blood testing, a good physical exam to see if you have weight gain, hair loss, brain fog, cold sensitivity, and also tracking your basal body temperature. I like the last one because it puts the patient in charge of their health, and they can see for themselves. I want people to know that headaches are a cardinal symptom of hypothyroidism."* See "Determining Basal Body Temperature." For more reading about this connection, refer to Dr. Brownstein's book, "Overcoming Thyroid Disorders" where it is more fully explained. You can also go to his website to sign up for his free newsletter, or get more information about thyroid, and also purchase his books www.drbrownstein.com.

Determining Basal Body Temperature

This is a simple, affordable way to evaluate thyroid function at home. You need to use the right thermometer. Buy a basal thermometer, (often sold to women seeking pregnancy). Such brands include "3M Nexcare," "Clearblue" or "BD." Here are the directions to follow:

> Wake up in the morning
> Put the basal body thermometer under your arm before getting out of bed (within 5 min of waking up)
> Thermometer beeps when done, usually after a minute
> Temperature should be between 97.8 - 98.2 (considered normal)
> If it's < 97.8, your thyroid is not working efficiently

Note: If you are still menstruating, do it while you are on your cycle. Adult woman (not menstruating) or man can do it anytime.

Some people put the thermometer under their tongue (instead of their armpit). If you do that, then a normal temperature would be 98.8 - 99.2 degrees. Below 98.8 and it's a strong indicator that you're hypothyroid.

Leptin Signaling Affects Thyroid Health

Leptin a hormone that has a strong bearing on how much thyroid hormone is produced by your thyroid gland. Leptin is technically a protein that's made in fat cells, and it's good for you. Leptin is your 'stop sign' for eating. When your body secretes leptin, you start to feel full . . . not that you stop eating (because there's always room for dessert right) but leptin gives you that sense of satiety and you should listen to it. When you get that sense of fullness caused by leptin, step away from the plate!

I know YOU don't do this, but some people over-eat. It happens. I get it. I was recently at an Indian buffet and I had 3 servings of Tandoori chicken, 2 curry chicken, an unidentifiable chickpea dish, a virtual bucket of vegetable korma (!) and 2 Samosas. Please don't tell Doug Kaufmann (that was so NOT Phase One) so I relieved my guilt by eating something green, the mint chutney. I felt my leptin release somewhere around the second plate of 'Aloo Gobi' cauliflower potatoes, (oops, I forgot to tell you about that) but like a Champ, I kept going. I almost knocked out a 10 year old kid, racing for the carrot pudding. I convinced myself that I should get my money's worth for this $12.95 buffet, leptin or not. Sam, amused by my lack of self control and poise, risked his life by taking some pictures of the event, but I allowed this because my mouth was full and I never talk with my mouth full. Well, like I said, it happens. For me, this display of carnage is rare.

If these indulgances happen frequently, so that you are eating too much on a consistent basis, then you will become "leptin resistant" and your skinny jeans dislpay an unwanted muffin top. Spandex works well here. In fact, spandex is what I'll wear when I go back to that Indian buffet.

Switch your regular table salt which only contains "sodium chloride" to sea salt which contains a full range of minerals. Your thyroid gland loves minerals.

People. Pay attention to leptin! If you don't, you become leptin resistant. Then, no matter how much leptin is secreted from your cells, your brain doesn't see the signal to stop eating, it thinks there's a famine going on. Just like Pavlov's dog, you become conditioned to see leptin and ignore it, and keep eating.

With leptin resistance, your brain thinks your body is starving. I know this sounds ridiculous to you, but it is very common, dare I say it is epidemic, and it affects your thyroid gland . . . badly! When you're thyroid gland gets involved, your risk for headaches goes up.

When leptin resistance happens in the body, it basically 'tells' your thyroid gland via complex signaling hormones to slow down metabolism and stop burning food for calories. In other words, it tells you to hold on to fat to survive the famine (remember it thinks you are starving to death). Leptin resistence = Fat storage. See a physician skilled in endocrinology, if you think you have leptin resistence.

Can Showering Reduce Thyroid?

Sadly, it might, but this is not your excuse to skip showers. Did you know that certain chemicals like chlorine, fluoride, bromine and perchlorates can attach to your thyroid and reduce your ability to absorb iodine. Chlorine is found in your tap water (like from your shower, or drinking water), your pool and jacuzzi. Chlorine goes through your skin.

Fluoride is in toothpaste, mouthwash and it attacks your pineal gland (which happens to make melatonin to help you sleep). You absorb fluoride through your skin and mucus membranes. Do you see how using *fluoride-free* personal care products might help you sleep better? Look up pineal gland and fluoride. It will stun you. Bromine is in hydrogenated vegetable oil, it's in citrus sodas and most breads.

What's the big deal? First of all those chemicals are pollutants and they're hard to get out of your system. These guys are bullies, and the halogens like chlorine, fluoride and bromine are always going to beat up iodine. Poor little iodine, darn! It's going to take a beating. And so will your thyroid production.

Without iodine you cannot make T4. There's no way to do it. The T stands for tyrosine and the 4 stands for 4 molecules of iodine. So that's 4 iodines to 1 tyrosine to make T4 or "thyroxine."

Nothing can replace those 4 molecules of iodine and make T4, but those three halogens can displace it, then you can't make T4. Then you're clinically hypothyroid, even if you have a perfect TSH. Measuring free T4 is important (so is measuring free T3). Doctors can't agree on what the best range is. I think you'll feel well if your T3 is between 3.5 – 4.2 but do as your physician says too, I'm only educating you, not advising you.

T4 is a precursor hormone to T3, which is your real, wake-me-up thyroid hormone. T4 must be converted in your body to T3 in order for you to feel well, have a normal body temp (hypothyroid patients almost always have a lower body temperature). The reaction takes place compliments of an enzyme you have. And so you know, T4 and T3 are exactly the same except that there are only 3 iodines on the molecule instead of 4. Your body craves and lives for T3. You can get this compounded at any pharmacy if you prefer to take that over natural dessicated thyroid (called NDT) or levothyroxine.

Compounded T3 isn't right for everyone, I just want you to know that you can get it with a prescription since most people do not know this. For some of you, especially those of you who have been on T4 drugs (levothyroxine) for many years, switching to compounded T3, about 5 or 10 mcg could be just what you need to breathe life into you. That discussion needs to take place with a doctor after proper testing because I do not know what's right for you. I just want you to know that the T4 drugs you take are inactive, they do nothing. Your body has to convert them to T3 for you to feel any effect, so if you can take T3 directly as a capsule, it might make a big difference for you.

Toxins found in bread, pools, and toothpaste could contribute to reduced thyroid production, reduced T3 (triiodothyronine) levels, as well as more antibodies against your precious little gland. TPO antibodies and others can be measured. If the toxins are fat-soluble, they'll cross your blood brain barrier and harm your hypothalamus. That means your hypothalamus gland can no longer detect thyroid or leptin signals correctly. Bummer, that means more thyroid problems, and that means higher risk of migraines and other types of 'brain pain.' Your brain doesn't actually feel pain, but I like the term.

Probiotics Influence Thyroid Levels

Probiotics can make a big difference because 20 - 30% of your inactive T4 is converted to active T3 in your gut. You always want to take a high-quality probiotic. Did you know that all medicines are drug muggers of intestinal flora? I recommend Dr. Ohhira's Probiotic because it helps you grow your own intestinal flora, the one you were born with, and plus, it's guaranteed to be alive and fresh. More on probiotics in Chapter 7. The following medications and conditions are among the worst offenders for mugging beneficial bacteria:

Antibiotics

Corticosteroids

Antacids

Acid blockers

Estrogen containing hormones

Blood pressure pill

Alcohol

Caffeine

Sugar and refined foods

Post-appendectomy

Celiac, Crohn's and IBS

As for your liver, this is primary detoxification organ. One snafu here, and you will hold onto poisons. Some T4 is converted to T3 on the cell membrane of your liver so if you consume a fat-soluble toxin (or you have a chronic infection), it will interfere with thyroid hormone activation at the level of the liver. Supplements that support liver health are important. Eating artichokes is useful too. Milk thistle is one option, careful though it has mild estrogenic effects, and there are many other liver detox supplements.

If your liver isn't fully functional, and busier dealing with fat-soluble toxins than activating thyroid hormone you are going to be tired and hypothyroid and all that goes with it. You are also going to find yourself stuffing toxins into your fat (white adipose tissue). Not good. This is an important time to remind you why losing weight helps so much.

You see, as you lose fatty tissue, all those stored poisons go out with the fat. You reduce biotoxin load. Before you get all the benefits of losing weight though, you might crash. Think about it. You break down fatty tissue, all those fat cells dump their poison right back into your bloodstream. Your kidneys and liver go crazy trying to deal with the toxic burden. Your thyroid might crash, and your brain might get very slightly 'inflamed' from all the pro-inflammatory cytokines released. You could feel achy, sore, tired, cranky and have diarrhea. Eventually, if you stay hydrated and keep exercising, sweating (far-infrared saunas are okay), clearing poisons, drinking, juicing, eating healthy, etc . . . you will get to a point where you feel better.

Eating fiber comes in handy here because it binds up and removes fat-soluble toxins. If you get to a 'crisis' place you should call your doctor, or weight loss practitioner, but most people do just fine. Consuming low doses of activated charcoal, or bentonite clay may be helpful for a crisis, but not long-term, just a day or two. These are constipating and you don't want that. One more option is "calcium D glucarate" supplements, this helps control hormones as an added benefit.

Hawaiian Spirulina by Nutrex-Hawaii can also bind up toxic waste and it isn't constipating, in fact, it has valuable health benefits and may help with detoxification. Spirulina supplements are natural dietary supplements derived from purified algae, and it's rich in trace minerals as well as precious iodine which your thyroid hormone needs. A brand new animal study just proved that Spirulina platensis (the kind found in Hawaiian Spirulina) is capable of reducing fluoride toxicity in offspring, if it's taken by the pregnant moms.[8] The study looked at neurodevelopment and oxidative stress in 30 pregnant rats and those who were given spirulina had babies that fared out better because the spirulina could displace the fluoride and protect the thyroid gland. We know how awful the effect of fluoride is on thyroid glands, so to find a natural supplement that may protect the thyroid from fluoride damage, that's pretty cool!

There's a group of you who take thyroid medicine but can't lose weight. It doesn't make a lot of sense. It could be because you are iodine deficient to begin with. You've probably wondered, *"Why do some people on thyroid medicine remain iodine deficient or gain weight?"*

Good question! According to Dr. David Brownstein, "The problem is that we don't have enough information. This group of people were probably not initially assessed for their iodine status, and you have to do that. When you give an iodine deficient person thyroid hormone medications, you will make the iodine deficiency more pronounced, and they won't experience a good outcome. This means that they may remain clinically hypothyroid, even though they are medicated, and perhaps that explains why people experience weight gain, despite taking thyroid hormone. The levothyroid makes the TSH decrease, but it doesn't address the underlying cause of iodine deficiency which worsens."

Dr. Brownstein continued, "There's a lot of iodophobic people out there, and they don't understand the physiology and biochemistry of iodine, Between my partner and I, we've tested 6,000 people, and over 95% are defient in iodine, and it could explain the epidemic of breast cancer, hypothyroid, autoimmune thyroid illness, thyroid cancer, ovarian, uterine and prostate cancer that we're seeing today. I've used iodine supplements in my patients for years, with good results, especially when combined with adaptogens that support adrenal function."

It's very important to get your iodine levels into normal range before beginning thyroid medicine. Normal range for iodine, between 6 and 50mg iodine per day.

Better to do urinary test- 24 hour urine. Dr. Brownstein recommend the Iodine loading test which is offered through Hakala Labs. www.HakalaLabs.com

---

Optimal Thyroid Measurements

This is where you should feel good, my suggestions are merely that, and may not reflect the current standard of care.

Lab	Optimal Level
TSH	0.1 - 1.0 mIU/l
Free T3	3.5 - 4.2 pg/ml also expressed as 350 - 420 ng/dL
rT3	Ideally < 16 ng/dl or 160 pg/ml

Get Rid Of of these Migrenades™!

Artificial sweeteners
Fluoride-containing mouthwash, toothpaste, etc
Clothes that require dry-cleaning (chemicals harm your thyroid)
MSG
Gluten and all grains if possible
White salt, only use Celtic, pink Himalayan or Real™
Vegetable oil, it contains bromine
Fancy dryer sheets

Alpha lipoic acid supplements relieve nerve pain. This could interfere with the amount of active T3 your body makes. Keep dosages low. If you really need high dosages of alpha lipoic acid, such as 600mg per day then your medication dose can be increased. Taking more T4 drugs (as in Synthroid) won't help because it's T4.

Avoid Fake Estrogens

Many commercially fragranced popular dryer sheets and laundry detergents contain xenoestrogens or fake estrogens that permeate your clothing when you wash and dry them. Then the clothes or towels come into contact with your skin and can disrupt endocrine function, leading to thyroid problems. Look for natural detergents at the health food store. One of my favorites is "Grab Green 3-in-1 Laundry pods." You can make your own dryer sheets by taking some cotton and putting a few drops of your favorite essential oil and tossing it in the dryer with your clothes. I like sweet orange or vanilla, but my daughter likes lavender or lemon. The possibilities are limitless and this luxury doesn't harm your thyroid or estrogen hormones.

> *Exercise regularly to improve lymphatic drainage and increase blood flow. This will give your body fresh nutrients and oxygen while burning fat. Exercises that increase flexibility are good, as are those which are aerobic (like walking jogging).*

Suzy's "Script" for Thyroid Balance

Please note the "script" for thyroid hormone balance is 100% contingent on your body's chemistry. You may need medication, you may not. This is all based upon your tests. Medications such as natural dessicated thyroid or "NDT," compounded T3 or Cytomel are options. I don't get overjoyed about Synthroid (levothyroxine) however this is another popular choice.

I can give you a few ideas on supplements that help support thyroid health. Keep in mind you need a healthy diet rich in leafy greens and even seaweed to provide the minerals which nourish your thyroid gland. Before you take any of the following supplements, you must ask your doctor(s) if they are right for you. My intention here is to educate you about possibilities and options. Do not misconstrue my ideas for medical advice. I have no idea what is right for every individual reading this so take my list to your practitioner(s) to ask if they're right for you with your medical history. In addition, you might benefit from the following:

Iodine

Selenium
Ashwagandha
Tyrosine
Mullein
Japanese Knotweed

How This Helps You Become Headache Free

Iodine.
Iodine is one of the components that helps make thyroid hormone. It starts out as thyroxine or T4 for short. The "4" refers to the number of iodine molecules bound on to the "T" which stands for tyrosine. Thyroid hormone is just iodine and tyrosine glued together. At some point, one of the iodine atoms leave, and you're left with T3 which is your body's fuel. T3 wakes you up and burns fat, it makes you pretty.

Selenium.
Selenium taken preventively as selenium citrate or selenium picolinate should be taken at about 50 to 100 mcg once daily. If your levels are low, however, I recommend shooting for 100 to 200 mcg daily with your doctor's supervision. In rare cases, excess selenium can cause spots on your nails, nausea, vomiting, and nerve damage and cardiac palpitations, so I always suggest talking to your doctor before beginning a new supplement and start at the lowest possible dose.

One more thing, selenium-rich foods include walnuts, tuna (not too much, mercury!), shrimp, eggs, cheese, turkey, beef and oatmeal. I like Brazil nuts because eating four per day gives you about 200 micrograms of selenium. Do not make home-made Brazil nut milk like I did, you will overload!

Ashwagandha.
It helps make thyroid hormone and provide antioxidant protection. One of my favorite supplements for thyroid (and adrenal) health is "winter cherry" or ashwagandha, known botanically as Withania somnifera. Yeah, I hear ya, it has a funny name, one that is hard to pronounce unless you get into multi-syllabic scientific jargon like this nerd extraordinairre.

But if you can get past the name, and consider that this herb supports thyroid andadrenal health, you'll keep it handly like I do. In fact, I often suggest it as an option for people who can't tolerate the T4 drugs such as levothyroxine (such as Synthroid). You see, ashwagandha has the ability to help hyper and hypo thyroid. In hypothyroid people, it helps you make more thyroid hormone. It supports hormone health, it is an adaptogen so it nourishes those poor, tired adrenals that you've burnt out from taking care of a loved one, or from watching from watching The Tonight Show with Jay Leno instead of sleeping. So now you know that ashwagandha (as well as selenium) are wonderful for improving the health of your thyroid gland, and protecting it from DNA damage which leads to cancer sometimes.

Tyrosine.

This is an amino acid that is sold as a dietary supplement. It is needed for production of thyroid hormone and is only useful to people with hypothyroidism, not hyper. You should avoid it if you have hyperthyroidism, or Graves' disease. Your body makes tyrosine all by itself (with the help of another amino acid called phenylalanine) but you may not have enough to produce adequate amounts of thyroid hormone. The dosage varies, I've seen it as high as 500 to 1,000mg three times daily but I really think that is way too much. I only recommend a small amount, perhaps 50 to 200mg total daily dosage. Other nutrients that assist your body in converting the tyrosine to thyroid hormone include B vitamins like B6 and folate, as well a small amount of copper.

Caution: Don't take this if you have high blood pressure, or cardiac palpitations.

Mullein.

Also known as Verbascum thapsus. Mullein is terrific for general health and thyroid health. I really love it, and want to raise awareness for this herb because it can not only help reduce migraine suffering, it can nourish the thyroid gland and create more thyroid hormone for you. Mullein herb is anti-bacterial, and may help treat tubercoluosis. It's sold in many formulas for lung health. Lab studies prove that mullein has some antitumor, antiviral, antifungal and antibacterial effects. I've read that mullein can help with earaches and ear pain. Remember, this is just one herb! You can find mullein herb as a liquid extract, as a tea, and in combination with other nutrients in my supplement, ThyroScript™ (www.ScriptEssentials.com).

Japanese Knotweed.

Polygonum cuspidatum or Japanese knotweed, is an invasive flowering plant, what others would call a weed. This herb is used by supplement makers to produce another supplement you're very familiar with, called "resveratrol." We know that it's an antioxidant, anti-inflammatory and antibacterial. There are also anti-fungal properties to it. This helps support thyroid health. I've recommend Japanese Knotweed, as opposed to plain resveratrol because I've heard that resveratrol is too strong, that it causes vasodilation for some of you and triggers a migraine. I've not ever heard that with polygonum cuspidatum.

Zinc.

You need zinc to convert T4 to active T3. This means that people with low zinc can't convert it, and are clinically hypothyroid. Zinc is zapped by the body by hundreds of medications, including acid blockers, estrogen containing hormones and corticosteroids. Zinc is also useful at the level of your cells, on receptor sites. You need zinc to get that thyroid hormone into the cell. Zinc is best known for it's ability to help reduce severity of a cold, most people don't realize it plays a huge role in thyroid health. Zinc is also needed to help you smell things, and to help you see. It's important for blood clotting, and immune function. White marks on your fingernails may be a sign you have low zinc. Metabolic rates increase with zinc supplementation which means you can burn fat better. One study found that 26mg of zinc gluconate increased levels of T3 as well as resting metabolic rate (a sign that thyroid function improved).[9]

Want to read more on the topic?
Read books by some experts . . .

There are other ideas to help you relieve headache pain in Appendix IV, "Facebook Friends Helping Friends." In addition, pick up a copy of these books on the topic of thyroid health:

> *Beautiful Inside and Out: Conquering Thyroid Disease with a Healthy, Happy Thyroid Sexy Life* written by my good friend and thyroid expert, Mary Shomon and former Baywatch star, Gena Lee Nolin.

> *Overcoming Thyroid Disorders* or this book devoted solely to iodine, *Iodine: Why You Need it, Why You Can't Live Without It* both written by my good friend David Brownstein, MD

Hashimoto's Thyroiditis: Lifestyle Interventions for Finding and Treating the Root Cause by my good friend (and Hashi thriver), Izabella Wentz, Pharm D and Marta Nowosadzka MD

Why Do I still Have Thyroid Symptoms When My Lab Tests are Normal? Datis Kharrazian, DC, MS.

The Thyroid Diet Revolution: Manage Your Master Gland of Metabolism for Lasting Weight Loss. Mary J. Shomon

Wake Up Your Thyroid by Eating Right, an Ebook written by me, available at www.DearPharmacist.com and www.ScriptEssentials.com

Your Plan of Action: A Dozen Ways to Minimize the Pain

We've talked about thyroid hormone imbalances. Here are some ideas.

1) Get competent help. You need a doctor to identify your exact thyroid imbalance, for example is it low T3, is it thyroid resistance, is it a nutrient deficiency? These are important questions to ask. If you're doctor hands you a prescription for levothyroxine, without first determining that you are need T4 run. You want a doctor who can tease out what is wrong with your thyroid gland, and exactly which drug you need based upon tests.

2) Eliminate gluten. Researchers have found a significant link between wheat gluten allergies and people with thyroid disease (especially Hashimoto's or Graves' disease).[8] Antibodies may come down within months of going gluten-free. You can take supplements that contain "DPPIV" which blocks gluten absorption to some degree. This enzyme DPPIV stands for "dipeptidyl peptidase four" and it may offer some protection to your thyroid gland if you do eat gluten.

    I'd much prefer you completely avoid grains altogether though. My dietary supplement called "ThyroScript™" contains this enzyme, along with other nutrients that support thyroid health. That is available at www.ScriptEssentials.com

3) Avoid dairy. If you take thyroid medication, do not drink milk or eat dairy, or take mineral-containing supplements containing calcium (and other minerals) it will bind your drug, and render it less effective. Space it 2 hours away.

4) Avoid bromine! White bread, and baked goods often contain bromine, a halogen that you should never consume. It displaces iodine and prevents you from making enough thyroid hormone.

5) Eat organic. Pesticides and herbicides sprayed on foods contain bromine and this suppresses your ability to utilize iodine. Besides that you may have a "PON1 gene snp," a genetic polymorphism that makes consumption of pesticides even more dangerous because you cannot clear it from your body well. 23andMe can test.

6) Reduce soy. Dramatically reduce intake of soy, or eliminate it since it may reduce thyroid activity. Often it is GMO (genetically modified).

7) Careful how your dose is determined. Never base your medication dose on your TSH, this is a brain hormone, it has nothing to do with the cellular utilization of thyroid hormone. You have to base your dosage on free T3 levels, along with clinical presentation and other markers. A good physician will understand this.

8) Don't inhale while driving . . . I'm just kidding. But seriously, that 'new car smell' could spell thyroid disaster. The nice aroma (and I love it too) is from off-gassing of bromine, and that hinders thyroid production.

9) Buy a chlorine filter. Install it in your shower. Chlorine is a halogen, similar to bromine that hinders thyroid production. You can buy a filter at any home building store. And on this note, if you're a swimmer, you may need to supplement with iodine because of the chlorine from the swimming pool. Chlorine goes right through your skin.

10) Get dental care. Routine dental check ups are important to identify infection. Some people have rotting teeth in their jaw, so it's possible an extraction is needed. I leave this decision up to you, but just want to point it out. Pathogenic bacteria are an overlooked cause of thyroid and adrenal illness. I've heard time and time again, how quickly thyroid (and adrenal) function normalized after an extraction.

11) Start methylating! Many thyroid disorders are tied to poor methylation, an important detoxification pathway in the body. Methylation problems mean you have trouble clearing toxins.

See Chapter 2 on "Migraine Headaches" as well as Chapter 8 "Detoxification Matters" to learn why you may need more methylfolate (a type of folic acid). You may have to lower your thyroid medication dose with your doctor's blessings because once the methylation pathway opens up, you need less medicine to achieve the same result.

12) Take probiotics. They help naturally activate your thyroid hormone by helping you convert T4 (inactive) to T3 or "triiodothyronine" (the active thyroid hormone).

There's a man is on a mission to transform the lives of 10 million people and I believe he can do it. He's my juice guru, and good friend Drew Canole. His recipes for natural milks, smoothies and juices are out of this world, and if you visit his Facebook you will instantly see how healthy he is from his lifestyle. Health is at our fingertips too. Drew gave me this juice recipe to help you with headaches. You can learn more about Drew here, www.Fitlife.tv and www.JuiceWithDrew.com.

Pain Relieving Juice by Drew Canole
1/2 pineapple
2 ribs celery
1 head Romaine lettuce
6 sprigs cilantro
Up to a thumb-sized piece of ginger

Chapter 12

Reduce Pain-Causing Cytokines

With this chapter, my hope is to turn on a light in a very dark room, a room I know you have been enduring constant darkness in for a long time. It is irrelevant whether you have had a pain condition for 2 days or 20 years, I'm going to teach you about more than the NSAID and opiate bandages needed 10 times a day.

Pain affects 1.5 billion of the population and 100 million living in the United States. One consequence of pain, no matter its cause, is inflammation. It happens as part of your body's normal (and necessary) self-protection. Inflammation in response to one or more specific triggers is not a problem, it's a useful part of healing, and many biochemical pathways are involved in producing a cascade of substances in your body. Inflammation itself is not a problem, it helps patch you up.

Inflammation is not a problem. Chronic inflammation is!

I'm a mom, a wife, a daughter, a licensed pharmacist, and I've been a student of Functional Medicine for more than 14 years. What is that? Briefly stated, by the Institute for Functional Medicine:

"Functional medicine addresses the underlying causes of disease, using a systems-oriented approach and engaging both patient and practitioner in a therapeutic partnership. It is an evolution in the practice of medicine that better addresses the healthcare needs of the 21st century. By shifting the traditional disease-centered focus of medical practice to a more patient-centered approach, functional medicine addresses the whole person, not just an isolated set of symptoms."

Functional medicine has taught me to look at the body as a whole, and become a bit like Nancy Drew. When you think that way, you realize that the pain you feel is by a systemic (whole body) fire, a fire that smolders all day long, and all night long, regardless of what analgesic you take. I think you should get a tree healthy from the roots up, because you wouldn't heal a sick tree by cutting off branches!

Introducing Your Body's Pain-Causing Chemicals!

The following is a quick overview of pain-causing chemicals that I've referred to in prior chapters of my book. Knowing what your cells are secreting all day (causing you to say "ouch") will help you understand once and for all: Reducing pain isn't about faking your body into thinking the pain is not there, it's about eliminating pain! It's about putting that smoldering fire out.

One word you will hear over and over is cytokines. There are many of them, and they are often inflammatory or "pro-inflammatory." They are sugar-proteins (termed "glycoproteins") and they're secreted all over your body, usually from cells in the immune system, and they have a direct effect on how you deal with infection, injury and allergies.

Like hormones, cytokines work really hard in small concentrations, so a little goes a long way. But unlike hormones, they are made all over your body, rather than by one gland. For example thyroid hormone is made in one spot in your body, your thyroid gland at your neck.

Cytokines travel in groups and thus, inflict more pain. When they become pro-inflammatory, they are always part of cascade, as one cytokine stimulates its target cells to make additional cytokines like a domino affect. They mean well at first, they are stimulating your cells to help you heal when you initially hurt yourself.

The problem is that some cytokines don't 'shut up' and they basically start yelling at you, imagine them getting louder and angrier (more intense pain sensations). That is when you develop chronic pain. The only way to stop the pain is to get these guys to back off. You can do that with medications and with natural analgesics, things like botanicals or spices, even teas. I've included those options throughout my book.

Cytokines certainly become very dangerous, in excess, and can harm your brain as you might see in Parkinson's disease, Alzheimer's disease, cancer, autoimmune disease, infectious diseases, multiple sclerosis and even autism. Neither your body (nor your brain) likes the pro-inflammatory cytokines.

Overview of the Nervous System

Your nervous system consists of two primary parts: the brain and the spinal cord, which combine to form the central nervous system (abbreviated as CNS) and the sensory and motor nerves, which form the peripheral nervous system (or PNS).

The names make it easy if you think about it, the CNS is "central" it's the hub, and the sensory and motor nerves extend from the central part all the way to the top of your head, and the tip of your toes, that's why they are called "peripheral."

Pain begins with nerves. Let's say you hit your elbow on the corner of your desk. How does a sensory nerve in the peripheral nervous system know this wasn't a fuzzy blanket? There are different sensory nerve fibers that are capable of responding to different sensations such as a delicate touch, versus pressure. Special pain receptors are called nociceptors. They are a group of very 'nosy' cells, they have to know what's going on at all times. A life without nociceptors is a life without sensation. Some tissues have nociceptors which do not trigger pain. In the lungs, for example, there are "pain receptors" which cause you to cough, yet there's no pain.

Your spinal cord tries to coordinate all the nerve impulses so that you can sip coffee, read this book, pet your dog with your foot and update your facebook status. If you have a blow-out with your teenager or boss, your response to pain may be stronger. Other thoughts occur during an injury too, sometimes they include four-letter words (naturally!) since let's face it, pain ranges from mild discomfort to #@$#$@#$$@#%! You may cry with the pain. The limbic system decides this for you and triggers other responses like sweating or racing heartbeat.

Keeping it simple, once an injury that caused acute pain has healed, the pain sensations stop. Why don't you feel the pain once you've healed? Because the nociceptors (remember they are nosy!) no longer detect tissue damage or injury.

Chronic pain on the other hand continues to cause you grief because (in part) there is continuous damage, thus continuous pain signals traveling to the brain. Reducing certain cytokines (pain-causing chemicals) can blunt pain to some degree. In order to pacify headache pain, it helps to know more about the actual cytokines that are high during pain conditions.

NFκβ The Sleeping Giant in your Cells

I taught you in Chapter 1 about "migrenades" which is my term for substances that go off like a grenade in your body and trigger a migraine. All the pain-causing cytokines can be considered migrenades, because they are responsible for the pain and inflammation associated with headaches. Almost all migrenades are launched from a bigger missile in your body called NF Kappa B, abbreviated as NFκβ.

Chronic pain is due to persistent NFκβ activation. NFκβ is a biochemical pathway in your body. When you wake this sleeping giant, you activate hundreds (if not thousands) of genes that launch migrenades™ causing tissue damage, free radicals, and AGEs (advanced glycation end products) which are really just pro-inflammatory molecules in the body. When you brown food at a higher temperature, it causes a glycation molecule to form (that's the area that get's browned). Normal aging of the human body can be thought of as a slow cooking process, since the same AGEs form in the arteries, eyes, cartilage, joints, skin and so forth.

Anyway, NFκβ releases cytokines and long story made very short, you get aches and pains that end in "itis" which means inflammation. Think arthritis, pancreatitis, bursitis, tendonitis, neuritis, and so forth. You can also get every headache in my book!

Trust me when I tell you prolonged NFκβ activation can slowly kill you. These nasty pro-inflammatory cytokines are the result of merciless NFκβ getting out of control. You see, it's normally inert, keeping itself together. Bad idea to disturb a sleeping giant.

You disturb the sleeping giant by eating trans fats (found in high amounts in frozen, fast foods and canned soups), or exposing yourself to heavy metals, synthetic toxins, pesticides, oxidative stress (like smoking, drinking). Infections upregulate (induce) this pathway too. It's normal to induce it, though abnormal to run full speed ahead.

Persistent NFκβ activation occurs in many pain syndromes including headaches and facial pain. It occurs with autoimmune diseases, depression, anxiety, attention deficit, diabetes, chronic infections, certain cancers, abdominal obesity and just the mere fact that you are aging. When NFκβ has its way with you, it's basically a hostile take over, and a lot of pain-causing chemicals are unleashed.

Fortunately, there are natural compounds that slow down this pathway, reducing NFκβ's torch upon your body. Among the best are probiotics, astaxanthin, green tea, omega 3 fatty acids, curcumin, alpha lipoic acid and resveratrol. There are a few others. The popular medication for diabetes "metformin" also happens to dampen down this pathway.

Meet the Pain-Causing Chemicals

There are dozens to introduce you to, but I'm only going to highlight a few of the most common pain-causing chemicals, basically the ones I consider to be the most pertinent to headaches.

Interleukins are the name given to a group of proteins, many of which cause pain for you. They are measurable in your bloodstream, though they fluctuate a lot. Inter means "between" or "among" and leukin means "from leukocytes" because that's where they were first discovered, in your white blood cells, called "leukocytes." So interleukins were originally thought of as messengers that communicated in-between or among your white blood cells.

Today, pain specialists know that the term interleukin is a relic, as these protein messengers are produced all over the body, from all different kinds of cells. The majority of interleukins are produced by T helper cells, specifically CD4 lymphocytes, as well as monocytes, macrophages and endothelial cells; they promote immune system function. I'm going to quickly list a handful of the most important interleukins now, in case you want to research on your own and find out which ones apply to your personal pain condition. Let's start at the top with Interleukin 1.

Interleukin 1 Beta or IL-1β

IL-1β belongs to the family of Interleukin 1. There are actually 11 in that family so IL-1β has 10 brothers and sisters but they're not quite as 'mean' as IL-1β. Interleukin 1 (generally speaking) is the supreme commander and is one of the most powerful chemicals in the human body as it can control nearly every organ; interleukins are the major commanders of the immune system.

This cytokine is elevated in many different pain conditions including migraines and clusters. Reducing IL-1β protects bone and cartilage in people who deal with Rheumatoid Arthritis. To become headache free, it will help to reduce IL-1β cytokines. This bad boy makes your COX enzyme work more furiously and that causes more pain compounds such as prostaglandin E2 (PGE$_2$) as well as MMPs, to be discussed shortly. Remember to think of pain as a cascade of cytokines and chemicals in the body, it's not just one. It's a domino effect. Cytokines like to travel together.

What reduces IL-1β? Astaxanthin, alpha lipoic acid, quercetin, curcumin, DHA (a part of fish oil)

Interleukin 2 or IL-2

IL-2 is a cytokine signaling molecule in the immune system. It is a protein that regulates the activities of white blood cells that are responsible for immunity. It also enhances activity of natural killer cells (good) and generates production of antibodies by your B lymphocytes (you want that). In excess it can cause pain, especially chronic neuropathic (around your nerves) pain. This cytokine is high in people with bone metastatic lesions. You might find high levels in people with neuropathies, I'm thinking sciatica, post-herpetic neuralgia, diabetic neuropathy, or multiple sclerosis, to cite some examples. The literature is very clear about cytokines in nerve pain. When it comes to migraines, clusters and tension headache, the science isn't that clear, but it suggests reduced levels of IL-2 occur, or perhaps it changes during different phases of the cluster episodes. This could happen for a number of reasons such as reduction in certain brain neurotransmitters such as catecholamines (norepinephrine, epinephrine) and/or serotonin.

IL-2 has also been linked to depression and high amounts may cause mental status changes, as in symptoms of schizophrenia such as hallucinations, delusions, confusion of time and place, and disorientation.

What increases IL-2? Astaxanthin and zinc. What reduces IL-2? Copper deficiencies, Vitamin D3 and CoQ10.

Interleukin 6 or IL-6

IL-6- one of the most important (and first to respond) cytokines in the body; it is an anti-inflammatory until your body cranks out too much and then it becomes pro-inflammatory. It frequently causes fever in the body. Elevated levels of IL-6 have been tied to many disorders such as diabetes, atherosclerosis, depression, lupus, prostate cancer and Rheumatoid arthritis.

IL-6 has found to be elevated during migraines. A study involving 30 children found a "significant increase" in IL-6 levels during the first hour of a migraine attack, suggesting that the inflammation IL-6 causes may be part of the inflammatory process underlying migraines. In other words, pesky old IL-6 will keep lighting matches in your head, fanning the flames of inflammation.

Another study looking at how the actual molecules of pain work (in the journal *Molecular Pain*) also points to IL-6 participating in the development of migraines. And a third study found migraine patients to have higher levels of a form of IL-1 and IL-6 in their blood than people without migraines.

What brings IL-6 down? Curcumin, DHA (a part of fish oil), resveratrol, statin cholesterol drugs, yoga (studies prove it)

Interleukin 10 or IL-10

This interleukin is among my favorites because it is not pro-inflammatory, just the opposite. It puts the breaks on the bad interleukins, namely IL-1, TNFα, and other pain-causing compounds like Interferon gamma (IFNγ) and GM-CSF (granulocyte-macrophage colony-stimulating factor).

Don't worry about these details too much, just think yay for IL-10. The goal for you is to do things or find ways that raise IL-10, as it 'puts out the fire.' So in summary, IL-10 (and also IL-13) reduce cytokine production. And this is real cutting edge, but I have to tell you: IL-10 lowers the amount of certain cells called "Professional MHC II antigen presenting cells." They are professional indeed, since they are expert cells in your immune system that make the decision to let a germ peacefully coexist in you, or attack it.

For example, when these MHC II cells spot L. acidophilus coming through you (from your probiotics or yogurt) they see a germ but they are professional enough to know that this is a good germ. On the other hand, when they see Salmonella, a full blown attack ensues by your immune system. We can thank IL-10 for this.

Reduced amounts of the anti-inflammatory IL-10 have been tied to symptoms of depression, like feelings of helplessness, sleep disturbances and of course pain perception. Low levels of IL-10 are also seen in pre-eclampsia, a potentially life-threatening condition that can happen to pregnant women. You see a reduction in IL-10 during migraine attacks.

What raises IL-10? Astaxanthin, resveratrol, vitamin D

What else? Exercise! In a study of 31 women with osteoarthritis in their knees, researchers found that the women who exercised had higher levels of IL-10 around those joints! This suggests to me that exercise confers some protective mechanism in patients with knee osteoarthritis and explains the beneficial effect that exercise has on various pain syndromes.

Interleukin 17 or IL-17

Although it is rarely discussed because it is cutting-edge research, IL-17 is one of THE most damaging inflammatory pain chemicals I can think of. Old thinking was that we had two arms in the immune system, Th1 and Th2 for (T helper cells), but now we know there are T17 cells. It is these cells, the T17 cells which pump out Interleukin 17, and it causes a massive tissue reaction in the body. You don't want IL-17 hanging around, it harms your brain. It's often associated with neurological problems and serious disorders including multiple myeloma, Lyme disease that causes neurological symptoms, such as headaches and pain all over your body, Guillain-Barré Syndrome, as well as Hashimoto's thyroiditis and autism. As far as other syndromes IL-17 is elevated in rheumatoid arthritis and asthma, psoriasis, and inflammatory bowel disease (IBD).

What brings down IL-17? Curcumin, Green tea (EGCG), Lactobacillus plantarum (part of high-quality probiotics like Dr. Ohhira's and others), dexamethasone (prescription steroid drug).

Tumor Necrosis Factor Alpha or TNFα

Don't let the name of this one scare you. It doesn't cause tumors, it actually tries to prevent them as well as other infectious bugs from harming you. Healthy, normal amounts of TNFα is a good thing because it helps you fight infection and cancer.

Elevated levels of TNFα mean you have an overactive immune system. Elevated TNFα levels are associated with migraines, type 2 diabetes, heart failure, COPD, Lyme disease, depression, narcolepsy, inflammatory bowel disease, ankylosing spondylitis, lupus, psoriasis and many other autoimmune disorders. Excessive amounts of TNFα are tied to wasting of muscles (cachexia).

Managing levels of TNFα should be the goal for any pain sufferer. This stimulates production of IL-1β, and recall, this is a strong pain compound too. Both IL-1β and TNFα are elevated in migraines. I find it fascinating that magnesium deficiency and CoQ10 deficiency will drive up levels of TNFα. This just tells you how important those nutrients are for energizing your mitochondria and protecting your body. CoQ10 deficiency can lead to increases in TNFα meaning you could develop widespread pain from the increase in that cytokine. Keep in mind you could have pain from the CoQ10 deficiency all by itself, it feeds your muscles and keeps them oxygenated. So taking a medication that depletes CoQ10 from your body is a one-two punch for pain. Drug muggers as I call them, are medications that mug nutrients from your body. In this example, drug muggers of CoQ10 are statin cholesterol drugs, estrogen containing hormones, some diabetes medications and acid reducers.

What brings TNFα down? Probiotics, Astaxanthin, omega 3 fatty acids, vitamin D, CoQ10, magnesium, Green tea (EGCG), resveratrol, silymarin, L-glutamine, Butterbur, Alpha lipoic acid

Interferon Gamma or IFNγ

You'll see this called a cytokine or an interferon in the literature. Whatever you decide to call it, it's made by your "Natural Killer cells" (that's the actual scientific name. I didn't make it up!), and it's a gift in that it helps you fight germs. Natural killer cells are amazing, because they have the unique ability to recognize stressed cells, and enable a much faster immune reaction. They were named "natural killers" because of the initial notion that they do not require activation in order to kill cells that are missing "self" markers.

It signals your macrophages to work harder for you swallowing up debris, dead cells, and germs. So your Pac Man cells (macrophages) get the call to action from IFNγ but like I mentioned before, excessive production causes backlash. It will make your cells produce IL-1, IL-6, TNF alpha and others, which, as we discussed earlier, can cause inflammation. The reality is that aberrant expression or excessive amounts of IFNγ are associated with many pain conditions; so bringing down IFNγ should be a goal if you live in chronic pain as it relates to chronic infection (such as Lyme or HIV, pneumonia, or auto-immune disorders). IFNγ is often high in people with depression or symptoms that look like that (ie you just feel lousy and tired, low appetite and no interest in things; you want to sleep more and have trouble concentrating).

What Reduces IFNγ? Vitamin D3 and White Willow Bark, in high enough doses, but in sensitive people, white willow bark may cause bleeding complications, it's similar to aspirin.

COX 1- Cyclooxgenase 1

Aspirin was developed from willow bark in the 1800s. It's an ancient remedy dating back to at least 400 BC when Hippocrates told his patients to chew on the bark to bring down fever and reduce body aches. The bark of the tree contains the chemical salicilin, a cousin to aspirin (acetylsalicylic acid). Studies show willow bark reduces pain and inflammation, but it may thin the blood. Brand new studies suggest intravenous aspirin as a treatment for migraines.

Cox 1 is sort of a housekeeper, it is made throughout your entire body and is present day to day, minute to minute in many metabolic pathways. One of its primary functions is to protect your stomach lining, and regulate platelet function as well as blood flow to the kidneys. Non-steroidal anti-inflammatory drugs (NSAIDs) are COX 1 inhibitors, and that comes at a price because you need COX 1 to protect your stomach. Ibuprofen and naproxen are COX 1 inhibitors. That's why there's a high risk associated with long term or improper use (or high dose) of NSAIDs. Moreover, on the extreme end, the US Food and Drug Administration (FDA) reported in 2011 that more than 16,500 people die in the United States each year from NSAID-related gastrointestinal bleeding.

COX 2 or Cyclooxygenase 2

This enzyme triggers production of the prostaglandins related to pain. COX 2 stands for cycloxygenase. If you really want to know it converts arachidonic acid to endoperoxide H2 or "PGG2" which stands for prostaglandin G2. Arachidonic acid isn't all bad, it's both anti and pro-inflammatory, depending on what pathway it follows.

It does not really occur throughout the body like COX1 which is all over the place. It is a little bit more discreet and only called to action when needed. In excess however, it causes pain, throughout the body; it may be elevated in migraines, clusters, premenstrual headaches as well as tension headaches.

COX 2 was discovered pretty recently (in terms of medical history), like about 25 years ago, and drugs are available to block the pathway, thus they are called COX 2 inhibitors. Only Celebrex is available, a similar drug named Vioxx was recalled from the market in 2004 after a clinical trial involving 2,600 patients revealed an increased risk of cardiovascular complications only18 months after patients started taking Vioxx. Celebrex is very popular, and considered safe and effective since it does not cause the complications as Vioxx, a drug in the same therapeutic category. Prostaglandins whose synthesis involves the cyclooxygenase 2 enzyme or COX 2 are responsible for inflammation and pain.

What reduces COX 2? Astaxanthin, resveratrol, curcumin, green tea, kava root, and omega 3 fatty acids and ecklonia cava (a brown algae), celecoxib (Celebrex).

MMP2 and MMP9 Matrix metalloproteases

See why we call them MMPs? These are the compounds partially responsible for nerve pain, such as that from diabetic neuropathy and post-herpetic neuralgia or "shingles" which is a viral-induced neuropathy. Levels of MMPs fluctuate, it's not as simple as bring this down and you're cured. Usually, MMP9 is high during acute pain and MMP2 is the one to focus on reducing if your pain is chronic. MMPs are frequently elevated when one has cancer or heart disease.

MMP reduction can help with one of the most maddening sensations, that of allodynia (a painful response to an otherwise light touch or the slightest movement).

Anything that reduces MMP has some potential to support your immune system. Discuss everything you read here with your practitioner(s); for instance, naringin (from grapefruit) listed below interacts with many medications, and can cause spikes in drug levels. Not everything you read about is right for you.

What Reduces MMPs? Axtaxanthin, alpha lipoic acid, naringin, magnolia bark extract. Statin cholestrol reducing drugs (like atorvastatin, lovastatin, simvastatin, pravastain, etc.)

Histamines

You've probably heard of an antihistamine, like diphenhydramine (Benadryl) or loratadine (Claritin). These chemicals are used to relieve allergic symptoms by reducing levels of histamines that your mast cells release. Did you know that there are 4 different kinds of histamines? You'll be pleasantly surprised that they are named very simply, as histamine 1, histamine 2, histamine 3 and histamine 4. (Can you believe they gave us a break, the scientists must have been heavily sedated during the naming of these histamines or it would have gotten much more complex). Allergy drugs work by reduce Histamine 1 and acid blockers reduce Histamine 2.

New studies have confirmed that histamine is very high in pain syndromes such as rheumatoid arthritis. Cluster headaches may be the result of sudden spikes in histamine (or serotonin). This has been shown in several studies; one showed increase in the number of mast cells in the brain (which make histamine), and we know that migraine and cluster patients have histamine intolerance evidenced by reduced DAO activity. This is why certain histamine-rich foods trigger headaches, like aged cheese and wine. The high histamine theory may also explain why some of you enjoy a complete disappearance of symptoms with a histamine-free diet or with low-dose antihistamines. So one strategy for pain relief would be to reduce histamine in the body and reduce histamine-rich foods you consume.

What reduces histamine? Quercetin, vitamin C, L-methionine, DAO (diamine oxidase).

Substance P

Substance P is a chemical messenger associated with increased pain perception. The more substance P, the more pain you feel.

When substance P is released, other amino acids are simultaneously dumped out, one of which is glutamate (also aspartate).

Glutamate is a neurotransmitter, present in very small amounts, that aids the brain in learning, as well as short and long term memory. But when it is secreted in excess, glutamate, literally called an "excitotoxin" excites and vibrates all the cells around it to death. Chasing down glutatmate is important in reducing nerve pain and neurological problems. So anything that reduces substance P helps control the sitting pit bull glutamate. (MSG contains some glutamate). High substance P and glutamate are "migrenades™."

Brain scans of fibromyalgia patients show elevated levels of substance P, up to three times the normal level. Higher than normal levels are seen in respiratory disorders even in "air hunger," which is the feeling that you simply can't get enough air into your lungs) associated with Babesia infections (see Chapter 6 on "Lyme Headaches"). Substance P is also associated with anxiety, eczema, nausea and vomiting.

What reduces Substance P?

Capsacin cream, magnesium, quercetin, probiotics, and medications (pregabalin, gabapentin, opiates).

Leukotrienes

Leukotrienes are a sub class of "eicosanoids" pronounced "I-koss-anoids" which when you say that out loud, the last syllables sound like the word "annoyed" and that's exactly what they do, they are very annoying and irritating in the body!

This compound is produced by your immune system cells and it sparks production of interleukins (ILs), interferon (IFNs) and other compounds involved in allergies, food sensitivities, autoimmune disorders and anaphylactic reactions.

Leukotrienes increase if you're allergic to food coloring, like yellow dye #5, tartrazine, or other substances. Primary care clinicians often prescribe non-steroidal anti-inflammatory drugs (referred to as "NSAIDs"), such as Ibuprofen (marketed with the names "Advil," and "Motrin," Naproxen (marketed as Aleve and Naproxyn) and Celecoxib (marketed as Celebrex).

Researchers have found that some natural compounds like Boswelia and quercetin can reduce those annoying eicosanoids. Here's something that I find thrilling: Since about 2001, the medical literature has shown that dark chocolate can reduce annoyance too, by reducing eiconanoids! How about that!

What brings leukotrienes down? Omega 3s, flaxseed oil, perilla seed oil, curcumin, Boswellia serrata, glycyrrhiza, quercetin, the medications Accolate and Singulair

Prostaglandins

Prostaglandins are a second type of "annoying" compounds so they too are a sub category under the bigger class of "eicosanoid" implicated in pain. Prostaglandins are made when you hurt yourself, or get infected and cause redness, swelling, pain and fever. Higher than normal levels of prostaglandins are seen in certain types of arthritis, heavy menstrual bleeding, PMS, multiple sclerosis, chronic lyme disease, as well as colon and breast cancer.

In chronic headaches, or any pain for that matter, there may be excess production of prostaglandins, and as long as the root cause of the pain is present, there will be an onslaught of prostaglandins summoning up all sorts of other pain-causing compounds (remember, cytokines and pro-inflammatory compounds travel in groups). The goal for pain sufferers is to reduce prostaglandin production to a normal healthy physiological level.

What substances reduce prostaglandins? Fish oils, white willow bark (salix alba), Ecklonia cava (a brown algae), meadowsweet (don't take if you're allergic to salicylates like aspirin), turmeric, skullcap, ginger root, and passionflower, medications like celecoxib, aspirin, the NSAID class including ibuprofen and naproxen.

Summary

After reading this chapter, you have a more thorough understanding of the pain-causing cytokines that are elevated with headaches and various pain syndromes.

Cytokines are small proteins that act as chemical messengers. They have activity all over the body. Certain cytokines may cause inflammation but that is not a problem, it's a natural consequence. Chronic inflammation becomes a problem because it leads to tissue destruction, inflammation and pain. Some cytokines activate nociceptors, making them more sensitive to the pain.

Certain strategies can be used to reduce the pro-inflammatory cytokines and increase the anti-inflammatory ones. It is far more complex than this, however, a typical strategy you could begin today would include a healthy lifestyle (as in no smoking, drinking, overeating), consuming clean diet free of additives and artificial ingredients, the elimination of allergenic foods, gentle stretching exercises, dietary supplements and/or medications. Turn to page 311 for the summary on how you can live headache free.

Live Headache F-R-E-E

Determining the cause of your headaches is crucial to curing them. So in these final pages, I'm offering a brief guideline for you (or your practitioner) to help organize your care. This "formula" for recovery will vary from doctor to doctor.

I subscribe to the following simple plan to living headache "free."

I'll give you a closer look at how to do that. Everything I'm about to say was covered in the prior pages of my book, so this is just a summary, intended to help you organize thoughts and a treatment plan for full recovery. Here is what I propose for you to live headache free:

Find the cause
Reduce toxins
Eliminate triggers
Energize mitochondria

Find the Cause.

To do that, you need to track your history including every detail about triggers, age of onset, severity, type of headache(s) and so on. It may highlight the underlying pathology. After taking a history, you will need to detect all the imbalances. Every biochemical pathway in your body has to stay in balance. When serotonin, dopamine or norepinephrine become imbalanced headaches occur. When estrogen and progesterone become imbalanced, headaches occur. When thyroid and probiotic status alters, headaches occur, when infections overrun your immune system, headaches occur. Do you see what I'm talking about? The imbalances must be addressed. Imbalances may occur in the neurological, hormonal, neurotransmitters, lifestyle, structural, environment and genetic. Clinical tests will be needed to paint the picture for your doctor. It's expensive to do all the tests needed to uncover imbalances so just do 1 or 2 at a time, little by little you take baby steps forward.

Reduce toxins.

The toxins that come to mind include: Household chemicals, dry cleaning chemicals, artificial ingredients in food (like sweeteners), artificial colors noted by "FD & C," unnecessary vitamins and supplements (many on the market are laden with chemicals), junk food, trans fats, fungus in your home like mold in your walls or carpet and environmental pollutants that you can control (HEPA filter anyone?). Heavy metals are another toxin you can reduce, either by quitting smoking (high in cadmium), and avoiding second hand smoke. Mercury is another heavy metal found in your dental work, in seafood such as "Sea bass" and tuna. Last but not least, foods with pesticides (non-organic) are a toxic burden to your body. There are many others discussed in Chapter 8 "Detoxification Matters."

Eliminate triggers.

What triggers you, does not trigger everyone. For example, when I smell perfume I do not get a headache, but if I work at my computer and expose myself to a lot of electromagnetic radiation, I may get one. Other common triggers are stressful situations or meetings with people you don't like. Stress management is huge when it comes to headache triggers. I call some of these triggers migrenades™, because they blow up in your body like a grenade causing a migraine (or other type of headache).

Many foods contain artificial sweeteners, a "migrenade™" that is not even evident on the label! Honestly, that is so rude. I think the use of artificial sweeteners, preservatives, colors and fake foods is pervasive in the food industry. This dirty little secret makes your head hurt, because you are ingesting a migrenade™ without evening knowing it. Until the amount of the artificial sweetener reaches a certain threshold, the food maker doesn't have to disclose it on the front label, so it's up to you to read the fine print on the back of the label. Aspartame and sucralose are just two artificial sweeteners that I covered in greater detail in this book.

You'll also need to avoid foods that spark a headache such as wine, beer, chocolate, cold-cuts for example, (whatever it is for you), temperature changes such as cold weather; pet dander, chewing gum with sugar-alcohols in it. This list is never ending, so you need to sit down with a pen and try to figure out what triggers your headache, and then eliminate it.

Energize mitochondria.

In order to ultimately feel your best and live headache free you'll have to energize your mitochondria, these are the powerhouses that are inside each and every cell of your body. We have 10 million-billion mitochondria, and they help us product ATP, your energy molecule. Emerging research (as I explained in the Migraine chapter) shows that mitochondrial dysfunction causes headache pain, so supporting mito health becomes key to getting well.

Your cells have a few hundred mito in them. Red blood cells and skin cells have few or no mitochondria, just as an interesting aside. Mitochondria comprise a staggering 10% of your body weight! If you weigh 100 pounds, you carry10 pounds of mitochondria and if you're 200 pounds, you carry 20 pounds of mito! Remember, these generate energy. The weight you carry means nothing about their function. People who are ill often have dead, partial or non-functional mitochondria, that is the problem! You need those mito to work!

Here's some basics for mito health. Take care of your precious adrenals, sleep well if you can (no all-nighters to watch TV or facebook), take care of your gut, restore probiotics and support liver, thyroid, adrenal and hormone pathways. Detox detox detox! Open up your methylation pathway, but do it slowly. Keep folate and niacin in balance. Do not let serotonin go up too high, or drop too low. Consider genetics. You may not realize this but your genetic mutations, termed "snps" happen to shine a flashlight on lifelong symptoms, including medical conditions, personality traits, pain syndromes, autoimmune diseases, food sensitivities and so forth. You can test your genes for under a hundred dollars.

Up next, are supplements that help support mitochondrial health. Not all of these were covered, but I want you to be aware they are options for you, and ask your doctor if they're okay. You don't want all, just one or two, perhaps three in combination. Introduce supplements one at a time.

Mitochondrial Health

Support Mito Function	Create Mito (Biogenesis)
* CoQ10	Quercetin
Acetyl L Carnitine	Resveratrol
Lipoic Acid	Lipoic acid
Magnesium	Berberine
D-ribose	Ketogenic diet
B vitamins	** Caffeine
Creatine	Pterostilbene
	§ BCAA supplements

* CoQ10 is fine, or "Ubiquinol" its downline metabolite; you see it sold both ways. The ubiquinol is considered more body ready.

** Caffeine is a trigger for some headache sufferers.

§ BCAA supplements consist of "branched chain amino acids" and are sold at health food stores, usually for body-builders and folks into fitness.

Cool Me Down Kale-Aid

by Suzy Cohen, RPh (yes me :-)

My juiced recipe gives you a lot of mito building nutrients in the form of quercetin, resveratrol and pterostilbene. You'll enjoy some energy and mind clarity from this. Make sure you buy organic.

Ingredients
1/2 cup fresh pineapple
1 cup papaya
1/4 cup blueberries
1 cup coconut water
2 cups tightly packed raw kale)
2 or 3 leaves of fresh spearmint
1/4 teaspoon Hawaiian Spirulina powder

Directions: Juice together, you can alter the ingredient amounts to taste. This is pretty sweet to my taste buds, but if you're new to juicing, your palate may not have adjusted so feel free to add honey, maple syrup or coconut nectar. Best when served chilled.

Dairy-Free Strawberry Cilantro Smoothie

By Amie Valpone of www.TheHealthyApple.com

My friend Amie is a Manhattan based personal chef, and she has an impressive website with hundreds of delicious recipes. Her facebook page is awesome too, go like it: www.Facebook.com/TheHealthyApple

Amie's recipe for the following smoothie is satisfying and it's good for mito health and energy. As an added bonus, cilantro is known to bind heavy metals from the gut.

Ingredients
1 cup fresh strawberries, stems removed
1 medium ripe banana, peeled
¼ cup cashews
½ cup gluten-free oats
1 cup Almond Breeze Almond Milk
½ tsp. powdered stevia
½ tsp. coconut flakes
¼ cup finely chopped fresh cilantro
¼ tsp ground cinnamon
½ cup ice cubes

Directions: Combine all ingredients in a blender; blend until smooth. Transfer to serving glasses. Serve chilled.

Two Dozen Reasons Why Your Headaches Won't Get Better!

You can take whatever supplements and medicines you want to, but your headaches may not get better:

1. Because there's an underlying reason like a tumor, or aneurysm (but this is rare)
2. Food sensitivity, for example, you're allergic to eggs and don't know it
3. Emotional stress from relationships you can't break, cortisol is high or flat-lined
4. Consumption of artificial sweeteners or additives, read labels closely
5. You need glasses and don't realize, see an optometrist
6. Environmental pollutants, dry cleaning, or mold, humid climates

7. Unknown allergen in your medicine like gluten in your ibuprofen
8. Muscle tension or trigger points which need releasing
9. Eye strain from reading the computer
10. Undiagnosed infection (viral, bacterial, parasitic, fungal)
11. Poor detoxification and lymph drainage
12. Sitting with your head in constant flexion can cause tension headaches
13. Fluorescent lighting is a trigger that is reported anecdotally
14. You're not drinking enough (dehydration)
15. Some medications you take cause headaches, pg 341
16. Caffeine consumption or withdrawal causing rebound headaches
17. Sinus problems and chronic allergies
18. Weather or change in altitude
19. Hormonal imbalance, usually excess estrogen relative to progesterone
20. Clenching or grinding your teeth
21. Thyroid imbalances
22. Nutrient deficiencies, for example low magnesium
23. Methylation pathway isn't working
24. Neurotransmitters remain imbalanced

Bonus Reason: Your husband wants to have sex (haha, I'm really kidding).

ThyroScript™

This dietary supplement supports a healthy thyroid gland, energy production and metabolism. I'm proud to say it is my own personal blend of natural herbs and vitamins. I developed ThyroScript™ based upon my studies and every ingredient has scientific research to support a beneficial effect. Read chapter 11 for more on the thyroid connection to migraines.

www.ScriptEssentials.com

Appendix I

Lab Tests and Imaging Studies

The following lab tests may be helpful to uncover hidden causes of pain or rule out serious causes for headache pain. This is just a brief overview of labs that you can look up on your own or speak to your practitioner about.

Headache History

This is the most important part of your entire evaluation is your history. It may help you and your doctor uncover the cause for them. There are easily a hundred questions, and some of the important ones to keep track of are:

How old were you when the headaches began?
Is there any connection to where you live, or work?
Is there a cycle to them?
Do certain situations or people trigger them?
Does eating certain foods have any effect?
Do your siblings, or parent have headaches too?
What time of day?
Is there an aura or halo?
Do any medications or supplement help, or make worse?
How do you sleep? Sleep deprivation is a common cause.
How much do you drink? Dehydration is a contributing factor.
What tests have been done for you already?

One of my friends, a medical consultant sent me this story which highlights just how important a history is. He uncovered her problem, and spared her more misery and expense just by asking key questions and doing a little research:

One lady 50 doctors. Could not lose weight to safe her life and she had migraines. Perfect diet, supplementation, thyroid, everything normal. Within a few minutes I asked her about her work place. Bingo! Two people died of cancer with in 6 months. When I researched her demographics, I found out her work place was built on an old land fill. She has never been right since working there. After 2 months she decided to quit her job. Within days her health began to improve, and over time her adrenals started working again. This helped her lose weight and reduce headache pain. No Doctor even mentioned "Sick Building Syndrome."

Every physician has their own intake form, or questionnaire, and it helps if you have one yourself. There are many apps available too, among the best is "My Pain Diary" and iHeadache. You can also refer to Appendix II where I've created a headache log for you. It's is downloadable at my website:

http://www.dearpharmacist.com/headachelog

Sinus X-ray or CT scans
Where: At hospitals and specialized imaging centers

If you have chronic tension type headaches (CTTH) and regular sinus infections, your physician may want to order this test to uncover chronic allergies, mucosal thickening and congestion that may be causing your mystery headaches. You may not need a scan, some physicians can peek in there and the inflammation is quite evident.

Brain Imaging
Where: At hospitals and specialized imaging centers

There are CT scans (computerized tomography) and MRIs (magnetic resonance images). These provide a nice cross-sectional view of your brain and can help uncover developing tumors before they get too big or inoperable. Other issues may be seen such as evidence of mild stroke, aneurysms, or plaque in the brain. An MRI is not able to diagnose migraines, however it can rule out other causes for head pain.

PET Scan
Where: At hospitals and specialized imaging centers

PET for Positron emission tomography uses radiation to produce a 3 dimensional color image to show what is happening inside you; how your body is functioning, rather than how it looks. Radioactive medicine is tagged onto either of these chemicals glucose, water or ammonia (the tagged chemical is known as the radiotracer). The radiotracer is then inserted into your body where it travels to areas of your body that use the chemical. The images are reconstructed by computer analysis.

PET scans can be used to diagnose a health condition, as well as for finding out how an existing condition is developing. PET scans are often used to see how effective an ongoing treatment is, usually in combination with other tests.

This test may be particularly helpful in people with cluster headache because that involves some kind of malfunction in the hypothalamus region of the brain which controls your body's biological clock. It's an imaging study.

Circle of Willis
Where: At hospitals and specialized imaging centers

This image is taken during an MRI. The "Circle of Willis" is an image of a specific section of your brain which is where a bunch of arteries meet at the base of the brain. Research has shown us that an "incomplete" circle has greater asymmetry in blood flow to the brain. Certain parts of the brain are well oxygenated while others are not. Abnormalities in both the Circle of Willis and cerebral blood flow were most prominent in the back of the brain, where the visual cortex is located. This may help explain why the most common migraine auras consist of visual symptoms such as seeing distortions, spots, or wavy lines.

Lithium Level
Where: Any lab and www.directlabs.com/suzycohen

Some of you take lithium for your condition, whether that's anxiety, bipolar, memory, migraines or cluster headaches. Levels are often gauged by blood tests, and the blood draw should be taken about 12 hours after the last dose. If there is a dosage adjustment made, you should wait 5 days after the change to test your blood levels (unless your doctor tells you otherwise). Side effects for lithium may include dry mouth, metallic taste, tremor or shakiness, weakness or diarrhea.

These side effects are supposed to wear off after a while, and long-term you may see hypothyroidism or weight gain. Medications include Eskalith or Lithobid. The supplement, which is much weaker, and sold at health food stores is called lithium orotate.

IL-6
Where: Many labs

This can be measured in the blood as a stand-alone marker, or you can evaluate a bunch of different cytokines all at once with a cytokine panel. Elevated IL-6 is a common denominator in many pain syndromes and inflammatory conditions. You can do this blood test (or panel) if you want to track your progress (and like hard evidence) but you certainly don't need this. Cytokines are supposed to be helpful compounds and we make them naturally, but in excess they can cause pain. Elevated IL-6 occurs in chronic infection, Lyme-related headaches, chronic tension headaches, migraines, autoimmune disorders, certain cancers and Alzheimer's disease. Fasting is not required for this blood test.

Adrenal Hormone Tests
Where: Doctors offices or home test kits that are physician-ordered

Because chronic headaches create a lot of mental stress, it's not a bad idea to have a lab test that evaluates your adrenal gland function, especially if you've been in pain for a long time. Your adrenals can't help but be weakened. Some clues that your adrenals are fatigued include muscle pain, weight gain, chronic fatigue, dizziness when you stand up, insomnia, light sensitivity or increased blood sugar. Until your adrenal hormones are balanced, you're more likely to experience headaches. See chapter 9 "Adrenal Hormones and the Headache Connection."

One little tip for evaluating adrenal function is to check blood pressure while sitting down. Then stand up, the blood pressure will usually drop 10 mm/hg upon rising from a lying down position. This isn't foolproof, just a little barometer, you still need to follow doctor's lab orders.

Another idea is to look in your eyes with a soft flashlight because pupil contraction is weak. As soon as you shine the light into your eyes, your iris cannot hold the contraction, it may contract quickly but then it goes back to normal very fast. Healthy adrenals are supposed to stay contracted for much longer. Have someone help you determine this because it's hard to do on your own.

There's another way to evaluate adrenal health, it's called "Sergeant's White Line" and you draw a line on your abdomen with a blunt instrument, the white line will remain there for several minutes if adrenal fatigued, but in a healthy person, the white line will normally turn pinkish-red within seconds. This only works in about 25% of people, it fails the rest so don't rely on it. Again, this is just a home method, it shouldn't delay you from labs your doctor wants to order.

Pain may (or may not) be present around the adrenal area, it's called a positive "Rogoff's sign" if you have it. Just press over the adrenal area on your mid-back, and see if it's tender. This doesn't work all the time, it's just one more barometer.

I recommend a "4 point" cortisol test, along with evaluations of other hormones such as DHEA for example. All of the following labs offer a 4 point test, which means you provide 4 saliva samples, one in the morning, noon, evening and midnight. Some of these companies also offer more comprehensive tests that include DHEA or other hormones, some are physician-ordered, others like ZRT can be ordered by you the consumer.

Diagnos-Techs	www.diagnostechs.com
ZRT Labs	www.zrtlab.com
Neuroscience	www.neurorelief.com
Genova Diagnostics	www.gdx.net

HHV-6 Testing
Where: Any lab

There are many tests that evaluate the presence of HHV-6, a herpes organism that often infects the trigeminal nerve. This is a blood test. I recommend a "Qualitative" PCR DNA test which uses blood. It can help differentiate if you have an active infection or have been exposed (like many years ago). Many people carry HHV-6, but they don't express it with bad symptoms. Some tests evaluate IgM antibodies. If you show higher than normal IgM antibodies, you might have an active infection. The antibody level goes down to normal after about 2 or 3 months so it's not as reliable as the qualitative PCR DNA test, but it's a choice if you think you've been infected recently.

Healthy persons usually have less than 20 copies/ml. If your viral load is > 200 copies per ml, (or 20 copies per microgram of DNA) consider that positive. You don't want a "quantitative" test because it only says positive or negative (no numerical value is given). The reason is most of us are exposed and carry this virus and seeing a "positive" doesn't say whether or not it is currently active and affecting your nervous system. I found a website devoted to this organism, www.HHV-6Foundation.org. You can have more herpes viruses tested for, with a larger panel that included cytomegalovirus and Epstein Barr and others.

Thyroid Profile
Where: Any lab

Thyroid tests are done as blood tests. All of the following should be included in your thyroid testing. You can do it once a year, unless you have hypo or hyperthyroidism, in which case you may need to do this more often. Elevated thyroid and hypothyroidism are both causes for headaches.

TSH	Thyroid Stimulating Hormone
Free T3	Free Triiodothyronine
Total T3	Total Triiodothyronine
Free T4	Free Thyroxine
rT3	Reverse Triiodothyronine or "Reverse T3"

Drugs that may increase your T3 levels:
Estrogen-containing birth control pills or shots
Clofibrate (brand Atromid-S)
Menopausal drugs containing estrogen
Methadone

Drugs that reduce T3 levels:
Amiodarone (brand Cordarone)
Testosterone
Anabolic steroids

Propylthiouracil (PTU)
Methimazole
Lithium carbonate or orotate
Anticonvulsants (many including phenytoin)
Propranolol
DHEA supplements and medications

Neopterin/Biopterin Profile
Where: Metametrix.com

This requires an overnight urine catch and the test measures neopterin and biopterin values. Neopterin and biopterin are by-products of chemical reactions involving tetrahydrobiopterin (BH4) which is a cofactor for the enzymes responsible for the making monoamine (MAO) neurotransmitters (ephinepherine, norepinephrine, dopamine, serotonin) and nitric oxide. This test is great for people with migraines, autism, Parkinson's, Alzheimer's, depression, neurological disorders, cardiovascular disease and inborn errors of metabolism (phenylketonuria).

Neopterin rises with infection, autoimmune disorders, psychiatric illness and sleep apnea. It's also high in kids with autism or autism spectrum disorders.

Electrolyte Panel
Where: Any lab

May be helpful if you take blood pressure medications which can disturb electrolytes. This is a blood test, usually it's a panel that includes the ions below, or you can order them separately as in "serum calcium" etc. The panel includes all of these:

Calcium
Chloride
Magnesium
Phosphorous
Potassium
Sodium

Methylation Pathway Panel

Where: http://www.seekinghealth.com/methylation-pathway-panel-vitamin-diagnostics.html

Vitamin Diagnostics

This is one of the very best panels for people with complex illness like Cluster headaches, migraines and Lyme headaches. I love this panel, it's worth every penny if you ever want to stop the nonsense in your head. It can help you uncover things that conventional doctors would not find for years and years. I found this panel available direct-to-consumer at SeekingHealth.com so you can order it on your own. The base price is around $395 (at time of this writing), and I would highly recommend you buy the add-on tests too, for all of the following, but again this is up to you. Here's what I'd love you to test for:

Nitric Oxide
Nitrotyrosine or "Peroxynitrite"
Histamine
Ammonia
Kryptopyrrole

Peroxynitrite and nitric oxide are sometimes elevated in migraines and clusters. Also in neurological Lyme disease, and other health issues. Now, the basic test may look unnecessary to you so let's talk about it. The basic test (without the add-ons) looks at levels of both oxidized and reduced glutathione, red blood cell levels of SAMe, S-adenosyl-homocysteine, tetrahydrofolate, 5MTHF, folic acid and others. You may not think you need those levels but trust me on this, if something is awry in your head, this will help uncover neurotransmitter imbalances. It will show whether or not you're detoxifying.

While researching all of this, I became friends with the naturopathic doctor who runs this site, Dr. Ben Lynch, and he's giving my fans a 15% discount with the coupon code "Headache Free" for this test or anything on his site.

MTHFR Test Molecular Laboratory Testing

Where: www.Seeekinghealth.com
http://www.seekinghealth.com/mthfr-test-seeking-health.html

This is an oral swab test, no blood. You can order it yourself, no doctor needed. When you get your results, you take them to your doctor for interpretation and to help you make a plan, but again, you can buy the test on your own. It detects methylation difficulties, specifically it can test for the 2 most popular gene snps that hinder methylation:

C677T
A1298

You can be heterozygous (meaning +/- because only 1 parent passed it to you), or you can be homozygous, which creates more detox problems (meaning +/+ because both parents passed it to you). Methylation is discussed in detail, in chapter 8 "Detoxification Matters." You can test any way you want to, if you buy the test off "Seeking Health" site, my fans get 15% off with "Headache Free" coupon code.

Other common Lab Values That Suggest MTHFR Mutations

I'm including this little section primarily for doctors who are familiar with specialized testing from labs such as Doctor's Data, Genova Metametrix, and Vitamin Diagnostics. You might see the following in a patient with a MTHFR defect, but it's not a given:

Elevated histamine
Elevated UMFA (unmetabolized folic acid)
Elevated folic acid or folinic acid
Low 5-MTHF
High ammonia (or symptoms it like brain fog, "strange smell")
Low glutathione
Normal to elevated homocysteine
Digestive problems
Low 5-HIAA
Elevated FIGLU or formiminoglutamic acid in urine
Reduced Histidine
Reduced Homovanilate

US Biotek

Where: www.usbiotek.com

This lab helps determine food allergies. For some of you, a sensitivity to eggs, corn, soy, dairy and yeast could spark a headache. Lab tests to determine hidden food allergies require a blood sample and usually take 2 to 4 weeks to get your results back to you.

I am a big fan of testing for gluten and Celiac disease, as well as casein (the protein in dairy), but generally speaking, I'm not strongly attached to food testing because you can drive yourself crazy. If you were going to test, even just once, I like US Biotek for this, I trust them.

I know people that test their food sensitivities every few months, to see what is happening with the antibodies. You'll end up on a highly restrictive diet if you're not careful, meaning you will see all these positive "reactions" to foods you eat every day, so then have to avoid those foods. Take another test, and more positive reactions show up due to elevated antibodies. Go off those foods . . . And so on. I've been there, you will go bonkers and wind up eating water and bok choy if you assume you're "allergic" to those foods. If you're gut is that "holey" that you are consistently reacting to different food proteins that end up in your bloodstream, it speaks to a larger problem of gut permeability, poor probiotic status, infection, SIBO (small intesting bacterial overgrowth) or dysbiosis, what we affectionately call "leaky gut."

Here's why, when you eat a lot of a particular food, say coconut, you are apt to come positive on a test for antibodies for that food because the proteins are leaking out of your leaky gut. It doesn't mean you're necessarily "allergic" (although you could be), these food sensitivity tests are really just showing you that your body has seen the protein of "coconut" and created antibodies to it. *And your body should do that, because coconut is not "self" it's a coconut, not you!* Unless you have a serious IgE reaction to a food, that causes a true allergy, I'd be careful not to restrict yourself to gnashing on toothpicks all day. It's misery. Use common sense, try to track what foods spark headaches and avoid those. If you do food sensitivity testing do it once in a while, not as your primary test. I know other health experts will disagree with me, but this is my book, and my opinion. Avoiding highly allergenic foods is right, avoiding everything under the sun is not.

Cyrex Labs

Where: www.cyrexlabs.com

Cyrex Labs is particularly good at gluten testing, and cross-sensitivities with gluten, but they do some food testing too. It's always my pick for gluten testing because they check for more than just alpha gliadin, they look at omega, gamma gliadin, deaminated gluten and others; Immunoglobulin G or IgG is not as specific to Celiac, but may still be useful in diagnosing the condition in people who are unable to make normal amounts of IgA antibodies. It's possible to become deficient in IgA antibodies, that's why the IgG test is helpful and it's offered through Cyrex Labs. Many of you have headaches, driven by underlying gluten allergies or Celiac disease. This test may be of value.

The test is called "Array 3 Wheat/Gluten Proteome Reactivity & Autoimmunity." Did you know that the proteins in coffee look to your body, just like gluten? They can test for cross sensitivities with "Array 4 Gluten-Associated Cross-Reactive Foods and Food Sensitivity." They have a new, rather remarkabe test that evaluate certain compounds if you have an autoimmune disease, this one is called "Array 5 Multiple Autoimmune Reactivity Screen." If you are sensitive to everything 'under the sun' as they say, and you think you have been exposed to chemicals, environmental pollutants or lots of formaldehyde from the foods you eat, take "Array11 Chemical Immune Reactivity Screen." All these "Array" tests are available from www.CyrexLabs.com. Your physician may have to call the lab(s) and set up an account to order the tests for you. It usually requires nothing more than a few minutes of their time and an active license.

Tissue Transglutaminase IgA
Where: Cyrex Labs and others

We call it TTG IgA for short. This blood test is useful in detecting autoimmune conditions, most notably celiac disease, the disorder associated with gluten. IgA is short for Immunoglobulin A, and is more telling since it's made in the small intestine, where gluten causes inflammation and irritation in sensitive people.

H. Pylori Stool Antigen Test
Where: Genova Labs or www.directlabs.com/suzycohen

Determines if you have H. pylori, a germ associated with both ulcers and migraines. The results are more reliable with this stool test than they are with the 'breath test' which is what most doctors suggest.

Insulin, fasting

Where: Any lab and www.directlabs.com/suzycohen

Insulin sensitivity is impaired in patients with migraines. I would expect this blood level to be elevated if you have headaches. High insulin isn't just tied to migraines, it is associated with a higher risk of heart attack and stroke. Exercising brings it down. Eating foods that are healthy for you can bring it down. Start with leafy greens. You want your fasting insulin levels to be somewhere around 5, or 10. Above 20 or 25 uU/mL it's pretty much a slam dunk for diabetes and other diseases tied to high pro-inflammatory cytokines.

Blood Pressure

Where: Any doctor's office, or use a home test kit

Elevated cortisol and elevated serum insulin will both cause blood pressure to rise. It's a good value to track in someone who has migraines. If you're a migraineur, this is one test you can do at home if you buy a machine at your local pharmacy. I'm up with the times so I can tell you with confidence that a spot blood pressure test is pretty much useless. It changes minute to minute, with stress, with hormones, with circadian rhythm, with supplements, medicine, food, with your position (lying, standing) . . . I recommend you measure your blood pressure at regular intervals over 24 hours. This is specialized testing. In fact, there are devices you can buy over the internet for 24 hour monitoring, but usually you get them from a physician. There are many progressive doctors, especially cardiologists that have the device at their clinic (for lending to their patients). It's worth seeking out, the reasons I prefer this type of testing:

* You avoid the "white coat effect" which will spike your pressure
* Can see if your blood pressure is high at night, or during sleep
* Can tell if your blood pressure pills are work
* Will show what happens if you experience a headache

You have to wear the device all day, and carry on with your normal routine. Just don't go swimming or take a bath with it on. After 24 hours, you take off the cuff and bring it back to your office (if your doctor lent it to you). The machine stores all your readings so you don't have to bother watching it.

GI Effects Stool Test

Where: www.metametrix.com

Gastrointestinal tests offers solution for complex cases. Even if your physician is not trained in Functional Medicine, she or he will be shown what nutrients are needed to support areas of concern for you. I know I spend a lot of time here 'in the gut' even though your head is what hurts but images of your head like MRIs and CT scans are usually "unremarkable" as we say in medicine, meaning there is nothing there (usually, and thank goodness) so allow me to show you that your gut may hold the key to your head pain.

For GI testing, I recommend using the company, GI Effects Stool Testing by Metametrix, because it only requires a single stool sample and you do it at home (they send you the home collection test kit). Also, their tests uses DNA analysis to identify organisms that were previously untraceable, giving you and your doctor a snapshot of the germs inside you, some of which are tied to headaches and brain fog. It's important for you to know this because you may assume that stool tests are just for digestive function. GI Effects can even spot genes within the organisms that cause antibiotic resistance, offering your doctor insight into which antibiotics will work, and which won't.

Without this type of testing, it's like throwing a dart in pitch blackness, hoping to make the bullseye. Right! Although the tests I've suggested in this section have to be ordered from your physician, you can pick up the kit from the doctor's office (make sure that she or he signs the requisition form) and conduct this personal test from home. So after you get your kit home, you follow all the instructions, collect the stool or urine sample(s) and put them in the test tubes, then you seal the kit up and let Fedex come get it from your front door. You need your doctor's signature on the requisition form, before you mail it though.

Lab tests to determine gastrointestinal integrity requires a single stool sample and/or urine sample. One that I often recommend is called the "Organix Comprehensive Profile" by Metametrix. This easy urine test helps uncover whether or not you have intestinal bacterial overgrowth, poor hepatic phase II detoxification, clostridia overgrowth, problems with methylation pathways and neurotransmitter imbalances all of which contribute to headaches.

Hormonal Problems (for men and women)
Where: www.Rheinlabs.com or
www.directlabs.com/suzycohen)

Many companies do hormone testing. I like Rhein because they are fast, they use urine metabolites and they're accurate in my opinion. I compared my estrogen level from Rhein with a blood test. I knew I was normal from the way that I feel but my blood test said I was low. When I tried to "fix" this supposed low estrogen with a bio-identical cream I became estrogen dominant, highly uncomfortable and developed zits and painful menses!!! It took months to get that out of my system, and taught me not to experiment for the sake of gathering data for a book. (You should know I try a lot of things in my books, so I was just playing guinea pig). Dumb me. When I just left myself alone, I felt great, normal and happy. Genova is another good lab that does urine testing for hormones. Either one of those, you have my blessings, and that's what Functional Medicine doctors use too. Order labs directly from the website above.

Hormonal imbalances are usually clear to women, especially if you have bad PMS, fibroids, clotting during your period, heavy cramping, hot flashes or other peri-menopausal and menopausal concerns. Your doctor can do blood or urine tests to evaluate your hormone status, there are even saliva tests available. Hormones are more thoroughly discussed in chapter 10 "The Estrogen & Progesterone Connection to Headaches."

Sometimes it is all you have to fix in order to live migraine-free. I recommend a phytonutrient-rich diet, as well as other natural hormone balancers such as I3C, Black Cohosh, sage, Shatavari extract and bio-identical hormones that your doctor has to have compounded for you. This topic is a book in and of itself, and so I will allow your physician to handle your hormones for you, the point is, testing is important if you have migraines, it is a very common underlying cause of chronic pain. Do read my chapter on this, chapter 10 "The Estrogen & Progesterone Connection to Headaches."

NutrEval with Nutrients and Toxic Elements
Where: Genova Labs (www.gdx.com) or
www.directlabs.com/suzycohen

This test requires blood and urine, you do the test at a lab. Genova (or Direct Labs www.directlabs.com/suzycohen) will send you the home test collection kit and you follow the instructions. The profile and results you get may worth the time and effort it takes you to make this test happen. It requires a good lab that can make sure they follow the instructions with your blood and urine. I've done the NutrEval and it's comprehensive, something like 25 pages of results! It evaluates your whole body, metabolically speaking, measuring 39 organic acids to evaluate GI function, cellular energy production, neurotransmitter processing and your needs for vitamins, minerals and co-factors.

The test also measures 38 amino acids to evaluate dietary protein adequacy,digestion, absorption, amino acid transport, metabolic impairments, and nutritional deficits including essential vitamins, minerals, and amino acids. We're not done yet (I told you it's comprehensive!) it also measures essential and metabolic fatty acids in the red blood cell membranes which affect the inflammatory cascade of cytokines (just what you might need to know); heavy metals and oxidative stress analysis, antioxidant reserves and the presence of oxidative injury. CoQ10 is evaluated too, which helps energize your mitochondria. In some cases, restoring CoQ10 levels sets you headache free. It's expensive. The best price I could find for you (unless you buy it as a practitioner was through Direct Labs, and even that was close to a thousand U.S. dollars. Insurance may not pay, you need to check your plan. Use my link above to buy direct.

Spinal Tap
Where: Hospital setting

Also referred to as a "lumbar puncture" it is exactly that. A thin needle is inserted into a numbed area between two vertebrae in your lower back to extract a sample of cerebrospinal fluid. This is not a common test, but is helpful if your doctor suspects meningitis or an infection that has spread beyond the bloodstream. I never recommend it unless your doctor feels it is an absolute must.

Lyme Disease

Contrary to other infections or disease-states, Lyme disease does not afford healthcare providers the luxury of a "Gold-Standard" test. Historically, healthcare providers have been limited to Lyme tests such as an ELISA and Western Blot, two laboratory techniques that measure a person's antibody response to an infection. Although these antibody-based tests have been used consistently over the past few decades, there are a number of well-known faults that decrease their accuracy.

Antibody-based tests (also known as B cell-based or humoral tests) rely on patients producing an adequate amount of antibodies to measure. Antibodies look at 'shadow' of an organism, not the actual organism which may have come and gone 30 years ago. Antibodies are noted as "IgG" for Immunoglobulin G for example, and IgGs will come up positive years after you've seen a pathogen.

Current Lyme testing methodologies are often not sensitive enough to detect the antibody response in many Lyme patients, studies have found these tests can misdiagnose a good percentage of folks, up to 50 to 70% of true Lyme-infected patients (i.e. you get a false negatives).

In addition, not only must you and your doctor consider false negatives when the patient is the poster child for Lyme disease, but you must also remain vigilant for false positives. Studies have found Western Blots can also produce false positives (because of cross-reactivity with other pathogens) in nearly 30% of patients that do not actually have the Lyme bacteria! What I'm saying is it's really hard to know if you have Lyme, if you take just one test.

This problem could result in you being treated aggressively (and unecessarily) with antibiotics that can cause extensive damage to the "friendly" beneficial flora, and cause horrid side effects head to toe.

Lyme bacteria are adept at confusing your immune system and make it difficult for your B cells to not only recognize the the pathogen, but also clear it. This produces an antibody response that while is present and measurable, is not considered positive on a Western Blot or ELISA. In addition, not all patients produce antibodies at a similar rate. Some of you may take up to 6 weeks to produce the required level of antibodies to be termed "Lyme positive" on a Western Blot, which delays treatment and allows for unchecked disease progression.

What the Lyme community requires is a more sensitive and specific test that can catch an infection early. "Minimizing the risk of contracting chronic Lyme disease requires prevention and early detection," said Keith Berndtson, MD who treats patients in the Lyme hotspot of Illinois. Agreed! There is no question that a Lyme diagnosis is difficult, no "Gold Standard" test exists and the clinical symptomatology of Lyme disease mimics that of a plethora of other common disease-states and infections. First up iSpot, the 'new kid on the block' and at the top of the list because I recommend it frequently.

iSpot Lyme™ by Neuroscience
Where: www.neurorelief.com

This is a Lyme test that requires a blood sample. I know several readers who said it uncovered Lyme when another test failed to. This test was developed by an ILADS member (www.ilads.org) named Chenggang Jin, Md, PhD and some colleagues at Pharmasan Labs. (They are a CLIA- approved lab with expertise in testing for tick-borne diseases).

The test utilizes a methodology already approved and sanctioned by the FDA and CDC for assessing a tuberculosis infection and simply applies it to the Lyme bacteria Borrelia burgdorferi. Where other lab tests are predicated on a B cell antibody response (looking for 'shadows'), the iSpot Lyme test is unique in that it examines the primary mediator of the cell-mediated branch of the immune system, your T cells.

T cells are critical mediators of the immune system in clearing intracellular pathogens such as the Lyme bacteria. Although antibodies are produced by B cells in response to bacteria (specifically extracellular bacteria), T cells are required to interact with B cells in order to produce a robust antibody response. Thus, by designing a test that assesses T cells, Pharmasan Labs created a test with an 84% sensitivity and one that can detect a Lyme infection in as early as 14 days after your tick bite. Good time to tell you some doctors think Lyme is transmitted by fleas, mosquitoes and biting flies. The iSpot Lyme™ test also only utilizes Lyme-specific antigens, which yields little to no cross-reactivity while avoiding false positives in 94% of true Lyme patients.

Doctors sometimes treat lyme in the absence of positive tests. Nevertheless, it can give you some peace of mind to actually see if you're positive or not. Confirming the diagnosis of Borrelia burgdorferi (the causative agent of Lyme disease) through a reliable lab is possible, and I think it's important.

The ELISA and Western Blot tests are the most common tests currently used to confirm the presence of Borrelia burgdorferi (Bb) antibodies. An antibody doesn't mean you have Lyme disease, it just means your body has seen the germ, and you may be asymptomatic. If you have symptoms to go with the antibodies then I'd go with the diagnosis.

The Lyme PCR (polymerase chain reaction) Test is pretty good, but it's not that well-known and it's not fool proof. It looks at your blood. The PCR is only positive if you have Lyme about 30 percent of the time because Lyme does not readily live in the blood, but when it is positive it is correct 100% of the time.

Conventional IgG blood tests through Quest and Labcorp, are currently unreliable in my opinion. It's also very hard, if not impossible to prove the presence of other tick-borne infections such as Bartonella (cat scratch disease) and Babesiosis (a malarial type illness that causes day sweats, night sweats, chills, air hunger and an unexplained cough).

If you insist on using a local laboratory, ask your doctor to order an IgM and IgG Lyme Elisa peptide, but those test(s) may still miss 50 percent or more cases. Don't completely rely on them.

The iSpot Lyme™ test serves as a great compliment to other diagnostic Lyme tests such as an ELISA, Western Blot, PCR, or culture.

IgeneX Labs
Where: www.Igenex.com
Email: customerservice@igenex.com

Among the best in Lyme testing, IgeneX offers a Babesia test, as well as Bartonella and Borrelia. This test requires blood, and you can call the lab directly and order the test. You need your doctor to sign off on the requisition. IgeneX offers a lot of different tests because (like Pharmasan and other labs in this section) they specialize in tick-borne disease.

Note - there are dozens of species of Babesia and Bartonella that if you take this test and it comes back negative, don't believe that you are free and clear of those pathogens. I used to recommend the Bartonella and Babesia test all the time through IgeneX, but lately, because I've seen so many people with a negative test (that clearly had signs and symptoms of those organisms), I'm not sure if it's worth it.

If you have the money, I recommend Panel 6050 which is a complete initial panel. This panel includes the IFA, IgM and IgG

Western Blots and PCRs for Borrelia burgdorferi. The IFA is a general Lyme disease screen. The complete co-infection panel is also offered, for an added fee. The Western Blots are to determine which antibodies the patient is making. If you only have a few hundred dollars, the following 2 panels would be ideal: Panel 188 and 189.

I got this information right off IgeneX's site:

> "If a patient's Western Blot is positive by either IgM or IgG and has only bands 31 and 41kDa, there is a chance that it is a false positive due to presence of antibodies to viruses or other spirochetes. Therefore, confirmation of band 31kDa is recommended. Test 488 for IgM and Test 489 for IgG. Addition of this test improves specificity to greater than 97%."

IgM Western Blot

Where: Any lab

Your Western blot blood test should check for specific bands on the Western Blot (outerdA, 34 kdA, 39 kdA, 41 kdA and the 83/93 kdA bands. Assuming you have the above classic multi systemic symptoms, and your Western Blot is positive for any two of the above bands (without having received LymeriX vaccine), I'd suspect Lyme.

If you get a positive IgM (with chronic symptoms) I think it could be positive confirmation, especially if you have positive symptoms of Lyme, however, you may be told it's a false positive by your practitioner. It's hard to know because there is so much cross-reactivity with pathogens, with Lyme and all it's co-infections. Patients have a positive IgM antibody frequently in chronic Lyme, while we can't say it's 100% Lyme, we can say that other tests are needed to confirm it. You can do the iSpot Lyme™ and see if those results are positive or not. The more tests you do, the better.

IgG Western Blot for Lyme disease

It's not my favorite but done all the time. This test just shows whether or not you have ever been exposed to a tick germ, and all by itself it does not mean you have full blown Lyme disease. It's showing the shadow. A positive IgG just means that your body saw the organism, and set out to fight it. Too often in Lyme disease, the immune system has been hijacked and it can't fight anymore, so the IgG antibody levels are low, or fall into normal range. Doing an IgG test however, is important to the overall picture. Your Western blot blood test should check for specific bands on the Western Blot (outer surface proteins of the bacteria) that are indicative of exposure to Borrelia. These include the 23 kdA, 31 kdA, 34 kdA, 39 kdA, and the 83/93 kdA bands.

Assuming you have classic multi-systemic symptoms, and your Western Blot is positive for any of the above bands (and you haven't received the Lyme disease "LymeriX" vaccine), I'd suspect Lyme. I would personally run a few more tests though, before jumping into aggressive antibiotic treatment.

CD57
Where: Labcorp or www.directlabs.com/suzycohen

This is a blood test commonly ordered if your doctor suspect Lyme disease because it helps you evaluate immune status. It provides an indirect evaluation of bacterial load and severity of illness.

Anything < 150 is considered low.

CD means "cluster designation" in case you want to know. The CD57 is a type of white blood cell, specifically a type of "natural killer" or NK cell that helps you fight infection. It is almost always low in people with lyme, about 80% of infected Lyme patients, and it will stay low throughout their treatment. Sometimes it goes up at the end of treatment. Sometimes people are told they have Lupus, Multiple sclerosis or rheumatoid arthritis and they really have Lyme. The CD57 will not be reduced with those other disorders, but it often is with Lyme. At the end of antibiotic treatment, the CD57 count may go up. That is not a guarantee that you'll not have a relapse with Lyme, you still might. A lot of doctors ignore the CD57 because a low count doesn't necessarily mean you're symptomatic and sick, and a high count doesn't necessarily mean you feel great. I do think it tends to go up as you regain your health. The CD57 can vary day by day. It's constantly swinging; two different researchers proved the CD57 can go up or down by 30 points on a given day. It's up to you and your doctor if you want to test. Even though this test is not that telling, I still recommend the CD57 as part of your testing for Lyme. It's not diagnostic but it's suggestive and may be one piece of the puzzle.

Advance Labs Borrelia

Where: www.Advance-Labs.com

This lab uses your blood (a collection kit is sent directly to your doctor's office). The test is paid for by the patient (check or credit card), and may be reimbursed partly by some insurance carriers. The lab will try to culture and grow Lyme (Borrelia burgdorferi) from your blood. I think this test is good, but if the organism is not active and present in your blood at time of the blood draw, you've spent money for nothing.

The company has on their website some pointers to try to help you. It suggests you show symptoms and/or signs of active disease at the time of blood draw. They recommend you ship the specimen back to them on the day you draw the blood, making sure you do not ship it on Friday or Saturday (to make sure your blood arrives "fresh" if that's the best word).

C6 Lyme Elisa peptide

Where: www.Immunetics.com

This particular test or an ELISA may be ordered, but I'm afraid it may still miss 50 percent or more cases. Don't completely rely on them. The assay should be used only on samples from patients with clinical history, signs or symptoms consistent with B. burgdorferi infection, including individuals who have received the licensed recombinant OspA Lyme disease vaccine (Lymerix). Positive or equivocal results should be double checked by testing with a standardized Western Blot (second step) method. Negative results should not be used to exclude Lyme disease.

Galaxy Labs

Where: www.galaxydx.com

This lab is devoted to testing for Bartonella, a co-infection of Lyme. I think they have state-of-the-art equipment, and they use a patented enrichment culture to significantly increase odds of detection of Bartonella species. Most other labs will miss this bug. If you have rheumatoid arthritis, I'd double check that diagnosis because maybe it's Bartonella infection (which looks like rheumatoid).

Galaxy's method is designed to minimize the likelihood of false negatives across all types of samples and patient cases. For that reason, they run PCRs (polymerase chain reactions) both before and after enrichment culture to ensure that we capture any viable or nonviable DNA present in the sample. They verify all positive PCR results to identify the species of infection, ensuring the highest level of specificity possible for Bartonella. Galaxy Labs offers two types of tests:

1) A single blood test
2) A trio which requires 3 different blood samples, drawn on 3 separate days.

I've seen the test kit, and experimented with it by testing a friend. I have to say the instructions are easy as pie, you just need to find a nice phlebotomist at a local lab who is willing to draw your blood and send off the kit.

Appendix II

Headache Log

Date: _____   Time Started: _____   Ended: _____

Day of Week, circle: MON   TUE   WED   THUR   FRI   SAT   SUN

Aura?   YES   NO

Vision Loss   YES   NO

Type of Pain, choose all that apply: Piercing   Moving   Throbbing   Pulsating

                                               Dull   Stabbing   Pressure   Just "weird"

Location: Eye(s)   Between Eyes   Back of Head   Temples   Forehead

Pick one: Unilateral (one-sided pain)   Bilateral (both sides)

Did you have abnormal yawning with this headache? YES   NO

Nausea   YES   NO

Vomiting   YES   NO

Feel 'drunk'   YES   NO

On a scale of 1 to 5 (where 5 is the most severe), circle: 1   2   3   4   5

Treatments
What supplements or medications were taken (list all) and then circle if it helped you:

_____	Improved	Worsened	I am not sure
_____	Improved	Worsened	I am not sure
_____	Improved	Worsened	I am not sure
_____	Improved	Worsened	I am not sure
_____	Improved	Worsened	I am not sure

How Many Hours of Sleep Last Night? _____ Was it Fitfull? YES   NO

What did you eat today?

Breakfast _____   I Skipped it

Lunch _____   I Skipped it

Dinner _____   I Skipped it

Snacks _____

Did anything you eat today (or yesterday) give you diarrhea?   YES   NO

Circle or highlight what you ate in the last 2 days:

Chewing gum   Soda pop   Diet Soda   Alcohol Coffee   Eggs

Bread, muffins, pasta (anything with gluten)

Ice cream, yogurt, butter (anything with dairy)

Synthetic colors & dyes: Did you eat foods or drinks that are brightly colored (ie

blue Gatorade, red Kool-Aid)   YES   NO

Chocolate?   YES   NO

Other: List any food or drink you suspect may be a trigger?_____

_____

Are you on your period?   YES   NO

How many more days until your period begins? (Approximate is fine) _____

Did you exercise or do strenuous activity prior to headache? YES   NO

Are you upset, worried or under more stress?   YES   NO

Details about situation? _____

_____

Describe the weather, in particular, any storms present or rolling in?_____

_____

Spray perfume, cologne/aftershave, or near someone who did?   YES   NO

Did you light up incense or do you use fragrant plug ins?   YES   NO

Wearing clothes that have been dried with synthetic fabric sheets?   YES   NO

What medications or supplements have you taken in the last week? Please list all
that you regularly take and new ones that you started (ie ibuprofen for your knee, vitamin D for immune, curcumin on friend's suggestion, nasal spray for sinus, etc....
anything and everything no matter how irrelevant you think it is.)

_____

_____

_____

_____

_____

How is today's headache BEST described? Check one:

_____ It moves around my head and changes in intensity, every few minutes/hours

_____ It stays in the same area of my head and builds in intensity

_____ It starts in the one area and radiates upward

_____ The headache is accompanied by eye pain, in or around, or behind eyes

Appendix III

Medications That May Cause or Contribute to Migraines

Sometimes non-prescription and prescription medicines can cause headaches, especially with routine use. Medications listed below may be causing your headaches, and it does not necessarily have to be with chronic use, or excessive dosage. It just depends on you as an individual and your reaction to these:

Antihistamines (allergy medicine)
Antidepressants in the SSRI class (paroxetine, fluoexetine, sertraline and others)
Birth control pills (oral contraceptive) or shots or patches
Blood-thinners (aspirin, warfarin or heparin)
Bupropion
Caffeine
Caffeine withdrawal
Certain types of chemotherapy (and radiation)
Cold medicine
Corticosteroids, such as prednisone, hydrocortisone, dexamethasone
Fluticasone
Ginkgo biloba herb
Hormone replacement therapy (estrogen-containing drugs)
Interferons
Nitroglycerin
Organ transplant rejection medications
Triptan migraine medicine due to overuse (rebound headache)
HIV medicine
Vitamin A
Vitamin D
Vinpocetine herb

Appendix IV

Facebook Friends Helping Friends

I love to ask others to share their personal stories. I asked my friends on Facebook (www.Facebook.com/SuzyCohenRPh) to share remedies and treatment options that helped them or a loved one with headaches. Here are some of the best tips that they shared on September 6, 2013. Anytime you see [comments inside brackets like this] it is me offering some clarification.

*****

Valen Marie- Massage therapy!! Kicks them to the curb, and if I get them regularly, keeps them at bay.

Stacy- MagnesiumStephanie- 1/4 cup apple cider vinegar mixed with water/juice ASAP after auras present.

Joshua- High flow oxygen. Flow Rate of 15-25 LPM (liters per minute) using a non-rebreather mask. I don't have cluster, but chronic daily headache. [The non-rebreather mask is also called a "reservoir mask."]

Sally- I swear by Tiger Balm, plus lots of fresh ginger in hot water and magnesium to relax the muscles. Plus lots of water, of course.

Robin- Marijuana. Haven't had a headache or migraines since I started smoking. It's way better to ingest, just more expensive for oil.

Christy- I had chronic migraines from the time I was 16. (My mom's Diet Coke addiction started, so I drank it too). About a year ago I stopped all artificial sweeteners, and I've only had 1 stress-induced migraine since.

Julia- I love to use peppermint oil!

Brenda- Ice-packs are my best remedy with Ibuprofen gels.

Jules- Drinking cold water and lying on cold quarry tiles help me after detoxing in a lukewarm Epsom salt bath.

Trish- Reiki is one of the very best remedies. I strongly recommend learning Reiki. You could also work with a Reiki practitioner. I have been a Reiki Master for 12 years and never take meds [medications] for headaches.

Earlene- BioFreeze on my temples and the back of my neck. Topamax or Corgard, an old beta blocker. [BioFreeze is sold at pharmacies and chiropractor offices. Topamax and Corgard are prescription drugs]

Charles- Chiropractic helps many types of headaches. Some estimate over 80% of headaches are from a source in the neck (cervicogenic). Acupuncture, not necessarily the energy balancing type by directly needling the paraspinal muscles at the back of the neck. Also scalp needling and possible needling for TMJ can help. Self massage and trigger point work on a regular basis is invaluable to most, but they seem to always make an excuse and not do it. People reading this right now are making excuses now as to why learning and doing self massage and trigger point therapy won't help THEM . . . sad because it is cheap or free and lots of free help on youtube. Tennis balls, backnobber, etc. Ice massage with a styrofoam cup filled with water and frozen. Just tear away the styrofoam and massage the scalp/neck etc with gentle pressure. Obviously avoiding "triggers" is HUGELY important too.

Michelle- Suzy, the biggest headache relief I have ever found without taking any meds is a cold compress or a warm one (depending on what is causing the head pain). I will always try one or the other B4 taking ANYTHING!!! Also, my daughter and I JUST discovered how the saline nose spray WILL relieve a sinus headache ALMOST instantly! We're both so shocked, lol, and happy!!! Love your work here and everywhere I have ever seen it! Thank you.

Allyson- As an Acupuncturist, I've found that most headache/migraine sufferers have experienced head trauma/s in the past. I treat the area where the pain is experienced locally adding other points, usually on the hands & feet for support. Circulation is always an important consideration, so the treating the Heart is always done. I use fire cupping and "gua sha" on the back and neck to relieve tension. Of course if they remain refractory, I refer them to rule out anomalies (tumors, aneurysm). [Gua sha or guasha is an East Asian healing technique that requires the therapist to scrape or rub your back, and I don't mean massage. It's more intense because you turn red from it. A small study suggests it could benefit certain types of chronic neck pain.]

Annette- My sunscreen was causing migraine headaches that progressed to vomiting and diarrhea. It had 20% nano particle zinc. I would have never suspected it, but finally realized that it only happened on the boat and out on ATV trails. That was when I wore sunscreen. The day I stopped using the sunscreen, migraines stopped.

Susan- Lavender essential oil dabbed above the lip helps my daughter better than her meds. Balanced Way- Corydalin (a.k.a. Chuan Xiong, Chinese herb) is where I start. Build a formula with this as the foundation.

Denise- Craniosacral therapy. To find a qualified person in your area go to www.ncbtmb.com, www.abmp.com, or www.upledger.com.

Mary- I don't usually have headaches but when I do, I reach for my Young Living Peppermint Essential Oil and put a few drops in the palm of my hand, inhale 3x's and rub on the back of my neck/brain stem. GONE like NOW !

Karen- Clusters are the hardest to cure. I've tried everything. The only thing that works for me is low dose Prednisone. Works EVERY TIME. [Prednisone is a steroid that requires prescription. I don't recommend it for Lyme disease-related headaches or other immunocompromised conditions.]

Syed- Sleeping always give me relief from migraine.

Kathy- Feverfew herb helped my daughter-in-law.

Nancy- For me, a really hot shower. For my husband, Excedrin Migraine. . . .within just minutes! [Sold over-the-counter in pharmacies nationwide]

Veenu- Tiger Balm! And when I was in Australia, a tablet called Veganin, now known as Aspalgin. 325mg Aspirin and 8mg Codeine. [In the United States, you cannot buy Aspalgin over-the-counter because it contains codeine].

Robert- EFT [Emotional Freedom Technique].

Beth- To keep them in check, magnesium citrate, sea salt, feverfew, gluten free, low dose atenolol. When migraine is real bad Fioricet w/codeine. I know this sounds like a lot, but I have Lyme. [Fioricet w/codeine is a prescription opiate drug available in generic too]

Brooke- Curamin seems to offer some relief, along with drinking some green tea as soon as I start feeling headachy. I also take magnesium 2x/daily. [www.curamin.com]

Doryce- Head-A-care mini Roll-on - aromatherapy peppermint lavender and marjoram to roll on temples. Also like roll-on muscle rub on the neck for tension and if it's sinus-related, the sinus soother mini roll-on [applied] above the brow helps. It has eucalyptus, lavender, and tea tree. And drink water! Not fizzy water or other drinks, pure water and deep breathing! Low light and calmness. Thank you, Suzy, for opening everyone's mindset !!

Charles- YOUR PILLOW! Often the posture during sleep aggravates the facet joints in the neck, causing a headache on arising. Changing the pillow situation or the sleeping position can help this. Stomach sleepers have it the worst but are hardest to change. Key: Tennis ball fixed in a nylon stocking and applied to the xyphoid process. Tie the nylon in a bow with the tennis ball in the back then slide it around where the bow is in back and the tennis ball is just below the breast bone on the tender spot. This will make you roll off of it when you move to your stomach during sleep. People should avoid multiple pillows because they stretch the ligamentous support in the back of the neck and cause head forward posture. If one is older she/he must be careful here not to do anything extreme because the spine is often very fixated in older people with head forward posture.

Benedicta- I take a warm bath, take tab amitriptyline 25mg and relax when I have migraine. [Amitriptyline is a prescription drug.]

Tony- Take a wash cloth put in freezer wet, wait 10 min, apply to head, feels great.

Jason- Butterbur extract, Magnesium, Enzymated B-Complex, Potassium citrate plus, raw cucumber smoothie.

Carrie- Since I am compound heterozygous with MTHFR, taking the methyl B12 and methylfolate, NAC [n-acetylcysteine] and in addition, a chelated mineral supplement have worked wonders at keeping me migraine-free.

Victoria- Eating real food, no nitrates or sulfites; the Candida low-carb Paleo diet.

Whitney- I eat a low-histamine diet.

Annie- Vitamin B12 shots once a week. Haven't had a headache in years.

Juli- Riboflavin and magnesium help my headache. The prescription I take if I have a severe headache is called Maxalt 10mg. I don't take it every day though.

Gay- Magnesium helps everything. If I eat aged cheese (Parmesan or Feta) I am assured of a headache. They didn't bother me years ago.

Appendix V

Triptans: Moderate to Severe Interactions

This is a partial list, for exact information ask your local pharmacist and your physician about your particular medications.

Medication Class	Onset	Effect
Other Triptans	Rapid	Additive vasoconstriction
Ergot derivatives	Rapid	Additive vasoconstriction
MAO inhibitors	Rapid	Reduced breakdown of triptan
Buspirone	Rapid	Additive vasoconstriction

All of the following have an additive pharmacologic effect on the brain and can lead to dangerous and even life-threatening "Serotonin Syndrome" which is excessive serotonin. The effect of combining one of these drugs with a triptan is delayed, in other words, the problem may not occur within minutes, it could take hours to days. I would never combine these drugs with a triptan.

Generic	Brand
Citalopram	Celexa
Escitalopram	Lexapro
Fluoxetine	Prozac
Fluvoxamine	Luvox
Moclobemide	Manerix
Paroxetine	Paxil
Sertraline	Zoloft
Trazodone	Desyrel
Venlafaxine	Effexor
Bupropion	Wellbutrin

References

Chapter 2
Migraine Headaches

[1] National Headache Foundation,
http://www.headaches.org/education/Headache_Topic_Sheets/Migraine

[2] Ibid.

[3] Ibid

[4] Scharff L, Turk DC, Marcus DA. Triggers of headache episodes and coping responses of headache diagnostic groups. Headache. 1995 Jul-Aug;35(7):397-403. PMID: 7672956.

[5] Somerville BW, Estrogen-withdrawal migraine. II. Attempted prophylaxis by continuous estradiol administration. Neurology. 1975;25(3):245. PMID 1167631

[6] Somerville BW, Estrogen-withdrawal migraine. I. Duration of exposure required and attempted prophylaxis by premenstrual estrogen administration. Neurology. 1975;25(3):239. PMID 1167630

[7] Almgren O, Snider SR, Carlsson A. Recovery of dopamine in peripheral adrenergic nerves after reserpine treatment. Naunyn Schmiedebergs Arch Pharmacol. 1976;292: 133-136.

[8] Moja PL, Cusi C, Sterzi RR, Canepari C. Selective serotonin re-uptake inhibitors (SSRIs) for preventing migraine and tension-type headaches. Cochrane Database Syst Rev. 2005 Jul 20;(3):CD002919. Review. PMID: 16034880.

[9] Perlmutter, D, and Vojdani, A, Association Between Headache and Sensitivities to Gluten and Dairy, Case Report, Integrative Medicine, Vol. 12, No. 2, April, 2013

[10] Faraji F, Zarinfar N, Zanjani AT, Morteza A Pain Physician. 2012 Nov-Dec;15(6):495-8,The effect of Helicobacter pylori eradication on migraine: a randomized, double blind, controlled trial. PMID: 23159967

[11] As with all of my suggestions and natural "scripts," check with your prescribing clinician to make sure the compounds I recommend don't interfere with your medications.

[12] Volpe, SL, Magnesium in disease prevention and overall health. Adv Nutr. 2013 May 1;4(3):378S-83S. PMID: 23674807

[13] Tarighat Esfanjani A, Mahdavi R, Ebrahimi Mameghani M, Talebi M, Nikniaz Z, Safaiyan A.The effects of magnesium, L-carnitine, and concurrent magnesium-L-carnitine supplementation in migraine prophylaxis. Biol Trace Elem Res. 2012 Dec;150(1-3):42-8. PMID: 22895810

[14] American Academy of Neurology 2004 Annual Meeting, San Francisco, April 28, 2004, Abstract S43.004.

[15] Sandor PS, et al. Efficacy of coenzyme Q10 in migraine prophylaxis: a randomized controlled trial. Neurology 2005;64:713-715.

[16] Rozen, TD, Oshinsky, ML, Gebeline, CA, Bradley, KC, Young, WB, Shechter, AL & Silberstein, SD. "Open label trial of coenzyme Q10 as a migraine preventive." Cephalalgia 22 (2) 137-141.

[17] Markley HG. CoEnzyme Q10 and riboflavin: the mitochondrial connection. Headache. 2012 Oct;52 Suppl 2:81-7. PMID: 23030537.

[18] Boehnke C, et al. High-dose riboflavin treatment is efficacious in migraine prophylaxis: an open study in a tertiary care centre, European Journal of Neurology (2004;11:475–7):

[19] Ibid.

[20] Magis DI, Ambrosini A, Sandor P, et al. A randomized, double-blind, placebo-controlled trial of thioctic acid in migraine prophylaxis. Headache. 2007;47:52-57. PMID: 17355494

[21] Thomet OA, Wiesmann UN, Schapowal A, Bizer C, Simon HU. Role of petasin in the potential anti-inflammatory activity of a plant extract of petasites hybridus. Biochem Pharmacol. 2001 Apr 15;61(8):1041-7. PMID: 11286996

[22] Levin M, Herbal treatment of headache, Dartmouth Hitchcock Medical Center, Lebanon, NH 03756-0001, USA. Headache. 2012 Oct;52 Suppl 2:76-80.

[23] Lipton RB, Göbel H, Einhäupl KM, Wilks K, Mauskop A. Petasites hybridus root (butterbur) is an effective preventive treatment for migraine. Neurology. 2004 Dec 28;63 (12): 2240-4. PMID: 15623680

[24] Agosti R, Duke RK, Chrubasik JE. Effectiveness of Petasites hybridus preparations in the prophylaxis of migraine: a systematic review. Headache Center Hirslanden, Münchhaldenstr. 33, 8008 Zürich, Switzerland. Phytomedicine. 2006.

[25] Frech EJ, Go MF, Treatment and chemoprevention of NSAID-associated gastrointestinal complications. Ther Clin Risk Manag. 2009 Feb;5(1):65-73. PMID:19436617

[26] Olsen AM, Fosbøl EL, Lindhardsen J, et al. Long-term cardiovascular risk of nonsteroidal anti-inflammatory drug use according to time passed after first-time myocardial infarction: a nationwide cohort study. Circulation. 2012 Oct 16;126(16):1955-63. PMID: 22965337.

[27] Eiland LS, Hunt MO. The use of triptans for pediatric migraines. Paediatr Drugs. 2010 Dec 1;12(6):379-89. Review; PMID: 21028917.

[28] Schürks M, Kurth T, Stude P, Rimmbach C, de Jesus J, Jonjic M, Diener HC, Rosskopf D. G protein beta3 polymorphism and triptan response in cluster headache. Clin Pharmacol Ther. 2007 Oct;82(4):396-401. PMID: 17361120.

[29] Hawkes N. Too frequent use of painkillers can cause rather than cure headaches. BMJ. 2012 Sep 18;345:e6281. PMID: 22991196.

[30] Hambach A, Evers S, Summ O, Husstedt IW, Frese A. The impact of sexual activity on idiopathic headaches: An observational study. Cephalalgia. 2013 Feb 19. PMID: 23430983.

[31] see: http://www.metametrix.com/test-menu/profiles/gastrointestinal-function/dna-stool-analysis-gi-effects

[32] Jacob SE, Stechschulte S. Formaldehyde, aspartame, and migraines: a possible connection. Dermatitis. 2008 May-Jun;19(3):E10-1. PMID:18627677

[33] Bigal ME, Krymchantowski AV, Migraine triggered by sucralose--a case report. Headache. 2006 Mar;46(3):515-7. PMID: 16618274

[34] Bashir A, Lipton RB, Ashina S, Ashina M. Migraine and structural changes in the brain: A systematic review and meta-analysis. Neurology. 2013 Aug 28. PMID: 23986301.

[35] Rainero, I. et al. Insulin sensitivity is impaired in patients with migraine. Cephalalgia. 2005 Aug.; 25(8): 593-7.

[36] Oelkers-Ax, R., et al. Butterbur root extract and music therapy in the prevention of childhood migraine: an explorative study. European Journal of Pain. 2008 Apr.; 12(3): 301-13.

[37] Esposito, M., Carotenuto, M. Ginkgolide B complex efficacy for brief prophylaxis of migraine in school-aged children: an open-label study. Neurological Sciences. 2011 Feb; 32(1): 79-81.

[38] Baad-Hansen L, Cairns B, Ernberg M, Svensson P. Effect of systemic monosodium glutamate (MSG) on headache and pericranial muscle sensitivity. Cephalalgia. 2010 Jan;30(1): 68-76. PMID: 19438927.

[39] Schürks M, Kurth T, Stude P, Rimmbach C, de Jesus J, Jonjic M, Diener HC, Rosskopf D. G protein beta3 polymorphism and triptan response in cluster headache. Clin Pharmacol Ther. 2007 Oct;82(4):396-401. PMID: 17361120.

[40] Oterino A, Toriello M et. al. The relationship between homocysteine and genes of folate-related enzymes in migraine patients. Headache. 2010 Jan;50(1):99-168. PMID: 19619240.

[41] Menon S, Lea RA, et al. Genotypes of the MTHFR C677T and MTRR A66G genes act independently to reduce migraine disability in response to vitamin supplementation. Pharmacogenet Genomics. 2012 Oct;22(10):741-9. PMID: 22926161.

[42] Nagaki, Y, Hayasaka S, Yamada T, Hayasaka Y, Sanada M, Uonomi T. Effects of astaxanthin on accommodation, critical flicker fusion, and pattern visual evoked potential in visual display terminal workers. Journal of Traditional Medicines 2002. Vol.19;No.5;170-173.

[43] Sawaki Keisuke, Yoshigi, H. et al. Sports Performance Benefits from Taking Natural Astaxanthin Characterized by Visual Acuity and Muscle Fatigue Improvement in Humans. Journal of Clinical Therapeutics & Medicines 2002. Vol.18;No.9;1085-1100.

[44] Nakamura, A. et al. Changes in visual function following peroral astaxanthin. Japanese Journal of Clinical Ophthalmology 2004. Vol.58;No.6;1051-1054.

[45] Shiratori Kenji, Ogami, K. et al. Effect of Astaxanthin on Accommodation and Asthenopia-Efficacy-Identification Study in Healthy Volunteers. Journal of Clinical Therapeutics & Medicines 2005. Vol.21;No.6;637-650.

[46] Nagaki, Yasunori, Mihara Miharu., Tsukahara Hiroki, Ono, Shigeaki. The supplementation effect of Astaxanthin on Accommodation and Asthenopia. Journal of Clinical Therapeutics & Medicines 2006. Vol.22;No.1;41-54.

[47] Takahashi, Nanako and Kajita Masayoshi. Effects of Astaxanthin on Accommodative Recovery. Journal of Clinical Therapeutics & Medicines 2005. VoL.21;No.4;431-436.

Chapter 3

Tension Headache

[1] World Health Organization Fact Sheet, October 2012 http://www.who.int/mediacentre/factsheets/fs277/en/

[2] Harden RN et al. Botulinum toxin a in the treatment of chronic tension-type headache with cervical myofascial trigger points: a randomized, double-blind, placebo-controlled pilot study. Headache. 2009 May;49(5):732-43.

[3] Fumal A, Schoenen J. Tension-type headache. Rev Neurol (Paris). 2005 Jul;161(6-7):720-2. Review. French. PMID: 16141970

[4] Gupta R, Pathak R, Bhatia MS, Banerjee BD. Comparison of oxidative stress among migraineurs, tension-type headache subjects, and a control group. Ann Indian Acad Neurol. 2009 Jul;12(3):167-72. PMID: 20174497

[5] Sarchielli P, Alberti A, Floridi A, Gallai V. L-Arginine/nitric oxide pathway in chronic tension-type headache: relation with serotonin content and secretion and glutamate content. J Neurol Sci. 2002 Jun 15;198(1-2):9-15. PMID: 12039657.

[6] Ashina M, Lassen LH, Bendtsen L, Jensen R, Olesen J (January 1999). "Effect of inhibition of nitric oxide synthase on chronic tension-type headache: a randomized crossover trial." Lancet 353 (9149): 287–9.

[7] Febbraio MA, Pedersen BK (2005). "Contraction-induced myokine production and release: is skeletal muscle an endocrine organ?" Exerc Sport Sci Rev 33 (3): 114–119.

[8] Koçer A, Koçer E, Memi•o•ullari R, Domaç FM, Yüksel H. Interleukin-6 levels in tension headache patients. Clin J Pain. 2010 Oct;26(8):690-3. PMID: 20664340.

[9] Ma LQ, Gao DY et al. Effects of overexpression of endogenous phenylalanine ammonia-lyase (PALrs1) on accumulation of salidroside in Rhodiola sachalinensis. Plant Biol (Stuttg). 2008 May;10(3):323-33. PMID: 18426479.

[10] Parisi A, Tranchita E, Duranti G, Ciminelli E, Quaranta F, Ceci R, Cerulli C, Borrione P, Sabatini S. Effects of chronic Rhodiola Rosea supplementation on sport performance and antioxidant capacity in trained male: preliminary results. J Sports Med Phys Fitness. 2010 Mar;50(1):57-63. PMID: 20308973.

[11] Fernández-de-Las-Peñas C. What do we know about chronic tension-type headache? Discov Med. 2009 Dec;8(43):232-6. Review. PMID: 20040276.

[12] Chacko SA, Song Y, et al. Relations of dietary magnesium intake to biomarkers of inflammation and endothelial dysfunction in an ethnically diverse cohort of postmenopausal women. Diabetes Care. 2010 Feb;33(2):304-10. PMID: 19903755

[13] Grotz MR, Pape HC, van Griensven M, Stalp M, Rohde F, Bock D, Krettek C. Glycine reduces the inflammatory response and organ damage in a two-hit sepsis model in rats. Shock. 2001 Aug;16(2):116-21. PMID: 11508863.

[14] Barbiroli B, Iotti S, Lodi R. Improved brain and muscle mitochondrial respiration with CoQ. An in vivo study by 31P-MR spectroscopy in patients with mitochondrial cytopathies. Biofactors 1999 September (2-4):253-60

[15] Milligan SR, Kalita JC, Heyerick A, Rong H, De Cooman L, De Keukeleire D. Identification of a potent phytoestrogen in hops (Humulus lupulus L.) and beer. J Clin Endocrinol Metab. 1999;84:2249–2252.

[16] Hemachandra LP et al. Hops (Humulus lupulus) inhibits oxidative estrogen metabolism and estrogen-induced malignant transformation in human mammary epithelial cells (MCF-10A). Cancer Prev Res (Phila). 2012 Jan;5(1):73-81.

[17] Inoue S, Hoshino S, Miyoshi H, Akishita M, Hosoi T, Orimo H, Ouchi Y. Identification of a novel isoform of estrogen receptor, a potential inhibitor of estrogen action, in vascular smooth muscle cells. Biochem Biophys Res Commun. 1996;219:766–772.

[18] Bruck R, Wardi J. et al.Glycine modulates cytokine secretion, inhibits hepatic damage and improves survival in a model of endotoxemia in mice. Liver Int. 2003 Aug;23(4):276-82. PMID: 12895268.

[19] Alarcon-Aguilar FJ, Almanza-Perez J et al. Glycine regulates the production of pro-inflammatory cytokines in lean and monosodium glutamate-obese mice. Eur J Pharmacol. 2008 Dec 3;599(1-3):152-8. PMID: 18930730.

[20] Klaas CA et al. Studies on the anti-inflammatory activity of phytopharmaceuticals prepared from Arnica flowers. Planta Med. 2002 May;68(5):385-91. PMID: 12058311

[21] Olsen AM, Fosbøl EL, Lindhardsen J et al. Long-term cardiovascular risk of nonsteroidal anti-inflammatory drug use according to time passed after first-time myocardial infarction: a nationwide cohort study. Circulation. 2012 Oct 16;126(16):1955-63. PMID: 22965337.

[22] Jackson JL et al. Tricyclic antidepressants and headaches: systematic review and meta-analysis. BMJ. 2010 Oct 20;341:c5222. PMID: 20961988

[23] Cohen, Suzy. Drug Muggers, Which Medications are Robbing Your Body of Essential Nutrients and How to Restore Them. Rodale February 2011. Available at Amazon in paperback and an expanded hardcover version from DrugMuggersBook.com

[24] www.fda.gov/drugs/drugsafety/PostmarketDrugSafetyInformationforPatientsandProviders/ucm125222.htm

[25] Tella BA, Unubum EV, Danesi MA. The effect of TENS on selected symptoms in the management of patients with chronic tension type headache: a preliminary study. J Hosp Med. 2008 Jan-Mar;18(1):25-9. PMID: 19062467.

[26] Bayat M, Azami Tameh A et al. Neuroprotective properties of Melissa officinalis after hypoxic-ischemic injury both in vitro and in vivo. Daru. 2012 Oct 3;20(1):42. PMID: 23351182.

[27] Nestoriuc Y, Rief W, Martin A. Meta-analysis of biofeedback for tension-type headache: efficacy, specificity, and treatment moderators. J Consult Clin Psychol. 2008 Jun;76(3): 379-96. PMID: 18540732.

[28] Sun-Edelstein C, Mauskop A. Complementary and alternative approaches to the treatment of tension-type headache. Curr Pain Headache Rep. 2012 Dec;16(6):539-44. PMID: 22968473.

[29] Migliardi JR, Armellino JJ, Friedman M, Gillings DB, Beaver WT. Caffeine as an analgesic adjuvant in tension headache. Clin Pharmacol Ther. 1994 Nov;56(5):576-86. PMID: 7955822.

[30] Anneken K, Evers S, Husstedt IW. Efficacy of fixed combinations of acetylsalicyclic acid, acetaminophen and caffeine in the treatment of idiopathic headache: a review. Eur J Neurol. 2010 Apr;17(4):534-e25.

[31] Geybels MS et al. Coffee and tea consumption in relation to prostate cancer prognosis. Cancer Causes Control. 2013 Aug 2. PMID: 23907772.

[32] Lee BJ, Huang YC, Chen SJ, Lin PT. Effects of coenzyme Q10 supplementation on inflammatory markers (high-sensitivity C-reactive protein, interleukin-6, and homocysteine) in patients with coronary artery disease. Nutrition. 2012 Jul;28(7-8):767-72. PMID: 22342390.

Chapter 4
Cluster Headaches

[1] Martelletti P, Granata M, Giacovazzo M. Serum interleukin-1 beta is increased in cluster headache. Cephalalgia. 1993 Oct;13(5):343-5; discussion 307-8. PMID: 7694804.

[2] Steinberg A, Sjöstrand C, Sominanda A, Fogdell-Hahn A, Remahl AI. Interleukin-2 gene expression in different phases of episodic cluster headache--a pilot study. Acta Neurol Scand. 2011 Aug;124(2):130-4.

[3] Chen PK, Chen HM, et al. Treatment guidelines for acute and preventive treatment of cluster headache. Acta Neurol Taiwan. 2011 Sep;20(3):213-27. PMID: 22009127

[4] Cohen AS, Burns B, Goadsby PJ., High-flow oxygen for treatment of cluster headache. JAMA. 2009 Dec 9;302(22):2451-7. PMID: 19996400

[5] Shevel E. A new minimally invasive technique for cauterizing the maxillary artery and its application in the treatment of cluster headache. J Oral Maxillofac Surg. 2013 Apr;71(4):677-81.

[6] Pfaffenrath V et al. The efficacy and safety of Tanacetum parthenium (feverfew) in migraine prophylaxis. Cephalalgia. 2002 Sep;22(7):523-32. PMID: 12230594

[7] Levin M., Herbal treatment of headache. Headache. 2012 Oct;52 Suppl 2:76-80. PMID: 23030536

8 Rozen TD, Fishman RS. Demand Valve Oxygen: A Promising New Oxygen Delivery System for the Acute Treatment of Cluster Headache. Pain Med. 2013 Jan 31. PMID: 23369112.

9 Capobianco DJ, Dodick DW (2006). Diagnosis and treatment of cluster headache. Seminars in Neurology, 26(2): 242–259.

10 Srinivasan V et al. 2012 Jun;10(2):167-78. Melatonin in antinociception: its therapeutic applications. Curr Neuropharmacol. PMID: 23204986

11 Ibid.

12 Ibid.

13 Ibid.

14 Ibid.

15 Pringsheim T, Magnoux E, Dobson CF, Hamel E, Aubé M. Melatonin as adjunctive therapy in the prophylaxis of cluster headache: a pilot study. Headache. 2002 Sep;42(8): 787-92. PMID: 12390642

16 Leone M, D'Amico D et al. Melatonin versus placebo in the prophylaxis of cluster headache. Cephalalgia. 1996 Nov;16(7):494-6. PMID: 8933994.

17 Liu JJ, Huang TS, Cheng WF, Lu FJ. Baicalein and baicalin are potent inhibitors of angiogenesis: inhibition of endothelial cell proliferation, migration and differentiation. Int J Cancer. 2003;106:559–65.

18 Miocinovic R, McCabe NP, Keck RW, Jankun J, Hampton JA, Selman SH. In vivo and in vitro effect of baicalein on human prostate cancer cells. Int J Oncol. 2005;26:241–6.

19 Waldenlind E, Gustafsson SA, Ekbom K, Wetterberg L. Circadian secretion of cortisol and melatonin in cluster headache during active cluster periods and remission. J Neurol Neurosurg Psychiatry. 1987 Feb;50(2):207-13. PMID: 3572435

20 Vukovi• V, Lovrenci•-Huzjan A, Budisi• M, Demarin V. Gabapentin in the prophylaxis of cluster headache: an observational open label study. Acta Clin Croat. 2009 Sep;48(3):311-4. PMID: 20055254.

21 Mandegary A, Saeedi A et al. Hepatoprotective effect of silymarin in individuals chronically exposed to hydrogen sulfide; modulating influence of TNFα-cytokine genetic polymorphism. Daru. 2013 Apr 8;21(1):28.

22 Ibid.

23 Individualizing treatment with verapamil for cluster headache patients. Blau JN, Engel HO. Headache. 2004 Nov-Dec; 44(10):1013-8.

24 Stallmach M. Prophylactic treatment of cluster headache with verapamil. 2003 Praxis (Bern 1994). 2003 Nov 12; 92(46):1951-3.

25 Capobianco DJ, Dodick DW (2006). Diagnosis and treatment of cluster headache. Seminars in Neurology, 26(2): 242-259.

26 Xu F, Wang C, Yang L, Luo H, Fan W, Zi C, Dong F, Hu J, Zhou J. C-dideoxyhexosyl flavones from the stems and leaves of Passiflora edulis Sims. Food Chem. 2013 Jan 1;136(1):94-9.

27 Luke J., Fluoride deposition in the aged human pineal gland. Caries Res. 2001 Mar-Apr; 35(2):125-8. PMID: 11275672

28 Robbins L. Intranasal lidocaine for cluster headache. Headache. 1995 Feb;35(2):83-4. PMID: 7737866.

29 Rozen TD, Fishman RS. Female cluster headache in the United States of America: what are the gender differences? US Cluster Headache Survey. J Neurol Sci. 2012 Jun 15;317(1-2):17-28. PMID: 22482825.

30 Mir P, Alberca R, et al. Prophylactic treatment of episodic cluster headache with intravenous bolus of methylprednisolone. Neurol Sci. 2003;24:318–21.

31 Mueller L, Gallagher RM, Ciervo CA. Methylergonovine maleate as a cluster headache prophylactic: a study and review. Headache. 1997;37:437–42.

32 Leone M, D'Amico D, Frediani F, Moschiano F, Grazzi L, Attanasio A, et al. Verapamil in the prophylaxis of episodic cluster headache. Neurology. 2000;54:1382–5.

33 Bussone G, Leone M. et al. Double blind comparison of lithium and verapamil in cluster headache prophylaxis. Headache. 1990;30:411–7.

34 Costa A, Pucci E, Antonaci F, Sances G, Granella F, Broich G, et al. The effect of intranasal cocaine and lidocaine on nitroglycerin-induced attacks in cluster headache. Cephalalgia. 2000;20:85–91.

35 Fehrenbacher JC, Taylor CP, Vasko MR. Pregabalin and gabapentin reduce release of substance P and CGRP from rat spinal tissues only after inflammation or activation of protein kinase C. Pain. 2003 Sep;105(1-2):133-41. PMID: 14499429.

36 R. Andrew Sewell, MD, John H. Halpern, MD and Harrison G. Pope Jr, MD. Response of cluster headache to psilocybin and LSD. Neurology June 27, 2006 vol. 66 no. 12 1920-1922

37 Fischer, M. et al. Brain-derived neurotrophic factor in primary headaches. J Headache Pain. 2012 Aug.; 13(6): 469-475.

38 Miao Y, Ren J, Jiang L, Liu J, Jiang B, Zhang X. •-lipoic acid attenuates obesity-associated hippocampal neuroinflammation and increases the levels of brain-derived neurotrophic factor in ovariectomized rats fed a high-fat diet. Int J Mol Med. 2013 Sep 5. PMID: 24008266.

39 Zhao YN, Li WF, Li F. et al. Resveratrol improves learning and memory in normally aged mice through microRNA-CREB pathway. Biochem Biophys Res Commun. 2013 Jun 14;435(4):597-602.

40 Tanure MT, Gomez RS, Hurtado RC, Teixeira AL, Domingues RB. Increased serum levels of brain-derived neurotropic factor during migraine attacks: a pilot study. J Headache Pain. 2010 Oct;11(5):427-30.

41 Aslanargun P, Cuvas O, Dikmen B, Aslan E, Yuksel MU. Passiflora incarnata Linneaus as an anxiolytic before spinal anesthesia. J Anesth. 2012 Feb;26(1):39-44. PMID: 22048283

42 Sarris J, Panossian A, Schweitzer I, Stough C, Scholey A. Herbal medicine for depression, anxiety and insomnia: a review of psychopharmacology and clinical evidence. Eur Neuropsychopharmacol. 2011 Dec;21(12):841-60.

[43] Medicinal plants for the treatment of generalized anxiety disorder: a review of controlled clinical studies. Faustino TT, Almeida RB, Andreatini R. Rev Bras Psiquiatr. 2010 Dec;32(4):429-36. Review. Portuguese. PMID: 21308265

[44] J. Izquierdo, D. Mon, M. Lorente, L. Soler Singla A randomized doubled blinded trial of treatment with diamino-oxidase (DAO) in patients with migraine and deficit of enzyme'/INS;s activity. Journal of the Neurological Sciences. October 2013 (Vol. 333) Supplement 1, Pages e505-e506.

[45] Leon R, Wu H, Jin Y, Wei J, Buddhala C, Prentice H, Wu JY. Protective function of taurine in glutamate-induced apoptosis in cultured neurons. J Neurosci Res. 2009 Apr;87(5):1185-94. PMID: 18951478.

[46] Buroker NE, Ning XH et al. Genetic associations with mountain sickness in Han and Tibetan residents at the Qinghai-Tibetan Plateau. Clin Chim Acta. 2010 Oct 9;411(19-20):1466-73. Jun 4. PMID: 20570668.

Chapter 5
Trigeminal Neuralgia

[1] Prasad, S; Galetta, S (2009). Trigeminal Neuralgia Historical Notes and Current Concept. Neurologist 15 (2): 87–94. PMID 19276786

[2] Bagheri, SC; et al (December 1, 2004). Diagnosis and treatment of patients with trigeminal neuralgia. Journal of the American Dental Association 135 (12): 1713–7. PMID 15646605.

[3] The Dana Foundation,The Dana Guide to Brain Health, March, 2007; http://www.dana.org/news/brainhealth/detail.aspx?id=9894

[4] Ibid. (same as above)

[5] Bałkowiec-Iskra E. The role of immune system in inflammatory pain pathophysiology. Pol Merkur Lekarski. 2010 Dec;29(174):395-9. Polish. PMID: 21298993

[6] Zhang X, Burstein R, Levy D. Local action of the pro-inflammatory cytokines IL-1β and IL-6 on intracranial meningeal nociceptors. Cephalalgia. 2012 Jan;32(1):66-72.

[7] As you know, I mention brands that I know about, but these do not mean I am formally endorsing them, just advising based on what I know.

[8] Liao WC et al. Methylcobalamin, but not methylprednisolone or pleiotrophin, accelerates the recovery of rat biceps after ulnar to musculocutaneous nerve transfer. Neuroscience. 2010 Dec 15;171(3):934-49.

[9] Yamashiki M, Nishimura A, Kosaka Y. Effects of methylcobalamin (vitamin B12) on in vitro cytokine production of peripheral blood mononuclear cells. J Clin Lab Immunol. 1992;37(4):173-82. PMID: 1339917.

[10] Scalabrino G, Nicolini G et al. Epidermal growth factor as a local mediator of the neurotrophic action of vitamin B(12) (cobalamin) in the rat central nervous system. The FASEB Journal. 1999 Nov;13(14):2083-90. PMID: 10544191.

[11] TNFα production inhibitor comprising kavalactone as an active ingredient. http://www.google.com/patents/US7199152 Publication number: US7199152 B2

[12] A. Pitkäranta, H. Piiparinen, L et al. Detection of Human Herpesvirus 6 and Varicella-Zoster Virus in Tear Fluid of Patients with Bell's Palsy by PCR. J Clin Microbiol. 2000 July; 38(7): 2753–2755.

[13] Chan KC, Mong MC, Yin MC. Antioxidative and anti-inflammatory neuroprotective effects of astaxanthin and canthaxanthin in nerve growth factor differentiated PC12 cells. J Food Sci. 2009 Sep;74(7):H225-31. PMID: 19895474.

[14] Ibid

[15] As always, my advice is to take the lowest effective dose of any medication.

[16] Olsen AM, Fosbøl EL et al. Long-term cardiovascular risk of nonsteroidal anti-inflammatory drug use according to time passed after first-time myocardial infarction. Circulation. 2012 Oct 16;126(16):1955-63. PMID: 22965337.

[17] Hüseyin Sert, et al. Successful Treatment of a Resistance Trigeminal Neuralgia Patient By Acupuncture. Clinics (Sao Paulo). 2009 December; 64(12):1225–1226.

[18] Trigeminal Neuralgia Fact Sheet, National Institute of Health: http://www.ninds.nih.gov/disorders/trigeminal_neuralgia/detail_trigeminal_neuralgia.htm

[19] Wilsey B, Marcotte T et al. Low-dose vaporized cannabis significantly improves neuropathic pain. J Pain. 2013 Feb;14(2):136-48. PMID: 23237736

[20] Liang YC, Huang CC, Hsu KS. Therapeutic potential of cannabinoids in trigeminal neuralgia. Curr Drug Targets CNS Neurol Disord. 2004 Dec;3(6):507-14. PMID: 15578967

[21] Kenner M, Menon U, Elliott DG. Multiple sclerosis as a painful disease. Int Rev Neurobiol. 2007;79:303-21. PMID: 17531847

[22] Mason, L. Topical Capsaicin for the Relief of Chronic Pain. Am Fam Physician. 2005 Feb 1;71(3):574-577.

[23] Mason L, Moore RA, Derry S et al. Systematic review of topical capsaicin for the treatment of chronic pain. British Medical Journal. 2004 328: 991-994.

[24] Epstein JB, Marcoe JH. Topical application of capsaicin for treatment of oral neuropathic pain and trigeminal neuralgia. Oral Surg Oral Med Oral Pathol. 1994 Feb;77(2):135-40.

[25] M Hadjivassiliou et al. Neuropathy associated with gluten sensitivity. J Neurol Neurosurg Psychiatry 2006;77:1262-1266

[26] Jelínková L, Tucková L, Cinová J, Flegelová Z, Tlaskalová-Hogenová H. Gliadin stimulates human monocytes to production of IL-8 and TNF-alpha through a mechanism involving NF-kappaB. FEBS Letters. 2004 Jul 30;571(1-3):81-5. PMID 15280021

[27] Beckett CG, Dell'Olio D, et al. Gluten-induced nitric oxide and pro-inflammatory cytokine release by cultured coeliac small intestinal biopsies. Eur J Gastroenterol Hepatol. 1999 May;11(5):529-35.

[28] Anna Sapone et al. Differential Mucosal IL-17 Expression in Two Gliadin-Induced Disorders: Gluten Sensitivity and the Autoimmune Enteropathy Celiac

Disease. Int Arch Allergy Immunol. 2010 April; 152(1): 75–80. 2010 April; 152(1): 75–80.

29 Hernández-Lahoz C, Rodrigo L. [Gluten-related disorders and demyelinating diseases]. Med Clin (Barc). 2013 Apr 15;140(7):314-9. PMID: 22998972.

30 http://www.cyrexlabs.com

31 Lotfi J, Chaemmaghami AB, Minagar A, et al. Avicenna and his description of trigeminal neuralgia. Neurology 2000;54.

32 http://www.merriam-webster.com/dictionary/idiopathic

33 Marracci GH, McKeon GP, Marquardt WE, et al. Alpha lipoic acid inhibits human T-cell migration: implications for multiple sclerosis. J Neurosci Res. 2004 Nov 1;78(3):362-70.

34 Marracci GH, Jones RE, McKeon GP, Bourdette DN. Alpha lipoic acid inhibits T cell migration into the spinal cord and suppresses and treats experimental autoimmune encephalomyelitis. J Neuroimmunol. 2002 Oct;131(1-2):104-14.

35 Tashiro A, Okamoto K, Bereiter DA. Chronic inflammation and estradiol interact through MAPK activation to affect TMJ nociceptive processing by trigeminal caudalis neurons. Neuroscience. 2009 Dec 29;164(4):1813-20. PMID: 19786077.

36 Multon S, Pardutz A, Mosen J, Hua MT, Defays C, Honda S, Harada N, Bohotin C, Franzen R, Schoenen J. Lack of estrogen increases pain in the trigeminal formalin model: a behavioural and immunocytochemical study of transgenic ArKO mice. Pain. 2005 Mar;114(1-2):257-65. PMID: 15733652.

37 Gu N, Niu JY, Liu WT, Sun YY, Liu S, Lv Y, Dong HL, Song XJ, Xiong LZ. Hyperbaric oxygen therapy attenuates neuropathic hyperalgesia in rats and idiopathic trigeminal neuralgia in patients. Eur J Pain. 2012 Sep;16(8):1094-105. PMID: 22354664.

38 Rupprecht TA, Birnbaum T, Pfister HW. Pain and neuroborreliosis: significance, diagnosis and treatment. Schmerz. 2008 Oct;22(5):615-23 PMID: 18688658.

39 Drummond EM, Harbourne N, Marete E, Martyn D, Jacquier J, O'Riordan D, Gibney ER. Inhibition of proinflammatory biomarkers in THP1 macrophages by polyphenols derived from chamomile, meadowsweet and willow bark. Phytother Res. 2013 Apr;27(4):588-94. PMID: 22711544.

Chapter 6

Lyme Headaches

1 Ricardo G. Maggi, B. Robert Mozayeni, Elizabeth L. Pultorak, Barbara C. Hegarty, Julie M. Bradley, Maria Correa, Edward B. Breitschwerdt. Bartonella spp. Bacteremia and Rheumatic Symptoms in Patients from Lyme Disease–endemic Region. Emerging Infectious Diseases, 2012; 18 (5)

2 http://www.lymediseaseassociation.org 2010 Lyme Disease Cases

3 Steere AC, Gross D, Meyer AL, Huber BT. Autoimmune mechanisms in antibiotic treatment-resistant lyme arthritis. J Autoimmun. 2001 May;16(3):263-8. PMID: 11334491.

4 Ciut C, Nechifor V, Tomac I, Miron A, Novac B. Lyme disease - unusual medical encounter for an urologist. Rev Med Chir Soc Med Nat Iasi. 2012 Oct-Dec;116(4):1101-5. PMID: 23700896.

5 www.TreatLyme.net, Dr. Marty Ross and Dr. Tara Brooke

6 Chen, John K., and Tina T. Chen. 2004. Chinese Medical Herbology and Pharmacology. City of Industry CA: Art of Medicine Press, Inc., p. 647

7 Fallon, B., et al., Psychiatric manifestations of Lyme borreliosis, Jour of Clin Psychiatry 1993;54(7):263-68.

8 Fallon, B., et al., Late-stage neuropsychiatric Lyme borreliosis. Differential diagnosis and treatment, Psychosomatics 1995;36(3):295-300.

9 Georglis, K., et al., Fibroblasts protect the Lyme disease spirochete, Borrelia burgdorferi, from ceftriaxone in vitro, Jour of Infectious Diseases 1992;166(2):440-44.

10 Girschick, H. et al., Intracellular persistance of Borrelia burgdorferi in human synovial cells, Rheumatology International 1996;16(3):125-32.

11 Halperin, J., et al., Lyme disease cause of a treatable peripheral neuropathy," Neurology 1987; 37(11):1700-06

12 Hammond, R., et al., Alzheimer's disease and spirochetes; a questionable relationship, Neuroreport 1993;4(7):840.

13 Hess, Al, et al., Borrelia burgdorferi central nervous system infection presenting as an organic schizophrenial-like disorder, Biological Psychiatry 1999;45(6):795.

14 Kohler, J., Lyme borreliosis in neurology and psychiatry, Fortschrift Med 1990;108(10): 191-93, 97.

15 Legigian, E., Peripheral nervous system Lyme borreliosis, Seminars in Neurology 1997; March, 25-9.

16 Miklossy, J., Alzheimer's disease, a spirochetosis? Neuroreport 1993;4(9):1069.

17 Pachner, A., et al., The triad of neurologic manifestations of Lyme disease: meningitis, cranial neuritis, and radioculoneuritis, Neurology 1985;35(1):47-53.

18 Pachner, A., Neurologic manifestations of Lyme disease, the new 'great imitator.' Review of Infectious Diseases 1989;11(Suppl 6):S1482-26.

19 Pachner, A., et al., Central nervous system manifestations of Lyme disease, Archives of Neurology 1989;46(7):790-95.

20 Pfister, H., et al., Catatonic syndrome in acute severe encephalitis due to Borrelia burgdorferi infection. Neurology 1993;43(2):433-35.

21 Preac-Mursic, V., et al, Survival of B. burgdorferi antibiotically treated patients with Lyme borreliosis. Infection 1989;17:355.

22 Reik, L, et al., Demyelinating encephalopathy in Lyme disease, Neurology 1985; 35(2):267-69.

23 Reik, L., et al, Neurologic abnormalities of Lyme disease, Medicine 1979;58:281-94.

24 Steere, A., et al., Lyme arthritis: A new clinical entity, Hospital Practice 1978;13(4):143-58.

25 Stein, S., et al., A 25-year-old woman with hallucinations, hypersexuality, nightmares, and a rash, Amer J of Psychiatry, 1996;153(4):545-51.

26 Waisbren, B., et al., Borrelia burgdorferi antibodies and amyotrophic lateral sclerosis, Lancet 1987;2(8554):332-33.

27 Zhang, J., et al., Antigenic variation in Lyme disease Borreliae by promiscuous recombination of VMP-like sequence cassettes, Cell 1997;89(2):275-85.

28 http://www.ilads.org

29 http://www.igenex.com/Website/#

30 http://www.ilads.org/lyme_disease/B_guidelines_12_17_08.pdf

31 Heo HJ, Lee CY. Protective effects of quercetin and vitamin C against oxidative stress-induced neurodegeneration. J Agric Food Chem. 2004 Dec 15;52(25):7514-7.

32 Aboulaila M, Yokoyama N, Igarashi I. Inhibitory effects of (-)-epigallocatechin-3-gallate from green tea on the growth of Babesia parasites. Parasitology. 2010 Apr;137(5):785-91. PMID: 20025823.

Chapter 7
Mystery Headaches Solved

1 Oelkers-Ax, R., et al. Butterbur root extract and music therapy in the prevention of childhood migraine: an explorative study. European Journal of Pain. 2008 Apr.; 12(3): 301-13.

2 Esposito, M., Carotenuto, M. Ginkgolide B complex efficacy for brief prophylaxis of migraine in school-aged children. Neurological Sciences. 2011 Feb; 32(1): 79-81.

3 Martin GV, Houle T, Nicholson R, Peterlin A, Martin VT. Lightning and its association with the frequency of headache in migraineurs: An observational cohort study. Cephalalgia. 2013 Apr;33(6):375-83. Jan 24.

4 King NS (1996). Emotional, neuropsychological, and organic factors: Their use in the prediction of persisting postconcussion symptoms after moderate and mild head injuries. Journal of Neurology, Neurosurgery, and Psychiatry 61 (1): 75–81. PMID 8676166.

5 Centers for Disease Control. Injury Prevention and Control. http://www.cdc.gov/traumaticbraininjury/causes.html

6 Broglio SP, Eckner JT, Paulson HL, Kutcher JS. Cognitive decline and aging: the role of concussive and subconcussive impacts. Exerc Sport Sci Rev. 2012 Jul;40(3):138-44. PMID: 22728452

7 Ahman S, Saveman BI, Styrke J, Björnstig U, Stålnacke BM. Long-term follow-up of patients with mild traumatic brain injury: A mixed-method study. J Rehabil Med. 2013 Sep 3;45(8):758-64. PMID: 24002311.

8 Selekler, HM. et al. Prevalence and clinical characteristics of experimental model of 'ice-cream headache' in migraine and episodic tension-type headache patients. Cephalalgia. 2004 Apr.; 24(4): 293-7.

9   Fuh, JL. et al. Ice-cream headache – a large survey of 8359 adolescents. Cephalalgia. 2007 Mar.; 27(3): 286.

10 Check JH, Cohen R. Dihydrotestosterone may contribute to the development of migraine headaches. Clin Exp Obstet Gynecol. 2013;40(2):217-8. PMID: 23971241.

11 Silva-Néto R, Peres M, Valença M. Odorant substances that trigger headaches in migraine patients. Cephalalgia. 2013 Jul 5. PMID: 23832131.

12 F Longo DL, et al. Harrison's Online. 18th ed. New York, N.Y.: The McGraw-Hill Companies; 2012.

13 Ibid.

14 Ekusheva EV, Filatova EG. Headache caused by sexual activity. Zh Nevrol Psikhiatr Im S S Korsakova. 2003;103(10):21-5. Russian. PMID: 14628582.

Chapter 8
Detoxification Matters

1   Martin GV, Houle T, Nicholson R, Peterlin A, Martin VT. Lightning and its association with the frequency of headache in migraineurs: an observational cohort study. Cephalalgia. 2013 Apr;33(6):375-83.

2   Jacob SE, Stechschulte S. Formaldehyde, aspartame, and migraines: a possible connection. Dermatitis. 2008 May-Jun;19(3):E10-1. PMID: 18627677.

3   Wallace, Lance. TEAM Study: http://nepis.epa.gov/Adobe/PDF/2000UC5T.PDF

4   http://www.webnat.com/articles/MucusAbout.asp

5   http://mthfr.net

6   Bigal ME, Krymchantowski AV, Migraine triggered by sucralose--a case report. Headache. 2006 Mar;46(3):515-7. PMID: 16618274

Chapter 9
The Adrenal Hormone Connection

1   Chung SC, Brooks MM, Rai M, Balk JL, Rai S. Effect of Sahaja yoga meditation on quality of life, anxiety, and blood pressure control. J Altern Complement Med. 2012 Jun;18(6):589-96. PMID: 22784346.

2   Patak P, Willenberg HS, Bornstein SR. Vitamin C is an important cofactor for both adrenal cortex and adrenal medulla. Endocr Res. 2004 Nov;30(4):871-5. PMID: 15666839.

3   Starks MA, Starks SL, Kingsley M, Purpura M, Jäger R. The effects of phosphatidylserine on endocrine response to moderate intensity exercise. J Int Soc Sports Nutr. 2008 Jul 28;5:11. PMID:18662395.

4   Darbinyan V, Aslanyan G, Amroyan E, Gabrielyan E, Malmström C, Panossian A. Clinical trial of Rhodiola rosea L. extract SHR-5 in the treatment of mild to moderate depression. Nord J Psychiatry. 2007;61(5):343-8. Erratum in: Nord J Psychiatry. 2007;61(6):503. PMID: 17990195.

5   Evdokimov VG. Effect of cryopowder Rhodiola rosae L. on cardiorespiratory parameters and physical performance of humans. Aviakosm Ekolog Med. 2009 Nov-Dec;43(6):52-6. Russian. PMID: 20169741.

6   Van Diermen D et al. Monoamine oxidase inhibition by Rhodiola rosea L. roots. J Ethnopharmacol. 2009 Mar 18;122(2):397-401. PMID: 19168123.

7   Edwards D, Heufelder A, Zimmermann A. Therapeutic effects and safety of Rhodiola rosea extract WS® 1375 in subjects with life-stress symptoms--results of an open-label study. Phytother Res. 2012 Aug;26(8):1220-5. PMID: 22228617.

8   Michalsen A, Traitteur H et al. Yoga for chronic neck pain: a pilot randomized controlled clinical trial. J Pain. 2012 Nov;13(11):1122-30. PMID: 23117107.

9   Ward L, Stebbings S, Cherkin D, Baxter GD. Yoga for Functional Ability, Pain and Psychosocial Outcomes in Musculoskeletal Conditions: A Systematic Review and Meta-Analysis. Musculoskeletal Care. 2013 Jan 9. PMID: 23300142.

10 Turner, Anne, et al. Overweight and Obesity Influence Cortisol Response to Food Ingestion in Men. Endocr Rev June 2013; 34.

11 Bigal ME, Lipton RB, Holland PR, Goadsby PJ. Obesity, migraine, and chronic migraine: possible mechanisms of interaction. Neurology 2007; 68: 1851–1861.

12 Bigal ME, Liberman JN, Lipton RB. Obesity and migraine: a population study. Neurology 2006; 66: 545–550.

Chapter 10
Estrogen Progesterone and More

1   Somerville BW, Estrogen-withdrawal migraine. II. Attempted prophylaxis by continuous estradiol administration, Neurology. 1975;25(3):245. PMID 1167631

2   Somerville BW, Estrogen-withdrawal migraine. I. Duration of exposure required and attempted prophylaxis by premenstrual estrogen administration. Neurology. 1975;25(3):239. PMID 1167630

3   Simona, S. et al. Migraine in women: the role of hormones and their impact on vascular diseases. J Headache Pain. 2012 Apr.;13(3):177-189.

4   Ibid.

5   Necdet, K. et al. Impact of sex hormonal changes on tension-type headache and migraine: a cross-sectional population based survey in 2,600 women. J Headache Pain. 2012 Oct.; 13(7): 557-565.

6   Aggarwal BB, Ichikawa H. Molecular targets and anticancer potential of indole-3-carbinol and its derivatives. Cell Cycle. 2005 Sep;4(9):1201-15.

7   Garikapaty VP, Ashok BT, Chen YG, et al. Anti-carcinogenic and anti-metastatic properties of indole-3-carbinol in prostate cancer. Oncol Rep. 2005 Jan;13(1):89-93.

8   Ashok BT, Chen Y, Liu X, et al. Abrogation of estrogen-mediated cellular and biochemical effects by indole-3-carbinol. Nutr Cancer. 2001;41(1-2):180-7.

9   Ashok BT, Chen YG, Liu X, et al. Multiple molecular targets of indole-3-carbinol, a chemopreventive anti-estrogen in breast cancer. Eur J Cancer Prev. 2002 Aug;11 Suppl 2S86-S93.

10   Yuan F, Chen DZ, Liu K, et al. Anti-estrogenic activities of indole-3-carbinol in cervical cells: implication for prevention of cervical cancer. Anticancer Res. 1999 May;19(3A): 1673-80.

11   Liu H, Wormke M, Safe SH, Bjeldanes LF. Indolo[3,2-b]carbazole: a dietary-derived factor that exhibits both antiestrogenic and estrogenic activity. J Natl Cancer Inst. 1994 Dec 7;86(23):1758-65.

12   Chang X, Tou JC, Hong C, et al. 3,3'-Diindolylmethane inhibits angiogenesis and the growth of transplantable human breast carcinoma in athymic mice. Carcinogenesis. 2005 Apr;26(4):771-8.

13   Sarkar FH, Li Y. Indole-3-carbinol and prostate cancer. J Nutr. 2004 Dec;134(12 Suppl):3493S-8S.

14   Patel RM, Sarma R, Grimsley E. Popular sweetener sucralose as a migraine trigger. Headache. 2006 Sep;46(8):1303-4. PMID: 16942478.

15   Hirsch AR. Migraine triggered by sucralose--a case report. Headache. 2007 Mar;47(3):447. PMID: 17371367.

16   Bigal ME, Krymchantowski AV. Migraine triggered by sucralose--a case report. Headache. 2006 Mar;46(3):515-7. PMID: 16618274.

17   Calcium-D-glucarate. Altern Med Rev. 2002 Aug;7(4):336-9. PMID:12197785.

18   Warnecke, G: Influencing of menopausal complaints with a phytodrug: successful therapy with Cimicifuga monoextract (in German). Medizinische Welt 36: 871-874, 1985.

19   Bigal ME, Lipton RB, Holland PR, Goadsby PJ. Obesity, migraine, and chronic migraine: possible mechanisms of interaction. Neurology 2007; 68: 1851–1861.

20   Bigal ME, Liberman JN, Lipton RB. Obesity and migraine: a population study. Neurology 2006; 66: 545–550.

Chapter 11

The Thyroid Connection

1   American Thyroid Association, http://www.thyroid.org/media-main/about-hypothyroidism/

2   He L, Li M, Long XH, Li XP, Peng Y. A case of Hashimoto's encephalopathy misdiagnosed as viral encephalitis. Am J Case Rep. 2013 Sep 13;14:366-9. PMID: 24046804.

3   Singh SK. Prevalence of migraine in hypothyroidism. J Assoc Physicians India. 2002 Nov;50:1455-6. PMID: 12583488.

4   Nambiar PR, Palanisamy GS et al. Reagan WJ. Toxicities Associated with 1-month Treatment with Propylthiouracil (PTU) and Methimazole (MMI) in Male Rats. Toxicol Pathol. 2013 Sep 25. PMID: 24067673.

5   Oatridge A, Barnard ML, Puri BK et al. Changes in brain size with treatment in

patients with hyper- or hypothyroidism. AJNR Am J Neuroradiol. 2002 Oct;23(9):1539-44. PMID: 12372744.

6   Virili C, Bassotti G, Santaguida MG et al. Atypical celiac disease as cause of increased need for thyroxine: a systematic study. J Clin Endocrinol Metab. 2012 Mar;97(3):E419-22. PMID: 22238404.

7   Mi•kiewicz P, K•pczy•ska-Nyk A, Bednarczuk T. Coeliac disease in endocrine diseases of autoimmune origin. Endokrynol Pol. 2012;63(3):240-9. PMID: 22744631.

8   Banji D, Banji OJ, Pratusha NG, Annamalai AR. Investigation on the role of Spirulina platensis in ameliorating behavioural changes, thyroid dysfunction and oxidative stress in offspring of pregnant rats exposed to fluoride. Food Chem. 2013 Sep 1;140(1-2):321-31. PMID: 23578649.

9   Maxwell C, Volpe SL. Effect of zinc supplementation on thyroid hormone function. A case study of two college females. Ann Nutr Metab. 2007;51(2):188-94. PMID: 17541266.

Chapter 12
Reduce Pain-Causing Cytokines

1   The Dana Foundation, A Future Without Chronic Pain, http://www.dana.org/news/cerebrum/detail.aspx?id=39160

2   From http://www.functionalmedicine.org/about/whatisfm/

3   Hattori Y, Suzuki K et al. Metformin inhibits cytokine-induced nuclear factor kappaB activation via AMP-activated protein kinase activation in vascular endothelial cells. Hypertension. 2006 Jun;47(6):1183-8. PMID: 16636195.

4   Hattori Y, Suzuki K, Hattori S, Kasai K. Metformin inhibits cytokine-induced nuclear factor kappaB activation via AMP-activated protein kinase activation in vascular endothelial cells. Hypertension. 2006 Jun;47(6):1183-8.PMID: 16636195.

5   Martelletti P, Granata M, Giacovazzo M. Serum interleukin-1 beta is increased in cluster headache. Cephalalgia. 1993 Oct;13(5):343-5; discussion 307-8. PMID: 7694804.

6   Smith, Ronald S. Cytokines and depression. Chapter 7. www.Cytokines-and-Depression.com

7   Abramson, SB. Blocking the effects of IL•1 in rheumatoid arthritis protects bone and cartilage. Rheumatology 2002 41(9):972-980

8   Ren K, Torres R. Role of interleukin-1beta during pain and inflammation. Brain Res Rev. 2009 Apr;60(1):57-64. PMID: 19166877.

9   Serum Concentrations of IL-2 and TNF-• in Patients with Painful Bone Metastases: Correlation with Responses to 89SrCl2 Therapy, Fang, N, Li, Y, Xu, YS, et al, J Nucl Med, February 2006 vol. 47 no. 2, 242-246

10 Uçeyler N, Rogausch JP, Toyka KV, Sommer C. Differential expression of cytokines in painful and painless neuropathies. Neurology. 2007 Jul 3;69(1):42-9. PMID: 17606879.

[11] Helmark IC et al. Exercise increases interleukin-10 levels both intraarticularly and peri-synovially in patients with knee osteoarthritis: a randomized controlled trial. Arthritis Res Ther. 2010;12(4):R126. PMID: 20594330

[12] Prabhala RH, et al. Elevated IL-17 produced by TH17 cells promotes myeloma cell growth and inhibits immune function in multiple myeloma. Blood. 2010 Jul 1;115(26): 5385-92. Apr 15. PMID: 20395418

[13] Shujuan Li, et al. IL-17 and IL-22 in Cerebrospinal Fluid and Plasma Are Elevated in Guillain-Barré Syndrome, Mediators of Inflammation, vol. 2012, Article ID 260473, 7 pages, 2012.

[14] Baek SH, Lee SG, Park YE, Kim GT, Kim CD, Park SY. Increased synovial expression of IL-27 by IL-17 in rheumatoid arthritis. Inflamm Res. 2012 Dec;61(12):1339-45. PMID: 22825627.

[15] Moseley TA, Haudenschild DR, Rose L, Reddi AH. Interleukin-17 family and IL-17receptors. Cytokine Growth Factor Rev. 2003 Apr;14(2):155-74. PMID: 12651226.

[16] Xie Lin, et al. Amelioration of experimental autoimmune encephalomyelitis by curcumin treatment through inhibition of IL-17 production. International Immunopharmacology International Immunopharmacology 2009 Vol. 9 No. 5 pp. 575-581; PMID: 19539560

[17] Sun Q, et al. Novel immunoregulatory properties of EGCG on reducing inflammation in EAE. Front Biosci 2013 Jan 1;18:332-42. PMID: 23276926.

[18] Wang J, Ren Z, et al. Epigallocatechin-3-gallate ameliorates experimental autoimmune encephalomyelitis by altering balance among CD4+ T-cell subsets. Am J Pathol. 2012 Jan;180(1):221-34. Nov 3. PMID: 22056360

[19] Rodriguez-Morán M, Guerrero-Romero F. Elevated concentrations of TNF-alpha are related to low serum magnesium levels in obese subjects. Magnes Res. 2004 Sep;17(3):189-96. PMID: 15724867

[20] Vivier, E., Raulet, D.H., Moretta, A., Caligiuri, M.A., Zitvogel, L., Lanier, L.L., Yokoyama, W.M. & Ugolini, S. (2011). Innate or Adaptive Immunity? The Example of Natural Killer Cells. Science. 331: 44–49

[21] University of Maryland Medical Center. Willow Bark. http://www.umm.edu/altmed/articles/willow-bark-000281.htm

[22] Ibid.

[23] Bonaterra, G.A, et al. Anti-inflammatory effects of the willow bark extract STW 33-1 in LPS-activated human monocytes and differentiated macrophages. The Free Library. Phytomedicine: International Journal of Phytotherapy & Phytopharmacology (2010)

[24] Kearney PM et al. Do selective cyclo-oxygenase-2 inhibitors and traditional non-steroidal anti-inflammatory drugs increase the risk of atherothrombosis? Meta-analysis of randomized trials. BMJ 2006;332:1302

[25] Wu D, Yu L, Nair MG, DeWitt DL, Ramsewak RS. Cyclooxygenase enzyme inhibitory compounds with antioxidant activities from Piper methysticum (kava kava) roots. Phytomedicine. 2002 Jan;9(1):41-7. PMID: 11924763

[26] Liu T, Ji RR. New insights into the mechanisms of itch: are pain and itch controlled by distinct mechanisms? Pflugers Arch. 2013 May 1. PMID: 23636773

[27] Ammon HP. [Boswellic acids (components of frankincense) as the active principle in treatment of chronic inflammatory diseases]. Wien Med Wochenschr. 2002;152(15-16): 373-8. PMID: 12244881

[28] Schramm, D, Wang, J, Holt, R, et al, Chocolate procyanidins decrease the leukotriene-prostacyclin ratio in humans and human aortic endothelial cells1,2,3. Am J Clin Nutr January 2001 vol. 73 no. 1 36-40

[29] Monagas, M, Khan, N, and Andres-Lacueva, C, Effect of cocoa powder on the modulation of inflammatory biomarkers in patients at high risk of cardiovascular disease. Am J Clin Nutr 2009 90: 1144-1150

[30] Rasley A et al. Anguita J. Substance P augments Borrelia burgdorferi-induced prostaglandin E2 production by murine microglia. J Immunol. 2004 May 1;172(9):5707-13. PMID: 15100316

[31] Calder, PC., Omega-3 polyunsaturated fatty acids and inflammatory processes: nutrition or pharmacology? Br J Clin Pharmacol. 2013 Mar;75(3):645-62. PMID: 22765297

[32] Esatbeyoglu T, Wray V, Winterhalter P., Dimeric procyanidins: screening for B1 to B8 and semisynthetic preparation of B3, B4, B6, And B8 from a polymeric procyanidin fraction of white willow bark (Salix alba). J Agric Food Chem. 2010 Jul 14;58(13):7820-30. PMID: 20533825

[33] Su JY, Tan LR et al. Experimental study on anti-inflammatory activity of a TCM recipe consisting of the supercritical fluid CO_2 extract of Chrysanthemum indicum, Patchouli Oil and Zedoary Turmeric Oil in vivo. Ethnopharmacol. 2012 Jun 1;141(2):608-14. PMID: 21920423

[34] Sanuki R et al. Compressive force induces osteoclast differentiation via prostaglandin E(2) production in MC3T3-E1 cells. Connect Tissue Res. 2010 Apr;51(2):150-8. PMID: 20001844 Sanuki R, et a., Connect Tissue Res. 2010 Apr;51(2):150-8. PMID: 20001844

[35] Yu YS, Hsu CL, Yen GC., Anti-inflammatory effects of the roots of Alpinia pricei Hayata and its phenolic compounds. J Agric Food Chem. 2009 Sep 9;57(17):7673-80. PMID:19685877

[36] Montefusco-Pereira CV et al. Antioxidant, Anti-inflammatory, and Hypoglycemic Effects of the Leaf Extract from Passiflora nitida Kunth. Appl Biochem Biotechnol. 2013 May 12. PMID 23666642

[37] Imler TJ Jr, Petro TM. Decreased severity of experimental autoimmune encephalomyelitis during resveratrol administration is associated with increased IL-17+ IL-10+ T cells, CD4(-) IFN-gamma+ cells, and decreased macrophage IL-6 expression. Int Immunopharmacol. 2009 Jan;9(1):134-43. PMID: 19022403

[38] Sharma M, et al. Circulating human basophils lack the features of professional antigen presenting cells. Paris, F-75006, France. Sci Rep. 2013;3:1188. Feb 1. PMID: 23378919

[39] Dworkin RH et al. A standard database format for clinical trials of pain treatments: an Acttion-Cdisc initiative. Pain. 2013 Jan;154(1):11-4. PMID: 23218970

[40] Lee SJ, Bai SK et al. Astaxanthin inhibits nitric oxide production and inflammatory gene expression by suppressing I(kappa)B kinase-dependent NF-kappaB activation. Mol Cells. 2003 Aug 31;16(1):97-105. PMID: 14503852

[41] Babcock TA, Helton WS, Hong D, Espat NJ. Omega-3 fatty acid lipid emulsion reduces LPS-stimulated macrophage TNF-alpha production. Surg Infect (Larchmt). 2002 Summer;3(2):145-9. PMID: 12519481

[42] Zhang Y et al. Vitamin D inhibits monocyte/macrophage proinflammatory cytokine production by targeting MAPK phosphatase-1. J Immunol. 2012 Mar 1;188(5):2127-35. PMID: 22301548

[43] Schmelzer C, Lindner I, Vock C, Fujii K, Döring F. Functional connections and pathways of coenzyme Q10-inducible genes: an in-silico study. IUBMB Life. 2007 Oct;59(10):628-633. PMID: 17852568

[44] Resta-Lenert S, Barrett KE. Probiotics and commensals reverse TNF-alpha- and IFN-gamma-induced dysfunction in human intestinal epithelial cells. Gastroenterology. 2006 Mar;130(3):731-46. PMID: 16530515

[45] Zhang L, Li N, Caicedo R, Neu J. Alive and dead Lactobacillus rhamnosus GG decrease tumor necrosis factor-alpha-induced interleukin-8 production in Caco-2 cells. J Nutr. 2005 Jul;135(7):1752-6. PMID: 15987860

[46] Jiang J, Mo ZC et al. Epigallocatechin-3-gallate prevents TNF-•-induced NF-•B activation thereby upregulating ABCA1 via the Nrf2/Keap1 pathway in macrophage foam cells. Int J Mol Med. 2012 May;29(5):946-56. PMID: 22367622

[47] Manna SK, Mukhopadhyay A, Aggarwal BB. Resveratrol suppresses TNF-induced activation of nuclear transcription factors NF-kappa B, activator protein-1, and apoptosis: potential role of reactive oxygen intermediates and lipid peroxidation. J Immunol. 2000 Jun 15;164(12):6509-19. PMID: 10843709

[48] Manna SK, Mukhopadhyay A, Van NT, Aggarwal BB. Silymarin suppresses TNF-induced activation of NF-kappa B, c-Jun N-terminal kinase, and apoptosis. J Immunol. 1999 Dec 15;163(12):6800-9. PMID: 10586080

[49] Wischmeyer PE, Riehm J, Singleton KD, Ren H, Musch MW, Kahana M, Chang EB. Glutamine attenuates tumor necrosis factor-alpha release and enhances heat shock protein 72 in human peripheral blood mononuclear cells. Nutrition. 2003 Jan;19(1):1-6. PMID: 12507630

[50] Zhang WJ, Frei B. Alpha-lipoic acid inhibits TNF-alpha-induced NF-kappaB activation and adhesion molecule expression in human aortic endothelial cells. FASEB J. 2001 Nov;15(13):2423-32. PMID: 11689467

[51] Worm M. 1,25-dihydroxyvitamin D(3) promotes IL-10 production in human B cells. Eur J Immunol. 2008 Aug;38(8):2210-8. PMID: 18651709

[52] Houssen ME et al. Natural anti-inflammatory products and leukotriene inhibitors as complementary therapy for bronchial asthma. Clin Biochem. 2010 Jul;43(10-11):887-90. 2010.04.061. PMID: 20430018.

[53] Okamoto M, Mitsunobu F, Ashida K et al. Effects of perilla seed oil supplementation on leukotriene generation by leucocytes in patients with asthma associated with lipometabolism. Int Arch Allergy Immunol. 2000 Jun;122(2):137-42. PMID: 10878492

[54] Jung WK et al. Ecklonia cava ethanolic extracts inhibit lipopolysaccharide-induced cyclooxygenase-2 and inducible nitric oxide synthase expression in BV2 microglia via the MAP kinase and NF-kappaB pathways. Food Chem Toxicol. 2009 Feb;47(2):410-7. PMID: 19111593.

[55] S. Bellosta, D. Via, M. Canavesi, et al. Arteriosclerosis, Thrombosis, and Vascular Biology. 1998; 18: 1671-1678

[56] Epstein J, Docena G, MacDonald TT, Sanderson IR. Curcumin suppresses p38 mitogen-activated protein kinase activation, reduces IL-1beta and matrix metalloproteinase-3 and enhances IL-10 in the mucosa of children and adults with inflammatory bowel disease. Br J Nutr. 2010 Mar;103(6):824-32. PMID: 19878610.

Index

About the Author

Suzy Cohen, America's Pharmacist™ is a licensed pharmacist and Functional Medicine practitioner. In addition to writing a syndicated health column, "Dear Pharmacist," which circulates to millions of readers each week, Suzy hosts a medical minute on "Know the Cause" television. You have seen her on The Dr. Oz Show, The View, The Doctors, 700 Club or Good Morning America Health. Get your free newsletter at www.SuzyCohen.com. Suzy is a member of the following organizations:

The American College for Advancement in Medicine (ACAM)

The Institute of Functional Medicine (IFM)

The American Academy of Anti-Aging Medicine (A4M)

American Pharmacist's Association (APhA)

International Lyme and Associated Diseases Society (ILADS)

The Academy of Comprehensive Integrative Medicine (ACIM)

Books by this author:

Headache Free: Relieve Migraine, Tension, Cluster, Menstrual and Lyme Headaches (Dear Pharmacist Inc. 2013)

Wake Up Your Thyroid by Eating Right (Dear Pharmacist Inc. 2013)

The 24-Hour Pharmacist: Advice, Options and Amazing Cures from America's Most Trusted Pharmacist (Collins 2009)

Diabetes Without Drugs, The 5-Step Program to Control Blood Sugar Naturally and Prevent Diabetes Complications (Rodale 2010)

Drug Muggers: Which Medications are Robbing Your Body of Essential Nutrients and How to Restore Them (Rodale 2011)

Eczema: Itchin' for a Cure (Dear Pharmacist Inc. 2012) *Kindle only*

Understanding Pancreatitis & Pancreatic Cancer (Dear Pharmacist Inc. 2012) *Kindle only*

Are you on the computer? Find me...

On Facebook www.Facebook.com/SuzyCohenRPh   click LIKE

Twitter: @SuzyCohen

www.ScriptEssentials.com for more information on HaloScript™ and ThyroScript™ supplements